1,001
PRESCRIPTION
DRUGS:

Side Effects, Dangerous Combinations and Natural Healing Alternatives
for SENIORS

By the Editors of
FC&A Medical Publishing

Publisher's Note

The authors have worked diligently to provide up-to-date and accurate information in this book. However, since pharmacology — the science of drugs — is such a rapidly expanding field, the publisher cannot be responsible for the results of any drug therapy program undertaken by anyone who has consulted this book for information. This publication does not constitute medical practice or advice. Its only intent is to provide the consumer with easy-to-understand information. Please consult carefully with your doctor before taking any drugs or discontinuing any medication.

Your body, you know, is the temple of the Holy Spirit, who is in you since you received Him from God. You are not your own property. You have been bought and paid for. This is why you should use your body for the glory of God.
1Corinthians 6:19-20

But I will restore you to health and heal your wounds, declares the Lord.
Jeremiah 30:17a

FC&A Medical Publishing
103 Clover Green
Peachtree City, GA 30269

Produced by the staff of FC&A
Cover Images: © PhotoDisc, Inc. 1995
© Digital Stock 1996

Third printing April 2001

ISBN# 1--890957-42-9

TABLE OF CONTENTS

INTRODUCTION

HOW TO USE THIS BOOK

The purpose of this book is to provide you with up-to-date, easy-to-understand information on the most frequently prescribed drugs. You'll find them listed alphabetically by their generic name.

Each drug entry has six sections. If one of the sections isn't used, it's because there was no information available on that topic.

Brand names: Here we list most of the common brand names of each drug. Sometimes you know your drug's brand name, but you don't know its generic name. That's why we included both in the big index at the front of the book.

Drug use: Next is a brief description of what condition each medication is designed to treat.

How to take this drug: If there are special instructions or tips that will make this drug work better for you, you'll find them here.

Possible side effects: Only the most common side effects are listed for each drug. You may not experience any of them at all — some depend on the size of the dose and will go away if the dose is lowered. Or you may experience different ones, perhaps reactions that are more rare or unexpected. Remember that older people sometimes experience side effects differently and may even have reactions that can be quite dangerous to them, like dizziness leading to falls. Call your doctor if you develop any side effect you're not comfortable with.

Possible interactions: Here you'll find the most common drugs, food, or lab tests that interact with each particular medication. Remember though that you might experience others, and the ones listed certainly won't apply to everyone.

Other important information: This section tells you when you should not take a drug, when you should take it with caution, and other information you should know. Discuss any concerns with your doctor.

In addition to these sections, you'll find each drug has a pregnancy category and perhaps a symbol or two. Here's what these mean.

KEY TO FDA PREGNANCY CATEGORIES

The Food and Drug Administration uses human studies as well as animal studies to determine the risk of prescription drugs to a developing human baby. The FDA has assigned one of the following five pregnancy categories to each drug. The categories rank each drug's potential to cause birth defects. (If you see the code NR, that means there is not enough research to allow the FDA to assign a risk category.)

Pregnancy category A. Studies of pregnant women have not shown a risk to the developing baby.

Pregnancy category B. This category can mean two things: (1) Animal studies have not shown a risk to the developing baby, but studies haven't been done in pregnant women, or (2) Animal studies have shown a risk to the developing fetus, but studies in pregnant women have not shown a risk.

Pregnancy category C. This middle category can mean two things: (1) Animal studies have shown a risk, and human studies are inconclusive because not enough have been done. The mother may gain enough benefit from the drug to make the risk to the developing baby acceptable, or (2) We really don't know the risk to the developing baby because there are no animal studies and not enough human studies.

Pregnancy category D. Studies in pregnant women have shown evidence of a risk to the developing baby. However, the mother may gain enough benefit from the drug to make the risk to the baby acceptable.

Pregnancy category X. Studies in animals or pregnant women have shown a definite risk to the developing baby. The drug has either caused birth defects or the developing baby has reacted badly to the drug in some way. The risk to the baby clearly outweighs any benefit the mother may gain from taking the drug.

Some of the same problems can occur when you breast-feed your baby. Be sure your doctor knows you are nursing before you take any medication.

KEY TO DRUG ENTRY WARNINGS

MAO warning means use caution with this drug if you are already taking any of the antidepressants called monoamine oxidase (MAO) inhibitors. In some cases you should not take the two drugs together, so consult your doctor. Combining an MAO inhibitor and this drug could cause dangerous, even fatal, side effects like changes in blood pressure, heart problems, high fever, convulsions, or even death.

No driving means don't drive a car or operate heavy machinery until you are sure the medicine isn't causing blurred vision or making you drowsy, dizzy, or less than alert.

Refrigerate means this medicine needs to stay cold and should be kept in the refrigerator. Do not freeze.

NATURAL ALTERNATIVES TO DRUGS

Prescription drugs play an important role in health care, but sometimes you can improve your condition just by making changes in your diet and lifestyle. To help you do that, we've included a section at the end of the book on natural alternatives to popping a pill. Here, you'll find helpful hints on ways to ease and heal everything from allergies and headaches to insomnia, ulcers, and weight problems.

If you're looking for a long-term solution, check this section first to see if you can help yourself without resorting to drugs. And, of course, always discuss all your options with your health care provider.

INSIDER'S GUIDE TO PRESCRIPTION DRUGS

It's important to keep abreast of the latest findings and decisions by researchers and the FDA. A drug you are taking today could very well be withdrawn from the market tomorrow due to newly discovered dangerous interactions. And tomorrow could see the approval of the latest wonder drug that does its job better, faster, and with fewer side effects.

New drugs are going before the FDA for approval all the time. That means more and perhaps better choices for depression or any other condition. You will always need the latest information on prescription drugs in order to make the healthiest decisions for yourself and those you love.

STATINS TAKE THE TROPHY — YOU WIN WITH LOWER CHOLESTEROL

There's a new statin in town and it just may be the best of the best. If you've got high cholesterol, you know all about statins. And fibrates. And niacin. And bile acid resins. They are all drugs used to lower cholesterol — in slightly different ways and with slightly different benefits and risks. But statins (HMG-CoA reductase inhibitors) usually edge out the competition by lowering total cholesterol more — by as much as 20 percent — and bad (LDL) cholesterol more — by as much as 40 percent. They have few side effects and dramatically reduce your risk of stroke.

Lovastatin, simvastatin, pravastatin, fluvastatin. It doesn't matter what you call them, they all do the job by suppressing a specific enzyme in the liver needed to make cholesterol. But now there's atorvastatin, brand name Lipitor. It not only lowers LDL and total cholesterol even more than the other statins, but it's the only one that is good for your triglyceride levels, too.

Compare all that to fibrates (fibric acid derivatives). Clofibrate (Atromid-S), gemfibrozil (Lopid), and fenofibrate (TriCor) are proven to lower triglycerides and increase HDL levels. However, experts are not as enthusiastic as you might think. Studies show that the risks of liver, testicular and pancreatic tumors, gallbladder disease, abdominal pain, and non-heart-related deaths from these drugs sometimes are great enough to outweigh the benefits.

Change your diet and lifestyle, then talk to your doctor about which drug treatment is best for you.

BEWARE THE HEART HAZARDS OF ORAL ANTI-DIABETICS

There is new evidence that sulfonylureas, drugs used to treat type II diabetes since the 1950s, may cause heart damage. The claim itself is not really new at all — 20 years ago a study found that a certain sulfonylurea, tolbutamide, increased the risk of heart-related death by two and one-half times — but there was controversy over that study process, and sulfonylureas weathered the storm. Very well, in fact. They went on to become the most widely used oral drug type for diabetes.

But now, new studies again show that sulfonylureas interfere with heart function by closing potassium channels and leaving your heart defenseless against heart attack. In fact, the Journal of the American College of Cardiology states that diabetic patients on sulfonylureas, hospitalized for coronary angioplasty, are at greater risk of dying than those not taking the drug.

All of these sulfonylurea drugs contain special warnings of "increased risk of cardiovascular mortality:"

- chlorpropamide (Diabinese)
- glimepiride (Amaryl)
- glipizide (Glucotrol)
- glyburide (Glynase, Micronase)
- tolazamide (Tolinase)

In addition, if you are on a sulfonylurea, you need to be especially watchful for symptoms of hypoglycemia (low blood sugar) — fatigue, restlessness, irritability and weakness. To avoid this dangerous condition, follow your prescribed diet and exercise plan, and be careful if you also take an anticoagulant, any sulfa drugs, or aspirin.

Other types of oral anti-diabetics carry their own problems:

metformin (Glucophage)	increased risk of heart-related death and a potentially fatal condition called lactic acidosis
acarbose (Precose)	a dose-related risk of liver injury
repaglinide (Prandin)	may develop dangerously low blood sugar (hypoglycemia)

Experts agree that weight control, exercise, and a healthy diet are the best ways to control type II diabetes. But if your doctor believes you need additional drug therapy, be sure to discuss all the risks and side effects.

FACT OR PHONY? NEW DRUGS FACE OFF IN THE WEIGHT-LOSS WAR

Meridia (sibutramine hydrochloride monohydrate) claims to be the latest weight-loss wonder drug. But if you're looking for miracles, you'll have to look through a cloud of controversy.

The good news is that the manufacturer, Knoll Pharmaceutical Company, lists the most common side effects as only dry mouth, anorexia, insomnia, and constipation. Besides fooling your brain into thinking that your stomach is full, Meridia also lowers your triglycerides, your bad (LDL) cholesterol, and your total cholesterol. It increases your good cholesterol and seems to improve glucose levels — especially helpful to diabetics.

The bad news? This drug can dangerously affect your heart rate and blood pressure. Because of this, people suffering from high blood pressure, heart disease, circulatory disease, congestive heart failure, stroke, heart rhythm disturbances, or high thyroid should not take this drug.

Xenical (orlistat) is the other big gun in weight control. It helps you shed pounds by keeping about one-third of the fat you eat from being absorbed into your body. In one recent study, researchers found that compared to other weight-loss treatments, Xenical:

- lowered blood pressure
- decreased waist circumference, a heart disease indicator
- improved cholesterol levels
- caused those in the study group to lose more weight
- caused those in the study group to better maintain their lower weight
- decreased blood insulin levels

Does this sound too good to be true? Then you should also consider that vitamin D and E levels decrease when taking Xenical and most people on the drug experience some kind of gastrointestinal upset — severe enough that many dropped out of the test.

It's hard to deny that Xenical seemed to work in this study. One question to consider though is whether this drug would have been as effective if the study group had not also been on a weight-loss diet. If you are prescribed Xenical in order to lose weight, but don't do anything except take the drug — no diet, no exercise program, etc. — will your results be as positive?

The moral to this weight-loss story is that there is no "magic pill." Exercise and a sensible diet are the best steps to a slimmer, healthier you.

CELEBREX PROMISES ARTHRITIS RELIEF WITHOUT STOMACH UPSET

You've got arthritis just like 40 million other Americans. You want pain relief, but you hate the stomach problems you get from aspirin and other anti-inflammatories. This is a serious issue if you are like most who suffer from this crippling disease and have to take an arthritis drug every day — for the rest of your life. More than 100,000 people are hospitalized each year for ulcers and internal bleeding caused by arthritis medications.

Now there's Celebrex (celecoxib), a new drug for the symptoms of osteoarthritis (OA) and rheumatoid arthritis (RA). While officially the drug still carries the same warning about gastrointestinal side effects, studies show that Celebrex does not seem to cause ulcers in the stomach or intestines like other NSAIDs.

SSRIs — A BETTER WAY TO DEFEAT DEPRESSION

There's a new class of drugs making life healthier and happier for millions of people suffering from depression.

Selective Serotonin Reuptake Inhibitors (SSRIs) seem to do the job without all the annoying and sometimes dangerous side effects that can come with other antidepressants.

Even though each case of depression is unique and each person's chemical make-up will respond to medication differently, experts have found that based on side effects, tolerance, and quality of life, people suffering from depression prefer the newer SSRIs over tricyclic antidepressants or the older class of antidepressants, monoamine oxidase (MAO) inhibitors. Here's how they measure up.

Tricyclic antidepressants are very effective, inexpensive drugs, but they are becoming less and less popular because of their long list of side effects, their numerous drug interactions, withdrawal symptoms, and the fact that most tricyclic overdoses are fatal.

MAO inhibitors suppress a chemical in your brain, monoamine oxidase, which then allows an increase in nerve impulse transmitters that maintain even mood and emotions. Some MAO inhibitors currently on the market are:

- furazolidone (Furoxone), antimicrobial
- isocarboxazid (Marplan), antidepressant
- selegiline HCL (Eldepryl, Carbex), anti-Parkinson's
- phenelzine sulfate (Nardil), antidepressant
- procarbazine (Matulane), Hodgkin's disease

- tranylcypromine sulfate (Parnate), antidepressant

These are usually prescribed for difficult or unusual depressions. But the side effects and food interactions make life with MAO inhibitors unpleasant. For instance, foods containing the amino acid tyramine can cause a dangerous, possibly fatal, rise in blood pressure when combined with MAO inhibitors. Although it's almost impossible to put together a complete list of these foods, here are some guidelines.

Tyramine occurs naturally in some foods and is produced in others as they age — so select fresh but not overripe produce and avoid strong or aged cheese. Certain methods of processing, like drying and pickling, produce tyramine. Therefore, avoid foods like sauerkraut; pickled fish; and smoked, dried, or tenderized meats. And when bacteria break down protein, it forms tyramine. That means many fermented alcoholic beverages, soy, and yeast products are full of this amino acid. Ask your doctor if you have specific questions about food interactions.

MAO inhibitors also can cause side effects that range from dizziness to potentially serious heart difficulties. They do work, but thankfully there are better, safer choices on the market.

SSRIs have fewer, less dangerous side effects than the older antidepressants, and so for the most part, patients taking SSRIs enjoy a better quality of life. They are becoming the drugs of choice for many patients.

Here's a list of some SSRIs that are currently available:

- fluoxetine (Prozac)
- sertraline (Zoloft)
- paroxetine (Paxil)
- fluvoxamine (Luvox)
- citalopram (Celexa)

These drugs are FDA-approved for depression, obsessive compulsive disorder (OCD), panic disorder, possibly bulimia, and several other anxiety-based problems. The most frequent side effects are intestinal problems and insomnia. Up to 62 percent of people on SSRIs have to take something to help them sleep.

But SSRIs are important because they are well tolerated. That means patients are comfortable taking these drugs and will stay on them long enough to get better.

LEARN THE ABCDS OF BLOOD PRESSURE DRUGS

All blood pressure medications are not created equal. The ads you read and the commercials you see on television are designed to do one thing — sell a drug. And that's why they may not be giving you the full story. Here's what you need to know to make the best choice for your health's sake.

ACE inhibitors. ACE stands for angiotensin converting enzyme. ACE inhibitors work by blocking a chemical called angiotensin in your body that causes blood vessels to tighten. As a result, ACE inhibitors relax your blood vessels. This lowers your blood pressure and increases the supply of blood and oxygen to your heart. A recent study found that ACE inhibitors also improve people's chances of surviving after a heart attack.

Beta blockers. These drugs lower blood pressure by blocking certain actions of your sympathetic nervous system. They expand blood vessel walls and slow down the contractions of your heart.

Calcium channel blockers. These drugs work by affecting the movement of calcium into the cells of your heart and blood vessels. They relax your blood vessels and increase the blood and oxygen supply to your heart.

Controversy surrounds the use of calcium channel blockers, mostly the short-acting ones. A recent study found that postmenopausal women who took calcium channel blockers were twice as likely to develop breast cancer as other women. Other studies have found an increase in deaths and heart attacks among people taking short-acting nifedipine, a calcium channel blocker.

The National Heart, Lung, and Blood Institute recommends to doctors that "short-acting nifedipine should be used with great caution (if at all), especially at higher doses in the treatment of hypertension (high blood pressure), angina, and MI (myocardial infarction)." The American Heart Association cautions people who are already taking this drug not to suddenly stop taking it without consulting their doctors.

Along with the short-acting drugs, the safety of longer-acting calcium channel blockers is also being questioned and studied. Other drugs may be safer for many people now taking calcium channel blockers.

Diuretics. Diuretics work on your kidneys to increase urination and get rid of excess fluid. They are probably the most commonly recommended high blood pressure medication — and the most inexpensive.

One problem with diuretics is that you may be flushing too many minerals out with your urine, including potassium, which is important for your heart's health. Sometimes potassium supplements are recommended if you are taking diuretics, or your doctor may prescribe a potassium-sparing diuretic.

Loop diuretics are another type of diuretic. They are so-named because they work in a part of the kidney called the Loop of Henle. This makes them more effective.

COMMONLY PRESCRIBED BLOOD PRESSURE MEDICATIONS

ACE inhibitors	benazepril (Lotensin), captopril (Capoten), enalapril maleate (Vasotec), fosinopril (Monopril), lisinopril (Prinivil, Zestril), quinapril (Accupril), ramipril (Altace)
Calcium channel blockers	amlodipine (Norvasc), diltiazem (Cardizem, Dilacor), felodipine (Plendil), isradipine (DynaCirc), nicardipine (Cardene), nifedipine (Adalat, Procardia), verapamil (Calan, Isoptin, Verelan)
Beta blockers	acebutolol (Sectral), atenolol (Tenormin), betaxolol (Kerlone), carteolol (Cartrol), labetalol (Normodyne, Trandate), metoprolol (Lopressor), nadolol (Corgard), penbutolol (Levatol), pindolol (Visken), propranolol (Inderal)

COMMONLY PRESCRIBED DIURETICS

Thiazides and related diuretics	chlorothiazide (Diuril), chlorthalidone (Thalitone, Hygroton), hydrochlorothiazide (Esidrix, Microzide, HydroDIURIL, Oretic), hydroflumethiazide (Diucardin, Saluron), methyclothiazide (Aquatensen, Enduron), metolazone (Mykrox, Zaroxolyn), bendroflumethiazide (Naturetin), trichlormethiazide (Naqua, Metahydrin, Trichlorex, Trichlormas), indapamide (Lozol)
Loop diuretics	bumetanide (Bumex), ethacrynic acid (Edecrin), furosemide (Lasix)
Potassium-sparing diuretics	amiloride (Midamor), amiloride HCTZ (Moduretic, Hydro-Ride), spironolactone (Aldactone), spironolactone HCTZ (Aldactazide), triamterene (Dyrenium), triamterene HCTZ (Dyazide, Maxzide)

DEADLY DRUG INTERACTIONS

GIVE WEIGHT LOSS PILLS A SECOND LOOK

Drugs that help you lose weight are enormously popular — as an entire nation continues its obsession with being thin — but they can be quite dangerous, too.

No one has forgotten the life-threatening consequences of "fen-phen," a combination of two central nervous system stimulants, fenfluramine and phentermine. Fenfluramine and dexfenfluramine (Redux) were withdrawn from the market because of their association with heart-valve disease, but phentermine is still widely prescribed for weight loss.

An MAO inhibitor, phentermine increases the amount of serotonin in your blood. While too much serotonin can damage heart tissue, as long as there are other ways for your body to remove this chemical from your bloodstream, phentermine shouldn't cause it to reach dangerous levels.

However, if you take phentermine with other drugs that also increase serotonin levels, you may cause a serotonin overload and heart problems such as primary pulmonary hypertension.

Antidepressants such as Prozac, Zoloft, and Paxil are drugs that keep serotonin from being reabsorbed into the brain. Therefore, combining any of these with phentermine could mean trouble for you and your heart.

Talk to your doctor before combining drugs like these. Losing a few pounds is not worth losing your health.

AVOID THIS DEADLY DUO: ANTIBIOTICS AND HEART DRUGS

Heart patients beware! If you pick up almost any kind of infection, from a respiratory infection to even an ulcer, the cure could endanger your life.

Why? Because some people need a specific, good bacteria in their digestive system to process and eliminate heart drugs like digoxin and disopyramide. And antibiotics prescribed for infections can kill off this good bacteria, causing blood levels of these drugs to climb dangerously high.

This happened to a 74-year-old woman in Germany. She had been taking disopyramide for a heart condition for several years without complications. But when she began antibiotic treatment for an ulcer caused by the *H. pylori* bacteria, the trouble began.

Within six days, she collapsed from disopyramide poisoning. It took two days in intensive care and nearly three weeks in the hospital to correct her body's chemical imbalance.

Another woman, 70 years old, already on digoxin, began taking clarithromycin for bronchitis. The antibiotic again affected how her body absorbed the heart drug, and within days she had to be hospitalized for digoxin toxicity. Her symptoms were weakness, vision changes, nausea, and vomiting.

Learn about these drug interactions, and don't let a doctor's quick medication fix spell deadly results for you.

MAP OUT A SAFER PRESCRIPTION PLAN

Antidepressants can literally save someone's life. But they can also spell danger when mixed with other medications. A 42-year-old woman was taking sertraline hydrochloride (Zoloft) for depression and added a prescription pain reliever, tramadol hydrochloride (Ultram). She developed chest pain, confusion, shaking, agitation, and accelerated heart rate.

Doctors believe that this combination of drugs interact to cause a dangerous increase in the chemical serotonin, called serotonin syndrome. If you experience any of these symptoms, see your doctor immediately.

DISCOVER THE TRAGEDY BEHIND ANTIDEPRESSANTS

Severe depression often leads to thoughts of death and dying. Hopefully, if you are this desperate you are getting help from a professional, who may prescribe one or more antidepressants. Tragedy can strike, though, when the newer antidepressants like Paxil or Prozac interact with older drugs, especially tricyclic antidepressants, and cause the very thing they are supposed to prevent.

A combination of these drugs can slow down your body's metabolism, causing too much of the tricyclic antidepressants to build up in your bloodstream — sometimes to toxic levels.

This happened to a 36-year-old man suffering from severe depression. He was prescribed a combination of amitriptyline (Elavil, Endep, Emitrip, or Enovil) and fluoxetine (Prozac) and died within six weeks.

Testing showed high concentrations of amitriptyline in his system — enough to cause a fatal heart attack.

If you are on Prozac or other SSRIs, be careful of adding other antidepressants to your daily regimen, especially amitriptyline, doxepin, nortriptyline, desipramine, imipramine, methadone, phenytoin, propranolol, or perphenazine.

GET TO THE HEART OF THIS DANGEROUS DRUG COMBINATION

Warfarin (Coumadin) is a serious drug for a serious heart condition. Unfortunately, even as necessary a medication as it is, there are possible dangers. Dozens of drugs interact with this anticoagulant (blood-thinner), and may cause everything from mild discomfort to death.

For example, antifungals, like terbinafine and fluconazole, suppress a liver enzyme that is important in processing warfarin out of your body. Without this important enzyme, warfarin builds up, thinning your blood to a dangerous level.

There may be no warning signs, but if you experience unusual bleeding, see your doctor immediately. While on terbinafine for a nail fungus, a 68-year-old woman had to have her warfarin dose constantly adjusted in order to keep dangerous bleeding under control.

Another combination to be careful of is warfarin and the antibiotics, clarithromycin or erythromycin. These drugs increase the blood-thinning effects of warfarin and could mean serious bleeding complications. Your doctor must monitor you very closely while you are on these drugs and even for several days after the medications are stopped.

SIDESTEP A DILANTIN DISASTER

Dilantin (phenytoin) is a drug that helps control seizures. It is often prescribed for symptoms suffered after a stroke. When a 61-year-old man on Dilantin was admitted to the hospital for bacterial pneumonia, doctors thought nothing of giving him ciprofloxacin (Cipro), an antibiotic. What the doctors didn't realize was that this antibiotic prevents Dilantin from being absorbed in the body. Within two days the drug's protective effect had diminished and the man had a seizure. The doctors increased his Dilantin.

As long as he was on the ciprofloxacin, the unusually large doses of Dilantin caused no problems. But once the man was taken off the antibiotic and discharged from the hospital, there was nothing to stop the Dilantin from flooding through his body and causing phenytoin intoxication. As a result, he developed ataxia, a severe loss of muscle control, suffered a head injury, and had to return to the hospital.

HIGH CHOLESTEROL? WATCH OUT FOR AN RX EMERGENCY

Rhabdomyolysis is a serious, sometimes fatal disease that attacks your skeletal muscles (those attached to bones and necessary for movement). It can also cause kidney damage. Some drug combinations can bring on rhabdomyolysis, especially ones including cholesterol-lowering agents.

This happened to an 83-year-old woman who was taking simvastatin (Zocor) for high cholesterol and began mibefradil for high blood pressure. Within three weeks, she developed muscle pain, dehydration, and finally kidney failure.

She was admitted to the hospital, where doctors stopped all her medication. For the next four weeks, she received intensive physiotherapy and underwent seven sessions of dialysis before she could be released. Unfortunately, her kidneys did not recover 100 percent.

This same dangerous interaction can occur between other cholesterol-lowering drugs and antibiotics like clarithromycin or azithromycin. Because of certain heart conditions, many people take antibiotics before dental procedures or surgery as a precaution against bacterial infections. One 73-year-old man on lovastatin did this, and as a result, developed rhabdomyolysis that eventually involved not only his kidneys, but his pancreas, intestines, and other internal organs as well.

DEMAND THE LOW-DOWN ON COUMADIN

If you have heart disease, warfarin (Coumadin) may be just the drug that saves your life. It is essential in thinning blood and preventing dangerous clots. However, this is one case where more is not better. If your blood doesn't have enough clotting factor, you can literally bleed to death.

Several drugs increase warfarin's blood-thinning power to life-threatening levels, including some antibiotics, arthritis remedies, aspirin, and even the ulcer drug, Tagamet. But nobody suspected the aspirin substitute, acetaminophen, of interacting with warfarin until recently.

Researchers out of Massachusetts General Hospital and Harvard Medical School discovered that warfarin and high doses or long-term use of acetaminophen can keep your blood from clotting, even when it needs to.

If you suffer from cancer and heart disease, you have even more prescription interactions to worry about. For one 59-year-old man, the drugs he was taking, warfarin and 5-fluorouracil for colon cancer, made him worse, not better. He was rushed to the emergency room for episodes of dangerous bleeding.

Another 73-year-old man was admitted to the hospital for bruising, bleeding, and fatigue. He had been taking warfarin for several years for deep vein thrombosis, but had recently added gemfibrozil (Lopid) to help control his cholesterol. When gemfibrozil was discontinued, his symptoms disappeared.

You may not notice symptoms of dangerously thin blood until it is too late. If you must take drugs like these together, make sure your doctor monitors your condition with frequent blood tests, and if you notice any unusual bleeding or bruising, see a doctor immediately.

USE CAUTION WHEN A NEW DRUG HITS THE SHELF

New drugs are often approved before all possible interactions are discovered. This was the case for one kidney transplant patient who was prescribed a promising new diabetes drug, troglitazone (Rezulin). It interacted with his transplant drug, cyclosporine, and caused a severe rejection episode. Because of a large number of kidney-related deaths, troglitazone was pulled from the market.

BYPASS THE PERILS OF PRESCRIPTION COMBOS

It all begins innocently enough. You fill a prescription for cisapride (Propulsid) a drug to relieve that awful heartburn you have every night. Then, because of strep throat, or a respiratory infection, or a urinary tract infection, you start taking an antibiotic like clarithromycin or erythromycin. Or perhaps you begin a drug, like diltiazem, to regulate your high blood pressure. Before you know it, you are heading to the hospital.

This happened to one 53-year-old woman. Because of the interaction between cisapride and other drugs, she lost consciousness while driving and was involved in two car accidents. She was lucky and lived, but you may not be so lucky.

Always talk to your doctor first before combining any types of drugs, including those sold over the counter. You may think it harmless to take an antidiarrheal remedy if a drug causes diarrhea, but you could make your condition dangerously worse. Let your doctor be the one to decide.

BEWARE THE HIDDEN ALCOHOL

Many prescription and over-the-counter products contain alcohol and can interact dangerously with other medicines you are taking.

One 45-year-old woman found this out when she went to the emergency room for peritonitis, an inflammation in her abdomen. Her doctors began treating her with a number of medicines, including Donnatal Elixir, a combination drug to quiet her abdominal spasms, and cefotetan, an injectable antibiotic to fight the infection.

Her condition, however, only got worse. She had difficulty breathing, her blood pressure dropped, her fever remained high, and her pain and nausea increased. It was three days before the hospital realized the alcohol in the Donnatal Elixir was interacting with the cefotetan, causing most of these symptoms. Once the alcohol-containing product was discontinued, the woman's symptoms improved, and she was discharged.

Several antibiotics will produce this kind of reaction when given with products that contain alcohol. You need to be aware that many over-the-counter medications are more than 5 percent alcohol, including Geritol Liquid, NyQuil Liquid, Formula 44 Cough Mixture, Dramamine Liquid, Comtrex, Adult Tylenol Liquid, Benadryl Elixir, Adult CoTylenol Liquid, and Donnatal Elixir.

7 WAYS TO SIDESTEP DEADLY DRUG ERRORS

Camilla Yates, a pregnant woman with gestational diabetes, picked up her first prescription for insulin at her usual drug store. Since she had just read an article on the importance of checking your prescription for errors, she compared the label to her prescription. Lucky for her that she did, because her instructions said to take 50 units, but her prescription was for 5 units. Her pharmacist had misread 5U as 50 — an honest mistake, but one that could have been deadly for Camilla and her baby.

Many people aren't so lucky. According to a study published in *The Journal of the American Medical Association*, more than 100,000 people every year die from adverse drug reactions. That makes it between the fourth and sixth leading cause of death in the United States.

But medications also save many lives every year. Here's how you can avoid becoming a victim to your prescription.

Write down the prescription. Copy the generic and brand names of your prescription, plus dosing information, while you're at your doctor's office. Then you'll have a record, in your own handwriting, to check against your actual prescription when you get it filled. Many times prescription errors occur because the pharmacist can't read the doctor's handwriting.

Inform your doctor. Make sure you tell your doctor about any other medications you're taking. Don't assume he knows, even if he prescribed your other medicines. Include any over-the-counter medications, herbs, or supplements. And remind him of any drug allergies you have. Often, people who are allergic to one drug may also be allergic to a related drug.

Stick with the same pharmacy. Most pharmacies now have computerized systems that will warn you if you've been prescribed two drugs that may interact. If you go to different pharmacies, however, you lose that advantage.

Check your pills. When you get a refill, check to make sure the pills look like the ones you're used to taking. If there is a change, ask your pharmacist about it.

Schedule a "brown bag" session. Put every medicine you're taking into a bag and let your doctor or pharmacist examine them for potential interactions, duplication, or expired dates.

Skip the alcohol. Alcohol is a drug that can interact with many prescription medications. To be safe, if you're taking medication, stay away from alcohol.

Don't be afraid to ask questions. Make sure you understand what you're taking and why. Your doctor and pharmacist want you to stay healthy, so they'll be glad to answer any questions you have.

LIFE-SAVING ADVICE FOR THE ELDERLY

Even properly prescribed medicine can be dangerous if you don't take it properly. That can be a particular problem for the elderly.

Older adults are more likely to take several types of medication, increasing the risk of interactions. And because their reading vision often declines as they age, they're more likely to misread the fine print on prescription labels. If vision is a problem for you, don't be embarrassed to ask your pharmacist to give your instructions in large print.

You also may have problems remembering whether or not you've taken your medication. This uncertainty might result in your taking too little or too much medicine, perhaps even causing an overdose. Containers that divide your dosages up for the week can be helpful.

Focusing on your pill while you take it is another good way to help yourself remember, according to psychologist Gilles Einstein. Don't just swallow it quickly; swish it around in your mouth, and make a mental note of it. You'll be more likely to remember you took it and maybe save yourself from a dangerous overdose.

PRESCRIPTION DRUG INDEX

Drugs listed in lower case letters are brand name drugs

Drugs listed in lower case letters are brand name drugs

Drugs listed in lower case letters are brand name drugs

Drugs listed in lower case letters are brand name drugs

Drugs listed in lower case letters are brand name drugs

Drugs listed in lower case letters are brand name drugs

Drugs listed in lower case letters are brand name drugs

Drugs listed in lower case letters are brand name drugs

Drugs listed in lower case letters are brand name drugs

Drugs listed in lower case letters are brand name drugs

PRESCRIPTION DRUGS

ACARBOSE

Pregnancy category: B
Refrigerate

Brand:
Precose

Acarbose treats type II diabetes when diet alone can't control high blood sugar levels.

How to take this drug:
- Take this medication with food.
- Often you will start with a low dose of this drug and work your way up to higher doses.

Possible side effects:
Abdominal pain   Diarrhea
Gas

Possible interactions:
- Acarbose could interact with these drugs to cause your blood sugar to fall too low: thiazides and other diuretics, corticosteroids, phenothiazines, thyroid products, estrogens, oral contraceptives, phenytoin, nicotinic acid, sympathomimetics, calcium channel blockers, and isoniazid.
- Check with your doctor if you are taking drugs to open your airways, like Sudafed, charcoal tablets, or digestive enzyme preparations.

Other important information:
- Use acarbose along with, not instead of, a good diet and healthy exercise program.
- It can be taken alone or with other diabetes medications.
- Don't use it if you have diabetic ketoacidosis, cirrhosis (a chronic degenerative liver disease), inflammatory bowel disease, colonic ulcers, or any kind of intestinal obstruction.
- Have your liver checked every three months for the first year of treatment. If you develop signs of liver toxicity (fever, rash, fatigue, jaundice, right-side pain), see your doctor immediately.

- Because it prevents the breakdown of table sugar, if you take acarbose with a sulfonylurea or insulin, be sure and have a source of glucose always at hand, in case you experience a drop in your blood sugar.
- Acarbose is not insulin and cannot be used in place of insulin.

ACEBUTOLOL HYDROCHLORIDE

Pregnancy category: B
No driving

Brand:
Sectral

Acebutolol is a beta blocker that controls high blood pressure and regulates heart rhythm.

Possible side effects:

Severe depression	Asthma
Tiredness	Dizziness
Headache	Difficulty breathing
Diarrhea	Constipation
Nausea	Gas
Frequent urination	Sleeplessness
Chest pain	Swelling
Abnormal dreams	Rash
Stuffy nose	

Possible interactions:
- Aspirin and other nonsteroidal anti-inflammatory drugs (NSAIDs) may decrease the effects of acebutolol.
- Other high blood pressure medicines, cold medicines, and nose drops may increase the effects of acebutolol.

Other important information:
- Don't use acebutolol if you have congestive heart failure, heart block, cardiogenic shock, or slow heartbeat.
- Use it cautiously if you have angina, diseases of the arteries, bronchitis, emphysema, or liver or kidney problems.
- If you have diabetes, use this drug cautiously because beta blockers can mask the signs of low blood sugar.
- Acebutolol can also mask signs of an overactive thyroid.
- Never quit taking this drug without talking to your doctor. It could increase your risk of angina or heart attack.
- You may have to discontinue this drug before having any surgery.

ACETAMINOPHEN WITH CODEINE

Pregnancy category: C
No driving

Brand:
Capital and Codeine   *Phenaphen with Codeine*
Tylenol with Codeine

This drug combines a narcotic painkiller with acetaminophen and is used to relieve pain.

How to take this drug:
*   Never take more medicine than you are prescribed.

Possible side effects:
Dizziness   Drowsiness
Shortness of breath   Nausea
Slow or irregular breathing

Possible interactions:
*   If you take this drug along with alcohol or tranquilizers, antihistamines, or muscle relaxants, the combination may dangerously depress your nervous system.
*   If you take this drug along with the tuberculosis drug isoniazid, the combination may cause liver damage.
*   ˙ If you take this drug along with the antiparkinson drug benztropine mesylate, the combination may cause paralysis of the intestines.

Other important information:
*   Use this drug with caution if you have a head injury, as it may increase fluid pressure on the brain.
*   If you have stomach pain, kidney or liver disorders, underactive thyroid, or narrowing of the urethra, use this drug cautiously.
*   You may become physically and psychologically dependent on this drug if you take high doses for long periods of time.

ACETAMINOPHEN WITH HYDROCODONE BITARTRATE

Pregnancy category: C
No driving

Brand:
Anexsia   *Co-Gesic*
Hydrocet   *Lorcet HD*
Lortab   *Vicodin*
Vicodin ES   *Vicodin HP*

This drug combines acetaminophen with a narcotic painkiller very similar to codeine and is used to relieve pain.

How to take this drug:

- Never take more medicine than you are prescribed.

Possible side effects:

Dizziness	Drowsiness
Nausea	Constipation
Mood changes	Mental clouding
Difficulty urinating	Slow or irregular breathing

Possible interactions:

- If you take this drug along with alcohol or tranquilizers, antihistamines, or muscle relaxants, the combination may dangerously depress your nervous system.
- Taking monoamine oxidase (MAO) inhibitors or tricyclic antidepressants with this drug can increase the effects of either the antidepressant or this drug.
- If you take this drug along with the antiparkinson drug benztropine mesylate, the combination may cause paralysis of the intestines.
- If you take this drug along with the tuberculosis drug isoniazid, the combination may cause liver damage.

Other important information:

- Hydrocodone suppresses the cough reflex, so people with lung disease should take this drug with caution.
- Use this drug with caution if you have a head injury, as it may increase fluid pressure on the brain.
- Older people and people with liver or kidney damage, an underactive thyroid, Addison's disease, or an enlarged prostate should take this drug with caution.
- You may become physically and psychologically dependent on this drug if you take high doses for long periods of time.

ACETAMINOPHEN WITH OXYCODONE

Pregnancy category: C
No driving

Brand:

Oxycet	*Percocet*
Roxicet	*Roxilox*
Tylox	

This drug combines acetaminophen with a narcotic painkiller similar to morphine and is used to treat pain.

How to take this drug:

- Never take more medicine than you are prescribed.

Possible side effects:

Dizziness	Sleepiness
Nausea	Rash
Itching	Constipation
Mood changes	Slow or irregular breathing

Possible interactions:

* If you take this drug along with alcohol or tranquilizers, antihistamines, or muscle relaxants, the combination may dangerously depress your nervous system.
* Taking monoamine oxidase (MAO) inhibitors or tricyclic antidepressants with this drug can increase the effects of either the antidepressant or this drug.
* If you take this drug along with the antiparkinson drug benztropine mesylate, the combination may cause paralysis of the intestines.
* If you take this drug along with the tuberculosis drug isoniazid, the combination may cause liver damage.

Other important information:

* Use this drug with caution if you have a head injury, as it may increase fluid pressure on the brain.
* Older people and people with liver or kidney damage, an underactive thyroid, Addison's disease, or an enlarged prostate should take this drug with caution.
* You may become physically and psychologically dependent on this drug if you take high doses for long periods of time.

ACETAMINOPHEN WITH PROPOXYPHENE NAPSYLATE

Pregnancy category: NR
No driving

Brand:

Darvocet-N 100   *Darvocet-N 50*

This drug combines acetaminophen with a narcotic painkiller similar to morphine to relieve pain and fever.

How to take this drug:

* Lie down after taking this drug to avoid some of the side effects.

Possible side effects:

Dizziness	Sleepiness
Nausea	Headache
Constipation	Hallucinations
Liver damage	Depression or anxiety
Rash	Stomach pain

Possible interactions:
- If you take this drug along with alcohol or tranquilizers, antihistamines, or muscle relaxants, the combination may dangerously depress your nervous system.
- Propoxyphene may increase the effects of anticoagulants and anticonvulsants.
- If you take propoxyphene with high doses of aspirin, the combination may cause kidney damage.

Other important information:
- People with liver or kidney problems may need a reduced dose.
- You may become physically and psychologically dependent on this drug if you take high doses for long periods of time.

ACETAZOLAMIDE

Pregnancy category: C
No driving

Brand:
Diamox

Acetazolamide is a diuretic that treats some kinds of glaucoma, fluid retention in congestive heart failure, epilepsy, and altitude sickness.

Possible side effects:

Tingling of extremities	Ringing in the ears
Loss of appetite	Nausea, vomiting or diarrhea
Confusion	Drowsiness
Frequent urination	

Possible interactions:
- If you take acetazolamide with high doses of aspirin, you could experience loss of appetite, rapid breathing, coma, and death.

Other important information:
- Don't use acetazolamide if you have liver or kidney problems.
- This drug may mask symptoms of some forms of glaucoma.
- Have regular liver and kidney tests while you're taking this drug.
- Acetazolamide can cause you to lose sodium and potassium. Eat extra potassium-rich foods like bananas.
- Weigh daily so you'll know if you're losing too much fluid, which can cause dehydration and possibly blood clots. Warning signs of dehydration include dry mouth, thirst, drowsiness, and weakness. Quit using the drug and contact your doctor if you stop urinating.

ACYCLOVIR

Pregnancy category: C
No driving

Brand:
Zovirax

This antiviral is used to treat the fever, pain, and other symptoms of Herpes Simplex Virus types 1 and 2 (genital herpes), shingles, chickenpox, and Epstein-Barr virus.

How to take this drug:
* Use a finger cot or a rubber glove to apply the ointment so you won't spread the infection. A one-half inch of ointment usually covers about four square inches.
* Never double a missed dose, instead take it as soon as you remember or skip it and go on with your regular schedule.

Possible side effects:
Skin rash	Bleeding gums
Headache	Dizziness
Nausea	Burning
Stinging	Itching

Possible interactions:
* The effects of acyclovir may be increased by the gout drug probenecid.
* If used with the AIDS drug zidovudine, acyclovir may cause intense tiredness and drowsiness.
* Interactions with kidney drugs may cause kidney problems.

Other important information:
* Because genital herpes is contagious, avoid sexual intercourse if you can still see blisters and inflammation.

ALBUTEROL

Pregnancy category: C
Refrigerate   MAO warning

Brand:
Proventil   *Ventolin*

Albuterol is a bronchodilator that relieves wheezing and the bronchial spasms that accompany asthma, bronchitis, and emphysema.

How to take this drug:
* This drug is available as an inhaler, syrup, or tablets.

- Never use this drug more frequently than your doctor recommends. The effects of each dose may last from six to eight hours or longer. Extended release tablets last for 12 hours or longer.
- An overdose can cause a heart attack or sudden death.
- The extended-release tablets must be swallowed whole with a liquid. You should not chew or crush the tablet.
- For the inhalation aerosol, the effect of the medicine may be decreased if the canister is cold. Shake well before using.

Possible side effects:

Tremors	Nervousness
Rapid or irregular heartbeat	Worsening of asthma symptoms
Headache	Sleeplessness
Dizziness	High blood pressure
Cough	Throat irritation
Stomach pain	Nausea

Possible interactions:

- Taking other bronchodilators or epinephrine while taking albuterol increases your risk of serious heart problems such as cardiac arrest.
- Taking beta blockers (a type of blood pressure drug) while taking albuterol can reduce the effectiveness of both drugs.

Other important information:

- If you have heart disease, an irregular heartbeat, high blood pressure, diabetes, or an overactive thyroid, talk to your doctor about your condition before using this drug.
- Your doctor should monitor your blood pressure and your heart while you are taking albuterol.

ALENDRONATE SODIUM

Pregnancy category: C

Brand:

Fosamax

This drug is prescribed for the treatment of osteoporosis and Paget's disease.

How to take this drug:

- Chewing or sucking on the tablet could cause mouth sores.
- Don't take this drug with food or other medications and wait at least 30 minutes to eat.
- Take it with a full glass of water first thing in the morning.
- Don't lie down for at least 30 minutes after taking it.
- Never double a missed dose, instead take it as soon as you remember or skip it and go on with your regular schedule.

Possible side effects:

Constipation
Diarrhea
Nausea or vomiting
Esophageal ulcers
Headache

Indigestion
Muscle, bone or joint pain
Abdominal pain
Gas
Difficulty swallowing

Possible interactions:

- Taking alendronate sodium with aspirin could cause stomach upset.
- Calcium supplements could interfere with your body's ability to absorb alendronate sodium.

Other important information:

- Avoid this drug if you are on hormone replacement therapy or have kidney problems.

ALLOPURINOL

Pregnancy category: C
No driving

Brand:

Lopurin   *Zyloprim*

Allopurinol treats gout by reducing the amount of uric acid your body produces.

How to take this drug:

- This drug may be less upsetting to your stomach if you take it with food.
- While you're taking this drug, drink 10 to 12 glasses of fluid per day to help prevent kidney stones.
- Never double a missed dose, instead take it as soon as you remember or skip it and go on with your regular schedule.

Possible side effects:

Severe gout attack
Fever
Joint or muscle pain
Diarrhea
Yellow skin or eyes
Bloody urine
Swollen lips and mouth

Skin rash
Chills
Nausea
Headache
Painful urination
Eye irritation

Possible interactions:

- Allopurinol may increase the effects of the anticoagulant dicumarol and the immunosuppressant azathioprine.

- Allopurinol may cause skin rash when taken at the same time as the antibiotics amoxicillin and ampicillin.
- Don't take allopurinol with high doses of vitamin C as it may cause kidney stones.

Other important information:
- People with preexisting kidney disease, liver disease, or high blood pressure should be carefully monitored.
- See your doctor immediately if you develop any of the listed side effects.
- You may not notice any improvement in your gout for two to six weeks.

ALPRAZOLAM

Pregnancy category: D
No driving

Brand:
Xanax

This benzodiazepine treats anxiety, anxiety associated with depression, and panic disorder.

Possible side effects:

Drowsiness	Lightheadedness
Headache	Depression
Confusion	Sleeplessness
Dry mouth	Constipation
Diarrhea	Nausea
Irritability	Memory loss
Change in sex drive	Change in appetite

Possible interactions:
- If you take this drug along with alcohol or tranquilizers, antihistamines, or muscle relaxants, the combination may dangerously depress your nervous system.
- Alprazolam may increase levels of the antidepressants imipramine and desipramine in your body.
- Effects of this drug may be increased by the ulcer drug cimetidine and by birth control pills.
- Talk to your doctor before drinking grapefruit juice while taking this drug.

Other important information:
- People with some kinds of glaucoma shouldn't use this drug. Ask your doctor.
- You can become dependent on alprazolam. To avoid seizures and other withdrawal symptoms, quit taking the drug gradually under your doctor's supervision.

- People with poor liver, kidney, or lung functions and obese people should use alprazolam cautiously.
- Have regular blood and urine tests if you are taking alprazolam for a long time.

AMANTADINE HYDROCHLORIDE

Pregnancy category: C
No driving

Brand:
Symmetrel

Amantadine reduces stiffness and improves muscle control for people with Parkinson's disease. It works as an antiviral to treat and prevent certain types of flu. Amantadine is also used to treat stiffness and shaking caused by some medicines.

Possible side effects:

Nausea	Dizziness
Sleeplessness	Depression
Anxiety	Irritability
Hallucinations	Confusion
Loss of appetite	Dry mouth or nose
Constipation	Swelling
Dizziness when standing suddenly	Headache
Drowsiness	Strange dreams
Diarrhea	Fatigue
Skin rash or mottling	

Possible interactions:
- Have your doctor monitor you if you take amantadine and other drugs that stimulate your central nervous system.

Other important information:
- Never stop taking this drug suddenly. It could bring on neuroleptic malignant syndrome (NMS) or "parkinsonian crisis." Symptoms of NMS are rigid muscles, uncontrollable movements, a rapid heartbeat, and high or low blood pressure.
- People with a history of mental problems are sometimes made worse by amantadine.
- People with a history of seizures sometimes have more seizures while taking amantadine.
- People with congestive heart failure, low blood pressure upon standing, a recurrent eczema rash, or liver problems should take this drug cautiously.
- Amantadine can lose its effectiveness for treating Parkinson's disease after you've taken it for several months.

AMILORIDE HYDROCHLORIDE

Pregnancy category: B

Brand:
Midamor

This diuretic is used to treat high blood pressure and congestive heart failure.

How to take this drug:
- Take this drug with food to avoid upset stomach.

Possible side effects:

Headache	Nausea
Loss of appetite	Diarrhea or constipation
Stomach pain	Mild rash
Weakness	Muscle cramps
Dizziness	Cough
Impotence	

Possible interactions:
- Anti-inflammatory drugs may lessen the effectiveness of amiloride.
- Amiloride is often used with other blood pressure drugs for beneficial effects, but some combinations may put you at risk for high levels of potassium in the blood. Amiloride should not be used with other potassium-sparing drugs.
- This drug may cause the antipsychotic drug lithium to accumulate to toxic levels in the body.

Other important information:
- People with diabetes, liver problems, or kidney problems should take this drug with caution.
- Stomach ulcer and liver damage are possible serious reactions.
- This drug can cause dangerously high, even fatal, levels of potassium in your body. Some warning signs are a prickling or tingling sensation, muscle weakness, tiredness, and slow heartbeat.
- Weigh daily so you'll know if you're losing too much fluid, which can cause dehydration and possibly blood clots. Warning signs of dehydration include dry mouth, thirst, drowsiness, and weakness. Quit using the drug and contact your doctor if you stop urinating.

AMIODARONE HYDROCHLORIDE

Pregnancy category: D

Brand:
Cordarone   *Pacerone*

Amiodarone is an antiarrhythmic used to correct irregular heartbeats.

Possible side effects:

Nausea or vomiting	Increased sensitivity to the sun
Lack of coordination	Constipation
Sleeplessness	Headache

Possible interactions:

- Amiodarone may increase the effects of anticoagulants and the effects of other drugs that regulate the rhythm of the heart.
- Amiodarone may cause toxic levels of the heart drug digoxin to build up in the blood.

Other important information:

- Toxic effects can be very severe, even fatal. Amiodarone should only be used as a last resort, after other heart-rhythm regulators have been tried.
- People with some types of heart rhythm disorders, such as people with second- or third-degree AV block not being treated with a pacemaker or people with a slow heartbeat that has caused fainting, should not use this drug.
- This drug will increase your skin's sensitivity to the sun. Always use a sunscreen and wear protective clothes when you will be exposed to the sun.

AMITRIPTYLINE HYDROCHLORIDE

Pregnancy category: NR
No driving   MAO warning

Brand:

Elavil

This drug treats the symptoms of depression.

How to take this drug:

- Since amitriptyline has a sedative effect, you may want to take the largest dose in the late afternoon or at bedtime.
- This drug is very likely to cause dry mouth and constipation, so you should drink plenty of fluids and eat a high-fiber diet.

Possible side effects:

Dizziness	Dry mouth
Headache	Increased appetite
Nausea	Unpleasant taste or a black tongue
Diarrhea	Increased sweating
Ringing in the ears	Breast enlargement in men and women
Hair loss	Sensitivity to light

Possible interactions:

- Any of the type of antidepressants called selective serotonin reuptake inhibitors (fluoxetine, sertraline, and paroxetine) can cause amitriptyline to reach dangerously high levels in your body. Don't quickly switch from fluoxetine to a tricyclic antidepressant like amitriptyline. You may need to wait five weeks for the fluoxetine to clear out of your body.

- Some blood-pressure-lowering drugs may not work as well if you also take amitriptyline.
- If you take amitriptyline along with tranquilizers, alcohol, antihistamines, or muscle relaxers, the combination may dangerously depress your nervous system.
- Taking disulfiram, a drug that helps you overcome alcohol addiction, and amitriptyline at the same time can cause delirium.
- Your doctor should supervise you closely for side effects if you take amitriptyline along with any anticholinergic drugs, such as some antihistamines and muscle relaxants or along with any sympathomimetic drugs, such as some decongestants.
- Cimetidine, an ulcer drug, can increase the levels of amitriptyline in your body.
- Taking ethchlorvynol, a drug for insomnia, and amitriptyline at the same time can cause delirium.

Other important information:
- Don't use this drug if you are recovering from a heart attack.
- If you have a history of seizures, liver problems, urinary retention, thyroid problems, increased pressure in the eye, or heart problems, talk with your doctor about your condition before you take amitriptyline.
- When possible, quit taking amitriptyline several days before surgery.
- If you suddenly quit taking this drug, you could have nausea, headache, and a general feeling of fatigue. If you gradually quit taking the drug, you may still experience irritability, restlessness, and dream and sleep disturbances.
- Be careful in hot weather. This drug could make you sweat less in high temperatures, so you're more likely to get a high fever or heatstroke.

AMLODIPINE BESYLATE

Pregnancy category: C

Brand:
Norvasc

Amlodipine is a calcium channel blocker. It lowers blood pressure and treats some forms of angina.

Possible side effects:
Swollen ankles and feet	Headache
Flushing	Rapid heartbeat
Tiredness	Nausea

Possible interactions:

- The ulcer drug cimetidine may increase the effects of amlodipine.
- Using amlodipine with beta blockers may result in very low blood pressure or heart irregularities.
- Don't suddenly stop taking beta blockers before or during treatment with calcium channel blockers.

Other important information:

- Use this drug cautiously if you have had a heart attack, liver disease, narrowing of the aorta, or congestive heart failure.
- Tell your doctor immediately if you have any signs of congestive heart failure, such as night cough; swelling and fluid retention in your legs, feet, or hands; or difficulty breathing, especially when lying down or after physical exertion.
- Have your blood pressure checked regularly while you're taking this drug.
- Don't stop taking your medicine without your doctor's approval, even if you feel better.
- When you withdraw from the drug, your chest pain may get worse for a while, a condition called rebound angina.

AMLODIPINE BESYLATE AND BENAZEPRIL HYDROCHLORIDE

Pregnancy category: C/D

Brand:

Lotrel

This drug, used to treat high blood pressure, is a combination of an ACE inhibitor and a calcium channel blocker.

How to take this drug:

- Never double a missed dose, instead take it as soon as you remember or skip it and go on with your regular schedule.

Possible side effects:

Cough   Swollen lips and face

Possible interactions:

- This drug may interact with diuretics, potassium supplements, and lithium.

Other important information:

- Monitor your blood pressure so it doesn't fall too low. Beware of the symptoms of hypotension (low blood pressure).
- Talk to your doctor before taking this drug if you have kidney or liver disease. Your liver and kidney functions should be monitored while you are on this drug.

- If you have severe congestive heart failure, this drug may affect your kidney function.
- If you have heart failure, you must use any calcium channel blocker cautiously.

AMOXAPINE

Pregnancy category: C
No driving   MAO warning

Brand:
Asendin

Amoxapine treats the symptoms of depression and depression accompanied by anxiety. It is a tricyclic antidepressant with mild sedative effects.

Possible side effects:

Drowsiness	Dry mouth
Constipation	Blurred vision
Anxiety	Sleeplessness
Shakiness	Rapid heartbeat
Confusion	Excitement
Nausea	Dizziness
Headache	Tiredness
Weakness	Increased appetite
Increased sweating	Skin rash
Fever	

Possible interactions:
- Any of the type of antidepressants called selective serotonin reuptake inhibitors (fluoxetine, sertraline, and paroxetine) can cause amoxapine to reach dangerously high levels in your body. Don't quickly switch from fluoxetine to a tricyclic antidepressant like amoxapine. You may need to wait five weeks for the fluoxetine to clear out of your body.
- If you take amoxapine along with tranquilizers, alcohol, antihistamines, or muscle relaxers, the combination may dangerously depress your nervous system.
- Your doctor should supervise you closely for side effects if you take amoxapine along with any anticholinergic drugs, such as some antihistamines and muscle relaxers.
- Cimetidine, an ulcer drug, can increase the levels of amoxapine in your body.

Other important information:
- Don't use this drug if you are recovering from a heart attack.
- If you have a history of seizures, urinary retention, increased pressure in the eye, or heart problems, talk with your doctor about your condition before you take amoxapine.

- Use this drug with caution if you have heart disease, certain kinds of glaucoma (ask your doctor), or urinary retention.
- If you have a history of seizures or convulsions, use this drug with extreme caution.

AMOXICILLIN AND CLAVULANATE POTASSIUM

Pregnancy category: B

Brand:
Augmentin

This penicillin antibiotic is used to treat a wide variety of infections of the ears, nose, throat, skin, lungs, and bladder by killing the bacteria that cause the infections.

How to take this drug:
- Most penicillins shouldn't be taken with food, but you can take amoxicillin with food to help prevent upset stomach.

Possible side effects:
Nausea or vomiting   Diarrhea
Rash

Possible interactions:
- This drug may decrease the ability of birth control pills to prevent pregnancy.

Other important information:
- Don't use this drug if you're allergic to penicillin or cephalosporin antibiotics. Call your doctor if you develop rash, itching, or fever.
- People with diabetes may have false-positive sugar tests.
- Take all of the prescription, even after the infection goes away.

AMOXICILLIN TRIHYDRATE

Pregnancy category: B

Brand:
Amoxil   *Trimox*
Wymox

This penicillin antibiotic is used to treat a wide variety of infections of the ears, nose, throat, skin, lungs, and bladder by killing the bacteria that cause the infections.

How to take this drug:
- Most penicillins shouldn't be taken with food, but you can take amoxicillin with food to help prevent upset stomach.

Possible side effects:
Nausea or vomiting   Diarrhea
Rash

Possible interactions:
- This drug may decrease the ability of birth control pills to prevent pregnancy.

Other important information:
- Don't use this drug if you are allergic to penicillin or cephalosporin antibiotics. Call your doctor if you develop rash, itching, or fever.
- People with diabetes may have false-positive sugar tests.
- Take all of the prescription, even after the infection goes away.

AMPICILLIN

Pregnancy category: B

Brand:
Omnipen

This penicillin antibiotic is used to treat a wide variety of infections of the ears, nose, throat, skin, lungs, and bladder by killing the bacteria that cause the infections.

How to take this drug:
- To improve absorption of the drug, take it on an empty stomach, at least one hour before or two hours after a meal.

Possible side effects:
Mild rash   Nausea or vomiting
Diarrhea

Possible interactions:
- This drug may decrease the ability of birth control pills to prevent pregnancy.

Other important information:
- Don't use this drug if you are allergic to penicillin or cephalosporin antibiotics. Call your doctor if you develop rash, itching, or fever.
- People with diabetes may have false-positive sugar tests.
- Take all of the prescription, even after the infection goes away.

ASPIRIN WITH DIHYDROCODEINE BITARTRATE AND CAFFEINE

Pregnancy category: C
No driving

Brand:
Synalgos-DC

This drug combines aspirin with a narcotic painkiller very similar to codeine.

How to take this drug:

- Take your medicine with food or a full glass of milk or water so it won't irritate your stomach.

Possible side effects:

Dizziness	Drowsiness
Nausea	Constipation
Slow breathing	Skin rash
Vision and hearing problems	Headache
Mental confusion	Rapid heartbeat
Sweating	Thirst

Possible interactions:

- If you take this drug along with alcohol or tranquilizers, antihistamines, or muscle relaxants, the combination may dangerously depress your nervous system.
- This drug may increase the effects of diabetic drugs and insulin (causing hypoglycemia), penicillin and sulfonamide antibiotics, antidepressant drugs called monoamine oxidase (MAO) inhibitors, other nonsteroidal anti-inflammatory drugs (causing stomach ulcers), and steroids.
- Don't take this drug if you are regularly taking anticoagulants. The combination could dangerously increase your bleeding time.
- This drug may decrease the effectiveness of the gout drugs probenecid and sulfinpyrazone.
- Furosemide (a diuretic) and vitamin C may cause aspirin to accumulate to toxic levels in your body.

Other important information:

- Don't take this drug if you are allergic to aspirin or codeine.
- If you have any bleeding disorder, a vitamin K deficiency, a stomach ulcer, or severe liver damage, don't take this drug.
- Don't use this drug to treat chickenpox or flu, as it could cause Reye's syndrome.
- People with the following conditions should use this drug with caution: liver or kidney damage, gallbladder disease or gallstones, breathing difficulties, irregular heartbeat, hypothyroidism, enlarged prostate, head injuries, or severe stomach problems.
- If you have liver or kidney damage, get regular liver and kidney tests while you are taking this drug.
- You may become physically and psychologically dependent on this drug if you take high doses for long periods of time. Never take more medicine than you are prescribed.

ASPIRIN WITH HYDROCODONE BITARTRATE

Pregnancy category: C
No driving

Brand:
Azdone

This drug combines aspirin with a narcotic painkiller very similar to codeine.

How to take this drug:
- Take your medicine with food or a full glass of milk or water so it won't irritate your stomach.

Possible side effects:
Dizziness
Nausea
Mood changes
Skin rash
Headache
Rapid heartbeat
Thirst

Drowsiness
Constipation
Slow breathing
Vision and hearing problems
Mental confusion
Sweating

Possible interactions:
- If you take this drug along with alcohol or tranquilizers, antihistamines, or muscle relaxants, the combination may dangerously depress your nervous system.
- This drug may increase the effects of diabetic drugs and insulin (causing hypoglycemia), penicillin and sulfonamide antibiotics, tricyclic antidepressants or antidepressant drugs called monoamine oxidase (MAO) inhibitors, other nonsteroidal anti-inflammatory drugs (causing stomach ulcers), and steroids.
- Don't take this drug if you are regularly taking anticoagulants. The combination could dangerously increase your bleeding time.
- This drug may decrease the effectiveness of the gout drugs probenecid and sulfinpyrazone.
- Furosemide (a diuretic) and vitamin C may cause aspirin to accumulate to toxic levels in your body.

Other important information:
- Don't take this drug if you are allergic to aspirin or codeine.
- If you have any bleeding disorder, a vitamin K deficiency, a stomach ulcer, or severe liver damage, don't take this drug.
- Don't use this drug to treat chickenpox or flu, as it could cause Reye's syndrome.
- People with the following conditions should use this drug with caution: liver or kidney damage, gallbladder disease or gallstones, breathing difficulties, irregular heartbeat, hypothyroidism, enlarged prostate, head injuries, or severe stomach problems.

- If you have liver or kidney damage, get regular liver and kidney tests while you are taking this drug.
- Hydrocodone suppresses the cough reflex, so people with lung disease should take this drug with caution.
- You may become physically and psychologically dependent on this drug if you take high doses for long periods of time. Never take more medicine than you are prescribed.

ASPIRIN WITH OXYCODONE

Pregnancy category: NR
No driving

Brand:
Percodan   *Percodan-Demi*
Roxiprin

This drug combines aspirin with a narcotic painkiller similar to morphine.

Possible side effects:
Dizziness	Sleepiness
Nausea	Ringing in the ears
Vision and hearing problems	Headache
Dizziness	Mental confusion
Rapid heartbeat	Sweating
Thirst	

Possible interactions:
- If you take this drug along with alcohol or a drug that depresses your nervous system, such as tranquilizers, antihistamines, or muscle relaxants, the combination may dangerously depress your nervous system.
- You shouldn't take this drug if you are regularly taking anticoagulants. The combination could dangerously increase your bleeding time.
- This drug may decrease the effectiveness of the gout drugs probenecid and sulfinpyrazone.

Other important information:
- Don't take this drug if you are allergic to aspirin or oxycodone. You could have an allergic reaction to aspirin that includes nausea, skin rashes or hives, asthma, swelling, and stomach pain.
- Don't use this drug to treat chickenpox or flu, as it could cause Reye's syndrome.
- People with the following conditions should use this drug with caution: liver or kidney damage, gallbladder disease or gallstones, breathing difficulties, irregular heartbeat, hypothyroidism, enlarged prostate, head injuries, or severe stomach problems.
- If you have liver or kidney damage, get regular liver and kidney tests while you are taking this drug.

- You may become physically and psychologically dependent on this drug if you take high doses for long periods of time. Never take more medicine than you are prescribed.

ASPIRIN WITH PENTAZOCINE HYDROCHLORIDE

Pregnancy category: NR
No driving

Brand:
Talwin Compound

This drug combines aspirin with a narcotic painkiller very similar to codeine.

How to take this drug:
- Take your medicine with food or a full glass of milk or water to help prevent stomach irritation.

Possible side effects:

Nausea	Dizziness
Sleepiness	Excitement
Headache	Confusion
Sweating	Vision or hearing problems
Rapid heartbeat	Thirst

Possible interactions:
- If you take this drug along with alcohol or tranquilizers, antihistamines, or muscle relaxants, the combination may dangerously depress your nervous system.
- This drug may increase the effects of diabetic drugs and insulin (causing hypoglycemia), penicillin and sulfonamide antibiotics, tricyclic antidepressants or antidepressant drugs called monoamine oxidase (MAO) inhibitors, other nonsteroidal anti-inflammatory drugs (causing stomach ulcers), and steroids.
- Don't take this drug if you are regularly taking anticoagulants. The combination could dangerously increase your bleeding time.
- This drug may decrease the effectiveness of the gout drugs probenecid and sulfinpyrazone.
- Furosemide (a diuretic) and vitamin C may cause aspirin to accumulate to toxic levels in your body.

Other important information:
- Don't take this drug if you are allergic to pentazocine, aspirin, or other salicylates.
- If you have any bleeding disorder, a vitamin K deficiency, a stomach ulcer, or severe liver damage, don't take this drug.
- Don't use this drug to treat chickenpox or flu, as it could cause Reye's syndrome.

- People with the following conditions should use this drug with caution: liver or kidney damage, gallbladder disease or gallstones, breathing difficulties such as asthma, irregular heartbeat or heart attack, hypothyroidism, seizures, enlarged prostate, head injuries, or severe stomach problems.
- If you have liver or kidney damage, get regular liver and kidney tests while you are taking this drug.
- You may become physically and psychologically dependent on this drug if you take high doses for long periods of time. Never take more medicine than you are prescribed.

ATENOLOL

Pregnancy category: D
No driving

Brand:
Tenormin

Atenolol is a beta blocker used to treat and control high blood pressure and angina. It also aids in recovery from some kinds of heart attacks.

Possible side effects:
Slow heartbeat	Leg pain
Dizziness	Depression
Difficulty breathing	Tiredness
Diarrhea	Nausea
Wheezing	Drowsiness
Cold, tingling fingers and toes	

Possible interactions:
- If you take both atenolol and the high blood pressure drug clonidine, you may have serious, even fatal, increases in blood pressure called rebound hypertension when you stop taking clonidine.
- Taking atenolol and the high blood pressure drug reserpine together may cause very low blood pressure.

Other important information:
- People with abnormally slow heartbeat, congestive heart failure, heart block, or cardiogenic shock should not take atenolol.
- People with circulatory disorders, bronchitis, emphysema, or liver or kidney problems should take atenolol with caution.
- If you have diabetes, use this drug cautiously because beta blockers can mask the signs of low blood sugar.
- Atenolol can raise your cholesterol and triglyceride levels.
- Atenolol can also mask signs of an overactive thyroid.
- Never quit taking this drug without talking to your doctor. It could increase your risk of angina and heart attack.

- Tell your doctor immediately if you have any signs of congestive heart failure such as night cough; swelling of your legs, feet, or hands; or difficulty breathing, especially when lying down or after physical exertion.

ATORVASTATIN CALCIUM

Pregnancy category: X

Brand:
Lipitor

Atorvastatin calcium lowers cholesterol. This statin is approved to reduce triglycerides as well as total and LDL cholesterol.

How to take this drug:
- Take this drug with or without food.

Possible side effects:

Constipation	Gas
Abdominal pain	Indigestion
Headache	Chest pain
Nausea	Bronchitis
Sleeplessness	Dizziness
Urinary tract infection	

Possible interactions:
- Atorvastatin calcium interacts with cyclosporine, digoxin, erythromycin, fluconazole, gemfibrozil, itraconazole, ketoconazole, niacin, and oral contraceptives.

Other important information:
- Have your liver checked periodically and don't take this drug if you have liver disease.
- Report muscle weakness or pain to your doctor immediately.
- Continue to exercise and eat a healthy diet in addition to taking this medication.

AZATADINE MALEATE WITH PSEUDOEPHEDRINE SULFATE

Pregnancy category: C
No driving   MAO warning

Brand:
Trinalin

This long-acting drug combines an antihistamine and decongestant to relieve congestion in the nose, sinuses, ears, and chest.

Possible side effects:

Sleepiness	Dry mouth
Dizziness	Lack of coordination
Stomach pain	Thickened mucus in your airways

Possible interactions:
- If you are taking digitalis or oral anticoagulants, let your doctor know before you begin taking this drug.
- While taking this drug, avoid alcohol and other depressants, such as sleeping pills and tranquilizers.
- Pseudoephedrine can reduce the effectiveness of beta blockers and other high blood pressure drugs, including methyldopa, mecamylamine, reserpine, and veratrum alkaloids.
- Antacids increase how quickly pseudoephedrine is absorbed.
- Kaolin decreases how quickly pseudoephedrine is absorbed.

Other important information:
- Don't use this drug if you have certain kinds of glaucoma (ask your doctor), urinary retention, bladder neck obstruction, obstruction of the pylorus (opening from the stomach to the intestine), diabetes, stomach ulcer, an enlarged prostate, severe high blood pressure, severe heart disease, or an overactive thyroid.
- If you have diabetes, asthma, or increased pressure in the eye, talk to your doctor before taking this drug.
- Don't use this drug to treat a lower respiratory disease, such as asthma, bronchitis, or pneumonia.
- Side effects of both antihistamines and decongestants can be worse for people over 60. You may want to test your reaction to a short-acting decongestant before trying the long-acting varieties.

AZATHIOPRINE

Pregnancy category: D

Brand:
Imuran

This drug is used to help suppress the immune system and prevent rejection in kidney transplants. It is also used to treat rheumatoid arthritis, ulcerative colitis, myasthenia gravis, Behçet's syndrome, and Crohn's disease.

How to take this drug:
- If you miss a dose, take it as soon as you remember. But if it is nearing time for your next dose, don't double up your doses (unless your doctor tells you to).
- Azathioprine may upset your stomach. Take it with food or milk.

Possible side effects:

Severe nausea or vomiting	Fever
Rash	Diarrhea
Muscle pain	

Possible interactions:
- Azathioprine may cause a drop in your white blood cell count if used with high blood pressure drugs called ACE inhibitors or with other drugs that lower the white blood cell count.
- Allopurinol, a drug used to treat gout, may increase the effects of azathioprine.

Other important information:
- You must try to avoid, and report immediately to your doctor, even mild infections such as colds, fever, sore throat, and general feelings of discomfort.
- Imuran can, in very rare cases, become toxic to the liver.
- It may take up to 12 weeks for the drug to become effective for rheumatoid arthritis.
- Be on the lookout for signs that this drug is depressing your immune system: fever, sore throat, tiredness, weakness, bruising, unusual bleeding. Have your blood tested regularly.

AZELASTINE HYDROCHLORIDE

Pregnancy category: C
No driving

Brand:
Astelin

Azelastine hydrochloride is an antihistamine nasal spray that relieves hay fever symptoms like sneezing and itchy, runny nose.

How to take this drug:
- Never double a missed dose, instead take it as soon as you remember or skip it and go on with your regular schedule.
- Prime the pump by depressing it until a fine mist appears.

Possible side effects:

Drowsiness	Headache
Sneezing	Sore throat
Burning nasal passage	

Possible interactions:
- You may experience extreme drowsiness if you take azelastine hydrochloride with antihistamines.
- This drug may interact with drugs that slow the nervous system, including codeine and phenobarbital.
- Talk to your doctor before combining it with cimetidine or ketoconazole.

Other important information:
- Talk to your doctor about this medication if you have kidney problems.

AZITHROMYCIN

Pregnancy category: B

Brand:
Zithromax

This antibiotic is used to treat some infections of the respiratory system and skin and some sexually transmitted diseases.

How to take this drug:
- Take one hour before or two hours after a meal. Don't take with food.
- If you miss a dose, take it as soon as possible. If several hours have passed or it is nearing time for the next dose, don't try to catch up by doubling your dose unless your doctor tells you to.

Possible side effects:

Nausea	Diarrhea
Stomach pain	Inflamed vagina
Rapid heartbeat	Chest pain
Headache	Dizziness
Sleepiness	Indigestion
Gas	Black and tarry feces
Rash	Sensitivity to sunlight

Possible interactions:
- This drug interacts dangerously with carbamazepine (Tegretol).
- Don't take aluminum-containing or magnesium-containing antacids with azithromycin. They may decrease the levels of this drug.

Other important information:
- Don't use this drug if you're allergic to any macrolide-type antibiotics, such as erythromycin.
- Use it with caution if you have liver or kidney problems.
- Azithromycin should not be used to treat syphilis or gonorrhea.
- Take all of your prescription, even after your symptoms have disappeared.

BECLOMETHASONE DIPROPIONATE

Pregnancy category: C

Brand:

Beclovent	*Beconase*
Beconase AQ	*Vancenase AQ*
Vancenase AQ Double Strength	*Vancenase PocketHaler*
Vanceril Inhaler	*Vanceril Double Strength*

Beclomethasone dipropionate is an anti-inflammatory steroid. Mouth-inhaled forms are used to treat and control asthma; nose-inhaled forms and sprays are used to treat congested, swollen nasal passages, often caused by allergies. They also treat nasal polyps (tumors in your nose).

How to take this drug:
- Avoid fungal infections in your mouth and throat by rinsing your mouth and gargling with warm water after using your inhaler. Don't swallow the water.
- Do your best to take your medicine at regular time intervals.

Possible side effects:
Inhaled forms:

Hoarseness	Dry mouth

Yeast infections in the mouth and throat (oral thrush)
Nasal forms:

Nasal irritation	Sneezing

Other important information:
- If you are switching to beclomethasone from steroid pills or shots, get off the other drug slowly. People have died after switching quickly from steroid pills to inhaled steroids. Report to your doctor any signs of corticosteroid withdrawal, including fatigue, weakness, painful joints or muscles, low blood pressure when you stand up, or difficulty breathing.
- In case of an emergency, carry a card that says you have used cortisone-related drugs in the past year.
- Because corticosteroid drugs can weaken your immune system, avoid exposure to people with chickenpox or measles. If you are exposed, let your doctor know right away.
- If you use inhaled steroids more often than your doctor recommends, you may suffer some serious side effects. Your adrenal glands may also quit producing natural steroids.
- Beclomethasone may begin relieving your stuffy nose or your asthma after three days or less, but it may take as long as two or three weeks.

BENAZEPRIL HYDROCHLORIDE

Pregnancy category: C/D

Brand:
Lotensin

Benazepril controls high blood pressure.

Possible side effects:

Headache	Dizziness
Fatigue	Drowsiness
Nausea	Cough

Possible interactions:
- Taken with diuretics, benazepril can cause very low blood pressure as well as a dangerous buildup of potassium in the body.
- Taken with the antipsychotic drug lithium, benazepril may cause a dangerous buildup of lithium, especially if you are also taking a diuretic.

Other important information:
- People with poor kidney function, diabetes, liver disease, heart failure, rheumatoid arthritis, or lupus should take this drug with caution.
- Benazepril may cause dangerously high levels of potassium in your blood. Don't use potassium-sparing diuretics or take potassium supplements or salt substitutes containing potassium without talking to your doctor.
- If you are allergic to this drug, you could experience a dangerous allergic reaction that includes mild swelling in the throat, face, lips, tongue, mucous membranes, hands, or feet. Swelling of the throat can be extremely dangerous. Contact your doctor immediately.

BENZONATATE

Pregnancy category: C

Brand:
Tessalon

This non-narcotic relieves coughing by temporarily deadening the nerves in the airway and reducing the cough reflex.

Possible side effects:

Sleepiness	Headache
Dizziness	Confusion
Hallucinations	Constipation
Nausea	Upset stomach
Itching	Skin eruptions
Stuffy nose	Chills
Burning eyes	Numbness in the chest

Possible interactions:
- Benzonatate may cause bizarre behavior or hallucinations when combined with some other prescribed drugs. Make sure you tell your doctor what other prescriptions you are taking.

Other important information:
- Don't chew or suck the soft capsules. This can completely deaden the nerves in your mouth and throat, possibly leading to difficulty breathing, choking, a spasm of the airway, or cardiovascular collapse.
- Don't use this drug if you are allergic to any related anesthetics (ester-type local anesthetics).

BENZTROPINE MESYLATE

Pregnancy category: NR
No driving

Brand:
Cogentin

Benztropine mesylate is used to treat Parkinson's disease and the stiffness and shaking caused by some medicines.

Possible side effects:
Difficulty urinating	Weak muscles
Constipation	Nausea
Dry mouth	Confusion
Memory loss	Hallucinations
Nervousness	Depression
Numb fingers	Blurred vision
Dilated pupils	Heatstroke
Fever	

Possible interactions:
- If you also take phenothiazines, haloperidol, tricyclic antidepressants, or other drugs that have drying side effects, make sure you report to your doctor any signs of fever or stomach complaints or any signs that you can't tolerate heat.

Other important information:
- This drug has drying side effects (it can keep you from sweating properly). Be very careful in hot weather, and watch for signs of heatstroke.
- People with certain kinds of glaucoma, a rapid heartbeat, or prostate problems should use this drug very carefully.
- This drug may cause or aggravate symptoms of tardive dyskinesia.
- If you are having a lot of trouble with nausea and dry mouth, talk to your doctor about a lower dose.

BETAMETHASONE DIPROPIONATE

Pregnancy category: C

Brand:
Alphatrex	*Diprolene*
Diprolene AF	*Diprosone*

This corticosteroid drug is used to treat itching, inflamed, and irritated skin.

How to take this drug:
- This drug comes as an ointment, cream, aerosol, and lotion.
- Don't wrap or bandage the area after you apply the medicine (unless your doctor tells you to).

- Avoid contact with your eyes.
- Apply a thin film and rub in gently and completely.

Other important information:
- Don't use this drug if you are allergic to other steroid creams.
- Don't use this drug for longer than prescribed. The high-potency formulations shouldn't be used for longer than two weeks.
- If you are covering a very large area of your skin and, therefore, using lots of medicine, have regular tests for hypothalamic-pituitary-adrenal axis suppression.

BETAXOLOL HYDROCHLORIDE

Pregnancy category: C
No driving

Brand:
Kerlone

Betaxolol is a beta blocker. It controls high blood pressure and regulates heart rhythm.

Possible side effects:

Tiredness	Dizziness
Headache	Difficulty breathing
Diarrhea	Constipation
Nausea	Gas
Frequent urination	Sleeplessness
Chest pain	Swelling
Depression	Abnormal dreams
Rash	Stuffy nose

Possible interactions:
- Betaxolol may decrease the effects of the allergic reaction drug epinephrine.
- Taking betaxolol with the blood pressure drugs diltiazem, nifedipine, reserpine, and verapamil may increase the effects of betaxolol and lead to very low blood pressure.

Other important information:
- Don't use betaxolol if you have congestive heart failure, heart block, cardiogenic shock, or slow heartbeat.
- People with angina, diseases of the arteries, bronchitis, emphysema, or liver or kidney problems should use betaxolol with caution.
- If you have diabetes, use this drug cautiously because beta blockers can mask the signs of low blood sugar.
- Betaxolol can also mask signs of an overactive thyroid.
- You may have to discontinue this drug before having surgery.

- Tell your doctor immediately if you have any signs of congestive heart failure such as night cough; swelling of your legs, feet, or hands; or difficulty breathing, especially when lying down or after physical exertion.
- Never quit taking this drug without talking to your doctor. It could increase your risk of angina and heart attack.

BISOPROLOL FUMARATE & HYDROCHLOROTHIAZIDE

Pregnancy category: C

No driving

Brand:

Ziac

This drug is a combination beta blocker and diuretic used to treat high blood pressure.

How to take this drug:

- You can take this drug with or without food.
- Don't stop taking it without talking to your doctor first. You may have to withdraw from it slowly.

Possible side effects:

Photosensitivity	Cough
Fatigue, weakness	Dizziness
Headache	Muscle pain
Diarrhea	Slow heartbeat
Stuffy nose	Upper respiratory infection

Possible interactions:

- Don't combine this drug with other beta-blocking agents.
- Have your doctor monitor you closely if you take it with catecholamine-depleting drugs like reserpine or guanethidine, myocardial depressants, antiarrhythmic agents like disopyramide, or calcium antagonists.
- The following drugs may interact with bisoprolol fumarate & hydrochlorothiazide: barbiturates, narcotics, antidiabetics, cholestyramine and colestipol resins, corticosteroids, pressor amines like norepinephrine, muscle relaxants, lithium, and NSAIDs.

Other important information:

- It may take two to three weeks to see the maximum benefit from this drug.
- Don't use this drug if you suffer from cardiogenic shock (a condition where your heart does not pump blood strongly enough throughout your body), heart failure, or bronchospastic pulmonary disease.
- If you suffer from congestive heart failure, your body won't absorb this drug as easily.

- If you are diabetic, talk to your doctor about the possibility of hypo-glycemia.
- Use extra caution if you have liver problems.
- Your heart rate at rest, as well as during exercise, will be slower while you are taking this drug. However, if you develop difficulty breathing or an extremely slow heart rate, see your doctor immediately.

BRINZOLAMIDE HYDROCHLORIDE

Pregnancy category: C
No driving

Brand:
Azopt

Brinzolamide hydrochloride is a sulfa drug used to treat increased pressure in the eye.

How to take this drug:
- Shake the dispenser before using.
- Do not allow the tip of the dropper to touch any surface because this may contaminate the medicine.
- If you wear soft contact lenses, remove them before using this drug. You may put your contacts back in 15 minutes after use.
- Wait at least 10 minutes after applying brinzolamide hydrochloride before using any other eye drop to lower the pressure in your eye.

Possible side effects:
Blurred vision	Unpleasant taste
Eye pain or discomfort	Red eyes
Dry eyes	Headache

Other important information:
- Although it is applied to the eye, this drug is absorbed by the body. Make sure you are not allergic to sulfa drugs.
- Talk to your doctor before using brinzolamide hydrochloride if you have serious kidney problems.

BROMOCRIPTINE MESYLATE

Pregnancy category: B
No driving

Brand:
Parlodel

This drug treats Parkinson's disease; it stops an unwanted flow of breast milk caused by pituitary gland tumors; it stimulates regular menstrual cycles; treats certain fertility problems; and treats acromegaly, a condition of middle age causing enlargement of the arms, legs, and head.

How to take this drug:
- Take this drug with food.

Possible side effects:

Nausea

Dizziness

Stomach cramps

Constipation

Drowsiness

Headache

Tiredness

Stuffy nose

Diarrhea

Loss of appetite

Possible interactions:
- This drug, when combined with blood-pressure-lowering drugs, can cause extremely low blood pressure.
- Be sure that you use an alternative form of contraception besides birth control pills while taking bromocriptine.
- Phenothiazines and butyrophenones may decrease the effectiveness of bromocriptine.

Other important information:
- Let your doctor know if you have high blood pressure or kidney or liver disease.
- Have regular liver, kidney, heart, and blood tests while taking this drug.

BROMPHENIRAMINE WITH PHENYLPROPANOLAMINE AND CODEINE

Pregnancy category: C

No driving   MAO warning

Brand:
Bromanate DC

Dimetane-DC

Myphenate DC

This combination of antihistamine, nasal decongestant, and cough suppressant works to relieve coughing and other symptoms of allergies and the common cold. It relieves congestion in the nose, sinuses, ears, and chest.

Possible side effects:

Sleepiness

Dizziness

Stomach pain

Constipation

Dry mouth

Lack of coordination

Thickened mucus in your airways

Possible interactions:
- If you are taking digitalis or oral anticoagulants, let your doctor know before you begin taking this drug.

- While taking this drug, avoid alcohol and other depressants, such as sleeping pills and tranquilizers.
- Phenylpropanolamine can reduce the effectiveness of beta blockers and other high blood pressure drugs, including methyldopa, mecamylamine, reserpine, and veratrum alkaloids.

Other important information:
- Don't use this drug if you have certain kinds of glaucoma (ask your doctor), urinary retention, bladder neck obstruction, obstruction of the pylorus (opening from the stomach to the intestine), diabetes, stomach ulcer, an enlarged prostate, severe high blood pressure, severe heart disease, and an overactive thyroid.
- If you have diabetes, asthma, or increased pressure in the eye, talk to your doctor before taking this drug.
- Don't use this drug to treat a lower respiratory disease, such as asthma, bronchitis, or pneumonia.
- You can become addicted to codeine if you use this drug for a long time.

BROMPHENIRAMINE WITH PSEUDOEPHEDRINE

Pregnancy category: NR
No driving   MAO warning

Brand:

Bromfed	*Bromfed-PD*
Dallergy-JR	*Lodrane*
Lodrane LD	*Respahist*
Ultrabrom	*Ultrabrom PD*

This drug combines an antihistamine and decongestant to relieve congestion in the nose, sinuses, ears, and chest.

Possible side effects:

Sleepiness	Nausea
Giddiness	Dry mouth
Blurred vision	Rapid heartbeat
Flushing	Irritability
Excitement	

Possible interactions:
- If you are taking digitalis or oral anticoagulants, let your doctor know before you begin taking this drug.
- While taking this drug, avoid alcohol and other depressants, such as sleeping pills and tranquilizers.
- Pseudoephedrine can reduce the effectiveness of beta blockers and other high blood pressure drugs, including methyldopa, mecamylamine, reserpine, and veratrum alkaloids.

- Antacids increase how quickly pseudoephedrine is absorbed.
- Kaolin decreases how quickly pseudoephedrine is absorbed.

Other important information:
- Don't use this drug if you have certain kinds of glaucoma (ask your doctor), urinary retention, bladder neck obstruction, obstruction of the pylorus (opening from the stomach to the intestine), diabetes, stomach ulcer, an enlarged prostate, severe high blood pressure, severe heart disease, and an overactive thyroid.
- If you have diabetes, asthma, or increased pressure in the eye, talk to your doctor before taking this drug.
- Don't use this drug to treat a lower respiratory disease, such as asthma, bronchitis, or pneumonia.

BUDESONIDE

Pregnancy category: C

Brand:
Rhinocort   *Pulmicort Turbuhaler*

Budesonide is an anti-inflammatory corticosteroid. As Rhinocort, it is a nasal spray used to clear up the stuffy nose associated with chronic or seasonal allergies. As Pulmicort Turbuhaler Inhalation Powder, it is a dry powder inhaled through the mouth to help prevent asthma attacks.

How to take this drug:
- Don't use the nasal inhaler longer than three weeks.
- Store both forms upright but shake the nasal spray before using. Follow package directions on the mouth inhaler.
- Use the inhaler within six months of opening the protective packing.
- Never double a missed dose, instead take it as soon as you remember or skip it and go on with your regular schedule.

Possible side effects:
Irritated nasal passage	Cough
Sore throat	Nosebleed
Dry mouth	Upset stomach
Respiratory infection	Sinusitis
Headache	Flu-like symptoms

Possible interactions:
- Talk to your doctor if you are taking prednisone or any other steroid, or ketoconazole.

Other important information:
- You may not feel relief for a few days.

- If you have been using an oral steroid to treat your allergies or asthma, switching to this medication may cause withdrawal symptoms such as joint or muscular pain, fatigue, or depression.
- If you are already taking prednisone, be careful adding budesonide. You increase your risk of developing hypothalamic-pituitary-adrenal (HPA) suppression.
- Be aware that corticosteroids depress your immune system, making you more susceptible to infections. Avoid exposure to viruses like chickenpox and measles.
- Large doses of budesonide can lead to hypercorticism, too much adrenal cortical hormones.
- Use this drug cautiously if you have tuberculosis; a fungal, bacterial or viral infection; or ocular herpes simplex.
- Budesonide can affect growth rate in children and teenagers.
- Talk to your doctor before taking this drug if you have liver problems.
- Don't use Pulmicort to relieve an acute asthma attack.

BUMETANIDE

Pregnancy category: C

Brand:
Bumex

Bumetanide is a diuretic used to reduce excess fluid in the body that may be associated with high blood pressure, congestive heart failure, or liver or kidney disease.

Possible side effects:
Muscle cramps or spasms	Dizziness
Headache	Nausea

Possible interactions:
- The effects of bumetanide may be decreased by the gout drug probenecid and nonsteroidal anti-inflammatory drugs (NSAIDs), such as indomethacin and aspirin.
- Bumetanide should not be used with thiazide diuretics as this can cause severe fluid loss and serious electrolyte problems.
- Bumetanide should not be used with the antipsychotic drug lithium as it may cause lithium to accumulate to toxic levels.

Other important information:
- Contact your doctor immediately if you experience allergic symptoms or stop urinating.
- People with liver problems who take this drug may experience irreversible hearing loss, increased sensitivity to light, impaired central nervous system function, or coma.

- If you have diabetes, bumetanide may raise your blood sugar levels.
- Bumetanide may increase levels of uric acid in the blood (this puts you at risk for gout) and may worsen symptoms of lupus.
- Bumetanide can cause dangerously low levels of potassium and other electrolytes. Eat extra potassium-rich foods like bananas.
- Weigh daily so you'll know if you're losing too much fluid, which can cause dehydration and possibly blood clots. Warning signs include dry mouth, thirst, drowsiness, and weakness. Contact your doctor immediately if you stop urinating.
- If you have high blood pressure, avoid using over-the-counter cold remedies or diet pills, which can increase blood pressure.

BUPROPION HYDROCHLORIDE

Pregnancy category: B
No driving   MAO warning

Brand:
Wellbutrin
Zyban

Bupropion hydrochloride relieves the symptoms of depression. Zyban helps people quit smoking.

How to take this drug:
- It's best to allow at least six hours between each dose.
- If you are having trouble sleeping, try not to take a dose right at bedtime.

Possible side effects:
Dry mouth	Headache
Nausea	Constipation
Shakiness	Anxiety
Restlessness	Sleeplessness
Weight loss	

Possible interactions:
- People taking antipsychotics or other antidepressants and people who have suddenly quit taking a benzodiazepine (a drug for anxiety) are at greater risk of seizures if they also take bupropion.
- Alcohol increases your risk of seizures.
- Drugs that affect liver function, such as carbamazepine, cimetidine, phenobarbital, and phenytoin, can increase or decrease the effectiveness of bupropion.
- If you take bupropion at the same time as levodopa, you may have more side effects.

Other important information:

- Bupropion hydrochloride is more likely to cause seizures than other antidepressants. To reduce this risk, don't take more than 450 mg of bupropion a day. Also, ask your doctor if you can divide your dose in half and take it twice a day.
- You have a higher risk of seizures if you have a history of bulimia, anorexia nervosa, head injury, or a tumor of the central nervous system.
- Use this drug cautiously if you are recovering from a heart attack or if your heart disease is unstable.
- People with liver or kidney damage probably need lower doses of bupropion and should be closely watched for any toxic effects.

BUSPIRONE HYDROCHLORIDE

Pregnancy category: B
No driving   MAO warning

Brand:
BuSpar

Buspirone hydrochloride treats anxiety.

Possible side effects:

Dizziness	Nausea
Headache	Nervousness
Lightheadedness	Excitement
Sleeplessness	Tiredness

Possible interactions:

- Due to lack of research, approach any combination of buspirone hydrochloride and other drugs for mental disorders with caution.
- Buspirone has been shown to increase levels of the antipsychotic haloperidol.

Other important information:

- If you are getting off a benzodiazepine drug or another sedative drug in order to begin taking buspirone hydrochloride, make sure you withdraw slowly from your previous drug. You can still suffer from withdrawal symptoms.

BUTABARBITAL SODIUM

Pregnancy category: D
No driving

Brand:
Butisol Sodium

This barbiturate is used to promote sleep and to relieve anxiety and tension.

Possible side effects:
- Daytime sleepiness

Possible interactions:
- If you take butabarbital sodium along with tranquilizers, alcohol, anti-histamines, or muscle relaxants, the combination may dangerously depress your nervous system.
- Butabarbital sodium may increase the effects of corticosteroids.
- This drug may decrease the effectiveness of anti-clotting drugs like warfarin, the anti-fungal drug griseofulvin, birth control pills, and doxycycline.
- Butabarbital sodium may increase the effects of phenytoin.
- Sodium valproate, valproic acid, and monoamine oxidase (MAO) inhibitors may increase the depressant effects of butabarbital sodium.

Other important information:
- You can become addicted to this drug. You must not increase your dose without talking to your doctor. Some symptoms of intoxication with barbiturates are walking unsteadily, slurred speech, confusion, and irritability.
- Withdraw from butabarbital slowly. If you quit taking the drug quickly, you may have nightmares, insomnia, anxiety, dizziness, or nausea. If you're addicted to the drug and you quit taking it suddenly, you may have delirium, convulsions, or death.
- Butabarbital loses its ability to promote sleep after two weeks of taking it regularly.
- Have regular blood, liver, and kidney tests if you take this drug for a long time.
- Use another type of contraception besides birth control pills while you're taking butabarbital sodium.

BUTALBITAL WITH ACETAMINOPHEN AND CAFFEINE

Pregnancy category: C
No driving   MAO warning

Brand:
Esgic-Plus   *Fioricet*

This combination drug is used to relieve mild to moderate pain, especially in tension (muscle contraction) headaches.

Possible side effects:
Dizziness	Drowsiness
Nausea or vomiting	Stomach pain
Shortness of breath	

Possible interactions:
- If you take this drug along with alcohol or tranquilizers, sedatives, sleep-inducing drugs, antihistamines, or muscle relaxants, the combination may dangerously depress your nervous system.

Other important information:
- People with suicidal tendencies or depression should use this drug with caution.
- People with liver or kidney disease should have regular liver and kidney tests while taking this drug.
- If you take this drug for a long time, you can become dependent on it, mentally and physically. It may take larger amounts to produce the same effects. When you stop taking the medicine, you may have withdrawal symptoms, such as rebound headaches.

BUTALBITAL WITH ACETAMINOPHEN, CAFFEINE, AND CODEINE
Pregnancy category: C
No driving

Brand:
Fioricet with Codeine

This barbiturate and analgesic combination is used to relieve mild to moderate pain, especially in tension (muscle contraction) headaches.

Possible side effects:
Dizziness	Drowsiness
Nausea or vomiting	Shortness of breath
Mental confusion	

Possible interactions:
- If you take this drug along with tranquilizers, alcohol, antihistamines, or muscle relaxants, the combination may dangerously depress your nervous system.
- This drug may decrease the effects of anticoagulants.

Other important information:
- People with suicidal tendencies or depression should use this drug with caution.
- If you take this drug for a long time, you can become dependent on it, mentally and physically. It may take larger amounts to produce the same effects. When you stop taking the medicine, you may have withdrawal symptoms, such as rebound headaches.

BUTALBITAL WITH ASPIRIN AND CAFFEINE

Pregnancy category: NR
No driving

Brand:

Butal   *Fiorinal*
Lanorinal

This barbiturate and analgesic combination relieves mild to moderate pain, especially in tension (muscle contraction) headaches.

Possible side effects:

Drowsiness   Dizziness

Possible interactions:

- If you take this drug along with tranquilizers, alcohol, antihistamines, or muscle relaxants, the combination may dangerously depress your nervous system.

Other important information:

- Take this drug with caution if you have peptic ulcer, blood clotting problems, suicidal tendencies, or depression.
- You may become physically and psychologically dependent on this drug if you take high doses for long periods of time.

BUTALBITAL WITH ASPIRIN, CAFFEINE, AND CODEINE PHOSPHATE

Pregnancy category: NR
No driving

Brand:

Fiorinal with Codeine #3

This barbiturate and analgesic combination relieves mild to moderate pain, especially in tension (muscle contraction) headaches.

Possible side effects:

Drowsiness   Dizziness

Possible interactions:

- If you take this drug along with tranquilizers, alcohol, antihistamines, or muscle relaxants, the combination may dangerously depress your nervous system.
- Monoamine oxidase (MAO) inhibitors may increase the side effects of this drug.
- This drug may increase the effects of anticoagulants, increasing your risk of bleeding.
- This drug may increase the toxic effects of methotrexate and 6-mercaptopurine.

- This drug may decrease the effects of probenecid and sulfinpyrazone, reducing their effectiveness in the treatment of gout.

Other important information:
- Don't use this drug if you have a stomach ulcer or blood clotting problem.
- If you have kidney or liver disease, your doctor should monitor you carefully while you take this drug.
- You may become physically and psychologically dependent on this drug if you take high doses for long periods of time. Never take more medicine than you are prescribed.

CALCITONIN-SALMON

Pregnancy category: C

Brand:
Calcimar
Miacalcin

This hormone is used to treat the symptoms of Paget's disease, to decrease bone loss, and to decrease calcium levels in the blood.

How to take this drug:
- Store this drug in the refrigerator.
- Giving the injection at bedtime may help prevent some of the nausea and flushing.

Possible side effects:

Nausea or vomiting	Inflammation at the point of injection
Flushing	Rash
Need to urinate at night	Itching earlobes
Fever	Eye pain
Poor appetite	Stomach pain
Swollen feet	Salty taste

Other important information:
- Don't use this drug if you are allergic to synthetic calcitonin. A severe shock reaction can result.
- This drug may cause a shortage of calcium in the blood.

CANDESARTAN CILEXETIL

Pregnancy category: C/D

Brand:
Atacand

Atacand is used to treat high blood pressure.

How to take this drug:
- You may take this drug with or without food.

Possible side effects:

Headache	Back pain
Dizziness	Upper respiratory infection
Sore throat	Stuffy nose

Other important information:
- If you are being treated with diuretics while on candesartan cilexetil, you may experience episodes of low blood pressure. Symptoms include dizziness and weakness.

CAPECITABINE

Pregnancy category: D

Brand:
Xeloda

Capecitabine is used to treat breast cancer that has spread to other parts of the body and does not respond to certain other chemotherapy treatment.

How to take this drug:
- Take capecitabine with food (or within 30 minutes after eating).
- Capecitabine is prescribed in 3-week cycles. Take it for 14 days followed by a 7-day rest period.

Possible side effects:

Diarrhea	Hand-and-foot syndrome
Nausea or vomiting	(tingling, numbness, pain,
Mouth or throat sores	swelling, or redness in the
Stomach pain	palms of your hands or
Loss of appetite	soles of your feet)
Dehydration	Rash
Tiredness	

Possible interactions:
- Antacids may interact with capecitabine.

Other important information:
- If you have liver problems, make sure your doctor monitors you carefully.
- Don't take capecitabine if you are allergic to 5-fluorouracil (5-FU) because capecitabine is converted by the body to 5-FU.
- Because severe diarrhea can be dangerous, if you have more than four bowel movements a day or diarrhea at night, stop taking this drug and contact your doctor.
- Elderly people may experience more gastrointestinal side effects.

- Contact your doctor if any of the listed side effects are severe enough to cause you discomfort.

CAPTOPRIL

Pregnancy category: C/D

Brand:
Capoten

Captopril is an angiotensin converting enzyme (ACE) inhibitor. It is used to control high blood pressure, to treat congestive heart failure, to slow down further weakening of the heart after a heart attack, and to treat kidney problems in some people with diabetes.

How to take this drug:
- Take captopril one hour before meals.

Possible side effects:

Cough	Rash
Itching	Loss of taste

Possible interactions:
- If you take captopril along with the antipsychotic drug lithium, the combination may cause lithium to accumulate to toxic levels.
- Aspirin and other nonsteroidal anti-inflammatory drugs (NSAIDs), such as indomethacin, may decrease the effects of captopril.
- Captopril can be used safely with other blood pressure drugs, like diuretics, but may cause too much fluid loss or very low blood pressure.

Other important information:
- Don't use this drug if you are allergic to any of the ACE inhibitor heart medicines.
- If you have poor kidney function, diabetes, heart failure, arthritis, or lupus, use this drug cautiously. If you have high blood pressure, heart failure, or poor kidney function, ask your doctor to test your kidneys regularly while you're taking this drug.
- People taking nerve-blocking drugs, diuretics, angina drugs, and people on dialysis should be watched closely by their doctors.
- Contact your doctor if you notice any swelling of the face, mouth, hands, feet, tongue, or larynx.
- If you develop jaundice (yellow eyes or skin), contact your doctor immediately.
- Be careful in hot weather and during exercise. Sweating can cause loss of fluid and low blood pressure, which can make you feel lightheaded.
- This drug can cause very low blood pressure, especially when you first begin taking it. Be careful when you rise quickly — you may feel lightheaded and dizzy.

- Never stop taking this drug without your doctor's approval.
- Captopril may cause dangerously high, even fatal, levels of potassium in the blood. Don't use potassium-sparing diuretics or take potassium supplements without talking to your doctor.

CARBAMAZEPINE

Pregnancy category: C
No driving   MAO warning

Brand:
Epitol   *Tegretol*

This drug treats depression and controls certain types of epileptic seizures. It is also used for pain associated with trigeminal neuralgia, a facial nerve disorder.

Possible side effects:
Dizziness   Drowsiness
Nausea

Possible interactions:
- The sedative phenobarbital and the seizure drugs phenytoin and primidone may lower your levels of carbamazepine.
- This drug may decrease the effects of the seizure drug phenytoin, the anticoagulant warfarin, the antibiotic doxycycline, the asthma drug theophylline, the antipsychotic drug haloperidol, and the anticonvulsant valproic acid.
- The antibiotic erythromycin, the ulcer drug cimetidine, the painkiller propoxyphene, the tuberculosis drug isoniazid, the antihistamine terfenadine, the antidepressant fluoxetine, and calcium channel blockers may increase blood levels of carbamazepine.
- Taking this drug with the antipsychotic drug lithium can cause toxic side effects.
- This drug can affect thyroid function if taken with other anticonvulsants.
- This drug can make birth control pills unreliable and can cause breakthrough bleeding if you're taking the pill.

Other important information:
- Don't use this drug if you have a history of bone marrow depression or allergic reactions to tricyclic antidepressants.
- Use this drug with caution if you have increased pressure in the eye, if you have had bone marrow depression as a reaction to medication in the past, or if you have heart problems or kidney or liver damage.
- Have your liver and kidney function tested regularly.
- Never stop taking this drug without your doctor's permission. Quitting suddenly can cause seizures.

CARBENICILLIN

Pregnancy category: B

Brand:
Geocillin

This penicillin antibiotic is used to treat infections of the skin, urinary tract, and prostate by killing the bacteria that cause the infections.

How to take this drug:
- To improve absorption of the drug, take it on an empty stomach — at least one hour before or two hours after a meal.

Possible side effects:
Nausea	Bad taste
Diarrhea	Gas
Inflamed tongue	

Possible interactions:
- Levels of this drug may be increased by probenecid, a drug used to treat gout.

Other important information:
- Call your doctor if you develop a rash, fever, or chills. You could be having an allergic reaction to the drug.
- Long-term use may lead to development of resistant bacteria in the body.
- People with kidney problems, liver problems, and blood disorders should take this drug with caution.
- Take all of the medication, even after you feel better.

CARBINOXAMINE WITH PSEUDOEPHEDRINE

Pregnancy category: C
No driving   MAO warning

Brand:
Rondec   *Rondec-TR*

This medication combines an antihistamine and decongestant to relieve a stuffy nose caused by allergies or a cold.

Possible side effects:
Sleepiness	Dry mouth
Dizziness	Lack of coordination
Stomach pain	Thickened mucus in your airways

Possible interactions:
- While taking this drug, avoid alcohol and other depressants, such as sleeping pills and tranquilizers.

- Pseudoephedrine can reduce the effectiveness of beta blockers and other high blood pressure drugs, including methyldopa, mecamylamine, reserpine, and veratrum alkaloids.
- Antacids increase how quickly pseudoephedrine is absorbed.
- Kaolin decreases how quickly pseudoephedrine is absorbed.

Other important information:
- Don't take this drug if you have certain kinds of glaucoma (ask your doctor), urinary retention, stomach ulcer, severe high blood pressure, and severe heart disease. Don't use this drug during an asthma attack.
- If you have diabetes, asthma, an enlarged prostate, an overactive thyroid, mild high blood pressure, mild heart disease, or increased pressure in the eye, talk to your doctor about your condition before taking this drug.
- Anyone over 60 should use this drug cautiously.

CARISOPRODOL AND ASPIRIN

Pregnancy category: C
No driving

Brand:
Soma Compound

This combination drug is used to relax certain muscles in your body and relieve the pain caused by strains, sprains, or other muscle injuries.

Possible side effects:
Drowsiness   Dizziness
Weakness

Possible interactions:
- If you take this drug along with alcohol or tranquilizers, antihistamines, or other muscle relaxants, the combination may dangerously depress your nervous system.
- Your doctor may need to adjust your dose of gout, arthritis, or diabetes medications.
- This drug may increase your risk of bleeding if you are taking anticoagulants.
- This drug may increase the toxic effects of methotrexate.
- This drug may reduce the effects of probenecid and sulfinpyrazone.
- If you take anti-diabetic drugs, your risk of hypoglycemia (low blood sugar) may be increased.
- Antacids may decrease the effectiveness of this drug.
- Corticosteroids may decrease the levels of this drug.

Other important information:
- People with kidney or liver problems should use this drug with caution.

- This drug can cause mild withdrawal symptoms if you stop taking it suddenly.

CARTEOLOL HYDROCHLORIDE

Pregnancy category: C

Brand:
Cartrol

This drug is a beta blocker used to lower high blood pressure.

Possible side effects:
Weakness
Muscle cramps

Possible interactions:
- Carteolol hydrochloride may interact with catecholamine-depleting drugs, like reserpine, general anesthetics, NSAIDs, calcium antagonists, oral anti-diabetic medications, or insulin.

Other important information:
- Talk to your doctor about this drug if you suffer from bronchospasms.
- You can take carteolol hydrochloride along with other antihypertensive drugs, like thiazide diuretics.
- Don't take it if you have bronchial asthma, extremely slow heart rate, serious heart block, cardiogenic shock, or congestive heart failure.
- Don't stop taking this drug suddenly if you have angina.
- If you are diabetic, you may have to adjust your insulin dose while on this drug.
- Have your doctor monitor you carefully if you have liver problems and are taking carteolol hydrochloride.
- This drug may interfere with glaucoma testing.

CEFACLOR

Pregnancy category: B

Brand:
Ceclor

This antibiotic is used to treat infections of the lungs, urinary tract, skin, and ears.

How to take this drug:
- You can take this drug with meals.
- You can store the reconstituted suspension in the refrigerator for 14 days.
- If you miss a dose, take it as soon as possible. If several hours have passed or it is nearing time for the next dose, don't try to catch up by doubling your dose unless your doctor tells you to.

Possible side effects:

Bloody diarrhea   Stomach cramps
Fever

Possible interactions:

- This drug may cause a false-positive urine glucose test, and it may increase the effects of anticoagulant drugs.
- Probenecid, a drug used to treat gout, can increase the effects of cefaclor.
- If taken with some other antibiotics, cefaclor may increase the side effects of those drugs.

Other important information:

- Don't use this drug if you are allergic to related antibiotics.
- People with impaired kidney function or a history of gastrointestinal disease, particularly colitis, should use this drug with caution.
- Take the full course of the antibiotic. Don't stop after symptoms go away.

CEFADROXIL MONOHYDRATE

Pregnancy category: B

Brand:

Duricef   *Ultracef*

This antibiotic is used to treat infections of the lungs, urinary tract, skin, and ears.

How to take this drug:

- You can take this drug with food or milk if it irritates your stomach.
- If you miss a dose, take it as soon as possible. If several hours have passed or it is nearing time for the next dose, don't try to catch up by doubling your dose unless your doctor tells you to.

Possible side effects:

Bloody diarrhea   Stomach cramps
Fever

Possible interactions:

- This drug may cause a false-positive urine glucose test, and it may increase the effects of anticoagulant drugs.
- Probenecid, a drug used to treat gout, can increase the effects of cefadroxil.
- If taken with some other antibiotics, cefadroxil may increase the side effects of those drugs.

Other important information:

- Don't use this drug if you are allergic to related antibiotics.

- People with impaired kidney function or a history of gastrointestinal disease, particularly colitis, should use this drug with caution.
- Take the full course of the antibiotic. Don't stop after symptoms go away.

CEFIXIME

Pregnancy category: B

Brand:
Suprax

This antibiotic is used to treat infections of the ears, throat, tonsils, lungs, and urinary tract. It is also used to treat gonorrhea.

How to take this drug:
- You can keep the reconstituted suspension in a tightly closed container for 14 days.
- You can take your medicine with food or milk.
- If you miss a dose, take it as soon as possible. If several hours have passed or it is nearing time for the next dose, don't try to catch up by doubling your dose unless your doctor tells you to.

Possible side effects:
Bloody diarrhea   Stomach cramps
Fever

Possible interactions:
- This drug may cause a false-positive urine glucose test.

Other important information:
- Don't use this drug if you are allergic to related antibiotics.
- People with impaired kidney function or a history of gastrointestinal disease, particularly colitis, should use this drug with caution.
- Take the full course of the antibiotic. Don't stop after symptoms go away.

CEFPODOXIME PROXETIL

Pregnancy category: B

Brand:
Vantin

Cefpodoxime proxetil is used to treat infections of the skin, urinary tract, and upper and lower respiratory tract. It is also used to treat sexually transmitted diseases.

How to take this drug:
- Take cefpodoxime proxetil with food to avoid upset stomach.

- If you miss a dose, take it as soon as possible. If several hours have passed or it is nearing time for the next dose, don't try to catch up by doubling your dose unless your doctor tells you to.

Possible side effects:

Diarrhea	Nausea
Yeast infection	Stomach pain
Rash	Headache

Possible interactions:
- Antacids can decrease the effects of this drug.
- Probenecid, a drug used to treat gout, can increase the effects of this drug.
- This drug may cause a false-positive result for the Coombs' test.

Other important information:
- Don't use cefpodoxime proxetil if you are allergic to related antibiotics. Allergic reactions can be life-threatening.
- People who have impaired kidney function or a history of gastrointestinal disease, particularly colitis, should use this drug with caution.
- Take the full course of the antibiotic. Don't stop after symptoms go away.

CEFPROZIL

Pregnancy category: B

Brand:
Cefzil

This antibiotic is used to treat infections of the skin, tonsils, throat, ears, and lungs.

How to take this drug:
- You can take this drug with food or milk.
- If you miss a dose, take it as soon as possible. If several hours have passed or it is nearing time for the next dose, don't try to catch up by doubling your dose unless your doctor tells you to.

Possible side effects:

Diarrhea	Nausea
Stomach pain	Dizziness

Possible interactions:
- Probenecid, a drug used to treat gout, can increase the effects of this drug.
- Using this drug with some antibiotics may cause kidney damage.
- This drug may cause a false-positive urine glucose test.

Other important information:
- Don't use cefprozil if you are allergic to related antibiotics. Allergic reactions can be life-threatening.

- People who have impaired kidney function or a history of gastrointestinal disease, particularly colitis, should use this drug with caution.
- Take the full course of the antibiotic. Don't stop after symptoms go away.

CEFUROXIME AXETIL

Pregnancy category: B

Brand:
Ceftin

This antibiotic is used to treat infections of the urinary tract, skin, bones, joints, tonsils, throat, ears, and lungs. It is also used to treat gonorrhea.

How to take this drug:
- Take cefuroxime axetil with food to enhance absorption.
- If you miss a dose, take it as soon as possible. If several hours have passed or it is nearing time for the next dose, don't try to catch up by doubling your dose unless your doctor tells you to.

Possible side effects:
Diarrhea	Nausea
Vomiting	Stomach cramps
Fever	

Possible interactions:
- This drug may cause a false-positive urine glucose test.

Other important information:
- Don't use this drug if you are allergic to related antibiotics.
- People with impaired kidney function or a history of gastrointestinal disease, particularly colitis, should use this drug with caution.
- Take the full course of the antibiotic. Don't stop after symptoms go away.

CELECOXIB

Pregnancy category: C

Brand:
Celebrex

Celecoxib is an NSAID used to relieve the symptoms of osteoarthritis and rheumatoid arthritis in adults.

How to take this drug:
- You can take celecoxib with or without food.
- If you take celecoxib with either high-fat foods or antacids containing aluminum or magnesium, the drug will not be absorbed as quickly or easily.

- Never double a missed dose. Instead take it as soon as you remember or skip it and go on with your regular schedule.

Possible side effects:
Headache   Indigestion
Upper respiratory infection   Diarrhea
Sinusitis   Stomach pain
Nausea

Possible interactions:
- Various medications may interact with NSAIDs, including celecoxib, so review all prescription and nonprescription drugs with your doctor.
- Your doctor may have to adjust your dose or monitor you closely if you take furosemide, fluconazole, lithium, or ACE-inhibitors for blood pressure like Capoten, Vasotec, and Prinivil along with this drug.

Other important information:
- Your doctor may have to adjust your dose if you suffer from mild liver problems.
- Don't take celecoxib if you have had an allergic reaction to sulfa drugs or have had asthma, hives, or an allergic reaction after taking aspirin or other NSAID, like diclofenac, Relafen, ibuprofen, naproxen, and ketoprofen.
- Talk to your doctor before taking this drug if you have had ulcers or stomach bleeding, have severe kidney problems, or are in the late stages of pregnancy.
- Watch for the warning signs of liver damage: nausea, vomiting, fatigue, loss of appetite, yellow coloring of skin or eyes, and dark urine.
- Celecoxib can cause fluid retention and swelling. Talk to your doctor if you retain fluids, have high blood pressure, or have heart failure.
- The longer you take this drug, the more likely you are to suffer from stomach problems, with symptoms such as gnawing or burning stomach pain, black or tarry stools, or vomiting.

CEPHALEXIN

Pregnancy category: B

Brand:
Keflex   *Keflet*

This cephalosporin antibiotic is used to treat infections of the ears, lungs, skin, bones, urinary tract, and genitals.

How to take this drug:
- Take with food or milk to help prevent upset stomach.
- If you miss a dose, take it as soon as possible. If several hours have passed or it is nearing time for the next dose, don't try to catch up by doubling your dose unless your doctor tells you to.

Possible side effects:

Diarrhea	Stomach pain
Rash	Hives
Genital, vaginal, or anal itching	Dizziness
Fatigue	Headache
Agitation	Confusion
Hallucinations	Arthritis

Possible interactions:

- This drug may cause a false-positive urine glucose test.

Other important information:

- Don't use cephalexin if you're allergic to related antibiotics.
- People with impaired kidney function or a history of intestinal disease, particularly colitis, should use this drug with caution.
- Be on the lookout for signs that this drug is depressing your immune system: fever, sore throat, tiredness, weakness, bruising, unusual bleeding. Have your blood tested regularly.
- Taking an antibiotic for a long time can cause bacteria or fungus to overgrow, leading to another infection, such as a yeast infection of the mouth or skin. If you get one of these "superinfections," you may need to stop taking cephalexin and start taking another antibiotic for the second infection.
- Take the full course of the antibiotic. Don't stop after symptoms go away.

CEPHALEXIN HYDROCHLORIDE

Pregnancy category: B

Brand:

Keftab

This antibiotic is used to treat infections of the lungs, skin, bones, urinary tract, and genitals.

How to take this drug:

- Take with food or milk to help prevent upset stomach.
- If you miss a dose, take it as soon as possible. If several hours have passed or it is nearing time for the next dose, don't try to catch up by doubling your dose unless your doctor tells you to.

Possible side effects:

Diarrhea	Stomach pain
Rash	Hives
Genital, vaginal, or anal itching	Dizziness
Fatigue	Headache
Agitation	Confusion
Hallucinations	Arthritis

Possible interactions:
- This drug may cause a false-positive urine glucose test.

Other important information:
- Don't use cephalexin hydrochloride if you are allergic to related anti-biotics.
- People with impaired kidney function or a history of intestinal disease, particularly colitis, should use this drug with caution.
- Be on the lookout for signs that this drug is depressing your immune system: fever, sore throat, tiredness, weakness, bruising, unusual bleeding. Have your blood tested regularly.
- Taking an antibiotic for a long time can cause bacteria or fungus to overgrow, leading to another infection, such as a yeast infection of the mouth or skin. If you get one of these "superinfections," you may need to stop taking cephalexin and start taking another antibiotic for the second infection.
- Take the full course of the antibiotic. Don't stop after symptoms go away.

CERIVASTATIN SODIUM

Pregnancy category: X

Brand:
Baycol

Cerivastatin sodium lowers total and LDL cholesterol and triglycerides and increases HDL cholesterol.

How to take this drug:
- You may take this drug with or without food.
- Never double a missed dose. Instead take it as soon as you remember or skip it and go on with your regular schedule.

Possible side effects:

Headache	Indigestion
Joint pain	Stuffy nose
Sore throat	

Possible interactions:
- Cerivastatin sodium can interact with immunosuppressive drugs, like Sandimmune and Neoral, fibric acid derivatives such as Atromid-S, niacin, erythromycin, and azole antifungals, like Diflucan and Nizoral.

Other important information:
- If you have kidney or liver disease, or use alcohol heavily take this drug with caution.
- Undergo liver tests before treatment and at six and 12 weeks into treatment.
- Use along with a controlled diet and regular exercise to control cholesterol.

- If you develop muscle pain or weakness, fever, and general tiredness, see your doctor immediately.

CETIRIZINE HYDROCHLORIDE

Pregnancy category: B
No driving

Brand:
Zyrtec

Cetirizine hydrochloride is an antihistamine used to treat the symptoms of allergies or chronic itchy skin and hives.

How to take this drug:
- Cetirizine hydrochloride comes in either tablet or syrup form.
- Take this drug with or without food.
- Never double a missed dose. Instead take it as soon as you remember or skip it and go on with your regular schedule.

Possible side effects:
Sleepiness	Tiredness
Dry mouth	Sore throat
Dizziness	

Possible interactions:
- Cetirizine hydrochloride may interact with large doses of theophylline.
- Don't take this medication with other drugs that may make you sleepy, like sedatives, muscle relaxants, etc.

Other important information:
- If you have liver or kidney problems or are on dialysis, you may need to adjust your dose.

CHLORAMBUCIL

Pregnancy category: D

Brand:
Leukeran

Chlorambucil treats various types of cancer.

How to take this drug:
- Eat small, frequent meals to help prevent nausea and vomiting.
- Drink seven to 12 glasses of water or other clear liquids every day.

Possible side effects:
Nausea or vomiting	Diarrhea
Mouth ulcers	Skin rash
Drug fever	Pneumonia

Possible interactions:
- Taking anticoagulants or aspirin with this drug may increase the chance of unusual bleeding or bruising.
- Use with extreme caution when you are taking any drugs that have a risk of seizure.

Other important information:
- This drug should only be taken by people with certain kinds of cancer.
- Have your blood checked weekly.
- Chlorambucil causes chromosome damage and may cause permanent sterility.
- Don't have any live virus vaccines while taking this drug.

CHLORAMPHENICOL

Pregnancy category: C

Brand:
Chloromycetin

This drug is available as a solution or an ointment and is used to treat serious eye infections.

How to take this drug:
- Don't allow the tip of the dropper to touch your eye or any surface because this may contaminate the medicine.

Possible side effects:
Burning or stinging eyes   Blurred vision

Other important information:
- Chloramphenicol may cause your bone marrow to stop producing enough red blood cells. This can lead to serious, even fatal, complications. Have your blood tested regularly.
- Taking an antibiotic for a long time can cause bacteria or fungus to overgrow, leading to another infection. If you get one of these "super-infections," you may need to quit taking chloramphenicol and start taking another antibiotic for the second infection.

CHLORDIAZEPOXIDE HYDROCHLORIDE

Pregnancy category: NR
No driving   MAO warning

Brand:
Librium

This benzodiazepine treats anxiety and alcohol withdrawal and acts as a mild pain reliever.

Possible side effects:
Drowsiness   Confusion
Lack of coordination

Possible interactions:
- If you take chlordiazepoxide along with other tranquilizers, alcohol, antihistamines, or muscle relaxers, the combination may dangerously depress your nervous system.
- Don't take chlordiazepoxide when you are taking other drugs for mental disorders, such as phenothiazines.
- Effects of this drug may be increased by the ulcer drug cimetidine and by birth control pills.

Other important information:
- You can become dependent on chlordiazepoxide. To avoid seizures and other less severe withdrawal symptoms, quit taking the drug gradually under your doctor's supervision.
- People with poor liver, kidney, or lung functions and obese people should use chlordiazepoxide cautiously. The drug may stay in your body longer and increase your risk of side effects.
- Have regular blood and urine tests if you are taking chlordiazepoxide for a long time.

CHLORHEXIDINE GLUCONATE
Pregnancy category: B

Brand:
Peridex   *Periogard*

This antibacterial drug is used to treat gingivitis.

How to take this drug:
- Use twice daily for 30 seconds after you brush your teeth.
- Don't eat or drink for several hours after using this drug.
- Don't swallow the oral rinse.

Possible side effects:
Change in taste   Increased plaque
Stained teeth, fillings, and mouth

Other important information:
- Have your teeth cleaned at least every six months.

CHLOROTHIAZIDE
Pregnancy category: C

Brand:
Diuril

This diuretic treats high blood pressure and the fluid retention and swelling associated with congestive heart failure, cirrhosis of the liver, kidney disease, estrogen therapy, and steroid therapy.

Possible side effects:

Weakness	Jaundice
Diarrhea	Vomiting
Breathing problems	Muscle spasms
Dizziness	Tingling
Skin irritation	Blurred vision
Impotence	

Possible interactions:

- Nonsteroidal anti-inflammatory drugs (NSAIDs), such as aspirin, may decrease the effects of chlorothiazide.
- If you take chlorothiazide with alcohol, depressants, narcotics, or other high blood pressure medicines, the combination may cause very low blood pressure.
- Corticosteroids combined with chlorothiazide may cause a dangerous loss of potassium from the blood.
- Chlorothiazide can increase the effects of muscle relaxers.

Other important information:

- Don't use this drug if you are allergic to diuretics or sulfonamide drugs.
- People with poor kidney function or liver disease should use this drug with caution.
- Since this drug may increase cholesterol levels, use it cautiously if you have moderate or high cholesterol levels.
- Chlorothiazide may increase levels of uric acid in the blood (this puts you at risk for gout) and may worsen symptoms of lupus.
- This drug may cause excess levels of calcium in the blood and may raise blood sugar levels.
- Chlorothiazide may cause dangerously low levels of potassium and other electrolytes. Eat extra potassium-rich foods, like bananas. Contact your doctor if you experience any of the symptoms of potassium loss: unusual thirst, tiredness, drowsiness, restlessness, muscle pains or cramps, nausea, or rapid heart rate.
- Be on the lookout for signs that this drug is depressing your immune system: fever, sore throat, tiredness, weakness, bruising, unusual bleeding. Have your blood tested regularly.
- Weigh daily so you'll know if you're losing too much fluid, which can cause dehydration and possibly blood clots. Warning signs include dry mouth, thirst, drowsiness, and weakness. Contact your doctor immediately if you stop urinating.
- If you have high blood pressure, avoid using over-the-counter cold remedies or diet pills, which can increase blood pressure.

CHLORPROPAMIDE

Pregnancy category: C

Brand:
Diabinese

This drug is used to treat noninsulin dependent (type II) diabetes by encouraging your pancreas to secrete more insulin.

Possible side effects:

Nausea	Diarrhea
Constipation	Dizziness
Drowsiness	Headache
Allergic skin reactions	Sensitivity to light

Possible interactions:
- Chlorpropamide is more likely to cause a drop in blood sugar if you are also taking nonsteroidal anti-inflammatory drugs (NSAIDs), some antibiotics, the gout drug probenecid, or some high blood pressure drugs.
- Loss of control of blood sugar may be caused by some high blood pressure drugs, corticosteroids, thyroid drugs, estrogen, birth control pills, seizure drugs, niacin (vitamin B3), and the tuberculosis drug isoniazid.

Other important information:
- Don't take this drug if you have diabetic ketoacidosis.
- While on this drug, you are at a higher risk of developing fatal heart problems.
- Tell your doctor if you have liver or kidney disease or are at high risk of heart attack.
- Check your blood and urine periodically for abnormal sugar levels while taking this drug.
- Wear identification that states you are diabetic.
- This drug may make your skin extra-sensitive to sunlight, so protect your skin if you'll be outdoors.
- Use along with a controlled diet and regular exercise to control diabetes.
- Since this drug can cause low blood sugar, especially when you haven't eaten enough, when you've exercised, or when you've consumed alcohol, learn to recognize the signs of hypoglycemia and know how to treat it.
- This drug can lose its effectiveness after you've taken it for a long period of time.
- Tell your doctor about any stressful events you experience, such as surgery, trauma, infection, or fever. You may need insulin or some other special treatment.

CHLORTHALIDONE

Pregnancy category: B

Brand:
Hygroton   *Thalitone*

This diuretic treats high blood pressure and the fluid retention and swelling associated with congestive heart failure, cirrhosis of the liver, kidney disease, estrogen therapy, and steroid therapy.

Possible side effects:

Loss of appetite	Upset stomach
Nausea	Cramping
Diarrhea	Constipation
Dizziness	Tingling
Headache	Vision problems
Sensitivity to light	Rash
Hives and other skin problems	Muscle spasms
Weakness	Restlessness
Impotence	

Possible interactions:

- Taking chlorthalidone along with other high blood pressure drugs may cause very low blood pressure.
- Chlorthalidone may increase or decrease the effects of insulin.
- If used with the antipsychotic drug lithium, chlorthalidone may cause lithium to accumulate to toxic levels.

Other important information:

- Don't use chlorthalidone if you are allergic to diuretics or sulfonamide drugs.
- If you have poor kidney function or liver disease, use this drug with caution.
- Chlorthalidone may increase levels of uric acid in the blood (putting you at risk for gout), may worsen symptoms of lupus, and may raise your blood sugar.
- This diuretic may cause dangerously low levels of potassium and other electrolytes. Eat extra potassium-rich foods, like bananas. Contact your doctor if you experience any of the symptoms of potassium loss: unusual thirst, tiredness, drowsiness, restlessness, muscle pains or cramps, nausea, or rapid heart rate.
- Be on the lookout for signs that this drug is depressing your immune system: fever, sore throat, tiredness, weakness, bruising, unusual bleeding. Have your blood tested regularly.
- Weigh daily so you'll know if you're losing too much fluid, which can cause dehydration and possibly blood clots. Warning signs include dry mouth, thirst, drowsiness, and weakness. Contact your doctor immediately if you stop urinating.
- If you have high blood pressure, avoid using over-the-counter cold remedies or diet pills, which can increase blood pressure.

CHLORZOXAZONE

Pregnancy category: C
No driving

Brand:
Parafon Forte DSC   *Strifon Forte DSC*

Chlorzoxazone is a muscle relaxant used to treat severe muscular pain associated with spasms, strains, sprains, and bruises.

Possible side effects:
Upset stomach	Drowsiness
Dizziness	Lightheadedness

Possible interactions:
* If you take chlorzoxazone along with alcohol or tranquilizers, antihistamines, or muscle relaxants, the combination may dangerously depress your nervous system.

Other important information:
* Call your doctor if you experience a rash or itching.

CHOLESTYRAMINE

Pregnancy category: C

Brand:
Locholest	*Locholest Light*
Prevalite	*Questran*
Questran Light	

Cholestyramine is used to reduce blood cholesterol levels.

How to take this drug:
* Increase your fluid and fiber intake to help avoid constipation.
* Take other drugs one to two hours before or four to six hours after taking cholestyramine. Ask your doctor about dosing schedules.

Possible side effects:
Constipation	Stomach pain
Gas	Nausea
Diarrhea	Indigestion
Belching	Loss of appetite
Flaky skin	Rash
Skin irritation	

Possible interactions:
* Cholestyramine may decrease the absorption of other drugs you take including the anti-inflammatory phenylbutazone, the anticoagulant warfarin, the blood pressure drugs chlorothiazide and propranolol, some

antibiotics, the sedative phenobarbital, some thyroid drugs, the heart drug digitalis, and phosphate supplements.

Other important information:
- People with bile duct obstruction should not use this drug.
- Cholestyramine may reduce your body's absorption of folic acid and the fat-soluble vitamins A, D, E, and K. A shortage of vitamin K can cause bruising and longer bleeding times. You may need vitamin supplements.

CILOSTAZOL

Pregnancy category: NR

Brand:
Pletal

Cilostazol is used to improve the symptoms of intermittent claudication.

How to take this drug:
- Take cilostazol about a half-hour before or two hours after breakfast and dinner.
- Take it at the same time every day.

Possible side effects:
Headache	Diarrhea
Abnormal stools	Rapid heartbeat

Possible interactions:
- Don't take this drug with grapefruit juice.
- These drugs may interact with cilostazol: erythromycin, ketoconazole (Nizoral), itraconazole (Sporanox), diltiazem (Cardizem), and omeprazole (Prilosec).

Other important information:
- Don't take this drug if you have congestive heart failure.
- You may not see improvement immediately, but if your symptoms are not better after three months on this drug, talk to your doctor about changing medication.
- Cilostazol won't relieve certain symptoms of other blood vessel diseases, such as leg pain at rest or skin breakdown.

CIMETIDINE

Pregnancy category: B

Brand:
Tagamet

Cimetidine decreases the amount of acid your stomach produces. It helps stomach ulcers heal, treats gastroesophageal reflux disease (severe heartburn), controls bleeding in the stomach or intestines, and treats Zollinger-Ellison disease.

Possible side effects:

Headache	Diarrhea
Sleepiness	Dizziness
Breast enlargement in men	Impotence

Possible interactions:

* Don't take antacids when you take your dose of cimetidine because they decrease its absorption.
* Cimetidine may increase levels, effects, or toxicity of nifedipine, the anti-anxiety drugs chlordiazepoxide and diazepam, the analgesic lidocaine, the antibiotic metronidazole, the seizure drug phenytoin, the beta-blocker propranolol, the asthma drug theophylline, and the anticoagulant warfarin.

Other important information:

* Don't take cimetidine if you are allergic to any anti-ulcer drugs.
* Take this drug cautiously if you have liver or kidney problems.
* Be on the lookout for signs that this drug is depressing your immune system: fever, sore throat, tiredness, weakness, bruising, unusual bleeding. Have your blood tested regularly.

CIPROFLOXACIN HYDROCHLORIDE

Pregnancy category: C
No driving

Brand:

Ciloxan   *Cipro*

This fluoroquinolone antibiotic is used to treat lower respiratory infections, bone and joint infections, urinary tract infections, skin infections, infectious diarrhea, and eye infections.

How to take this drug:

* Ciloxan is an ophthalmic solution used to treat eye infections (bacterial conjunctivitis).
* Cipro is the tablet form of this antibiotic.
* Although Cipro may be taken with food, it is best taken two hours after you eat.
* Drink plenty of fluids while taking Cipro.
* If you miss a dose, take it as soon as possible. If several hours have passed or it is nearing time for the next dose, don't try to catch up by doubling your dose unless your doctor tells you to.

Possible side effects:

Tablets:

Nausea	Diarrhea
Stomach pain	Headache

Restlessness	Rash
Bloody diarrhea	Stomach cramps
Fever	

Ophthalmic solution:

| Itching eyes | Irritation |

Possible interactions:
- Ciprofloxacin may increase the effects of caffeine, the asthma drug theophylline, and the anticoagulant warfarin.
- Antacids, some iron pills, and multivitamins containing zinc may decrease absorption of Cipro.
- Probenecid, a drug used to treat gout, may increase levels of ciprofloxacin in the blood.

Other important information:
- Don't use ciprofloxacin hydrochloride if you have any allergies to drugs in the quinolone class. Dangerous sensitivity reactions can occur, causing symptoms such as swelling of the face or throat, difficult breathing (such as an asthma attack), itching, hives, tingling, or loss of consciousness. Call your doctor at the first sign of rash or allergic reaction.
- If you have any condition that increases your risk of seizures, use this drug with caution.
- The dose may need to be adjusted for people who have poor kidney function. Kidney and liver function tests and certain blood tests should be done periodically while on this drug.
- This drug may make your skin extra-sensitive to sunlight, so protect your skin if you'll be outdoors.
- Taking an antibiotic for a long time can cause bacteria or fungus to overgrow, leading to another infection (such as a yeast infection of the mouth or skin). If you get one of these "superinfections," you may need to quit taking ciprofloxacin and start taking another antibiotic for the second infection.

CISAPRIDE

Pregnancy category: C

Brand:
Propulsid

Cisapride relieves nighttime heartburn by increasing the contractions of the stomach and the intestines.

How to take this drug:
- Cisapride begins working in 30 minutes to one hour.

Possible side effects:

| Headache | Diarrhea |

Abdominal pain	Nausea
Constipation	Gas
Stuffy nose	Sinusitis

Possible interactions:
- This drug can cause serious, possibly fatal heart rhythm disturbances when used with the following drugs: erythromycin, clarithromycin, troleandomycin, nefazodone, fluconazole, itraconazole, oral ketoconazole, indinavir, and ritonavir. Let your doctor know before you take any of these with cisapride.
- Cisapride doesn't cause sleepiness when you take it by itself, but if you take it along with drugs that depress your nervous system, such as tranquilizers, alcohol, antihistamines, or muscle relaxers, the combination may make you even more sleepy and sedated.
- Cisapride can make anticoagulants, such as warfarin, less effective.
- The ulcer drug cimetidine can increase the levels of cisapride.

Other important information:
- If you have any kind of heart rhythm abnormalities, heart disease or congestive heart failure, bleeding in the stomach, or any kind of intestinal blockage, don't use this drug.
- If you are taking any drugs that cause low potassium or magnesium levels, don't take cisapride.
- See your doctor right away if you experience dizziness, faintness, or irregular heartbeat after taking this drug.

CITALOPRAM HYDROBROMIDE

Pregnancy category: C
No driving   MAO warning

Brand:
Celexa

Citalopram hydrobromide is a selective serotonin reuptake inhibitor used to treat depression.

How to take this drug:
- Take this drug with or without food.

Possible side effects:

Sexual problems in male patients	Nausea
Dry mouth	Sleepiness
Increased sweating	Tremors
Diarrhea	Indigestion
Tiredness	Sleeplessness
Anxiety	Loss of appetite
Upper respiratory infection	

Possible interactions:
- Citalopram hydrobromide may interact with cimetidine, lithium, imipramine and other tricyclic antidepressants (TCAs).

Other important information:
- Before taking this drug, talk to your doctor if you suffer from mania, seizures, liver disease, or severe kidney problems.
- You may not see any improvement in symptoms before four weeks.

CLARITHROMYCIN

Pregnancy category: C

Brand:
Biaxin

This antibiotic is used to treat mild to moderate infections of the skin and the respiratory tract.

How to take this drug:
- You can take this drug with or without food. Take each dose with fluids, preferably more than 6 ounces.
- If you miss a dose, take it as soon as possible. If several hours have passed or it is nearing time for the next dose, don't try to catch up by doubling your dose unless your doctor tells you to.

Possible side effects:
Diarrhea	Nausea
Abnormal sense of taste	Indigestion
Stomach pain	Headache

Possible interactions:
- This drug may increase levels of carbamazepine (Tegretol), a drug used to treat seizures, and the asthma drug theophylline.

Other important information:
- Don't use if you're allergic to any of the macrolide antibiotics.
- People with severe kidney problems should use clarithromycin with caution.
- This drug may cause mild to severe colitis, inflammation of the colon. Tell your doctor if you have any of these symptoms: bloody diarrhea, stomach cramps, and fever.
- Take all the medicine you are prescribed, even after you begin to feel better.

CLEMASTINE FUMARATE

Pregnancy category: B
No driving   MAO warning

Brand:
Tavist

This 12-hour antihistamine relieves allergy symptoms, such as sneezing, runny nose, tearing eyes, itching, rashes, hives, swelling, and difficulty breathing.

Possible side effects:
Sleepiness
Dry mouth
Dizziness
Lack of coordination
Stomach pain

Possible interactions:
- While taking clemastine, avoid alcohol and other depressants, such as sleeping pills and tranquilizers.

Other important information:
- Don't take this drug if you have certain kinds of glaucoma (ask your doctor), bladder neck obstruction, obstruction of the pylorus (opening from the stomach to the intestine), stomach ulcer, or an enlarged prostate.
- Don't use clemastine if you have a lower respiratory disease, such as asthma, bronchitis, or pneumonia. Clemastine can dry out and thicken the mucus in your airways, making it more difficult to remove.
- Use clemastine cautiously if you have increased pressure in the eye, an overactive thyroid, heart disease, or high blood pressure.
- If you are over 60, you're more likely to feel dizzy and sedated and have low blood pressure while taking clemastine.

CLINDAMYCIN HYDROCHLORIDE

Pregnancy category: B

Brand:
Cleocin HCl

This drug is used to treat infections of the skin, lungs, digestive system, and female genitals.

How to take this drug:
- Take this drug with a glass of water to avoid irritating the esophagus.

Possible side effects:
Stomach pain	Nausea
Diarrhea	Rash
Itching	Yellow eyes or skin

Possible interactions:
- This drug may increase the effects of muscle relaxers.

Other important information:
- People with kidney disease, liver disease, or a history of intestinal disease, such as colitis, should not use this drug.

- This drug may cause severe or fatal colitis, inflammation of the colon. Call your doctor immediately if you develop bloody diarrhea, stomach cramps, or fever.
- Taking an antibiotic for a long time can cause bacteria or fungus to overgrow, leading to another infection (fungal infections of the mouth, anus, or vagina). If you get one of these "superinfections," you may need to quit taking clindamycin and start taking another antibiotic for the second infection.
- Be on the lookout for signs that this drug is depressing your immune system: fever, sore throat, tiredness, weakness, bruising, unusual bleeding. Have your blood tested regularly.

CLINDAMYCIN PHOSPHATE

Pregnancy category: B

Brand:
Cleocin T

This drug is an antibiotic prescribed to treat acne.

How to take this drug:
- This medication is available as a gel, solution, or lotion.

Possible side effects:
Redness
Dry skin
Itching
Burning
Peeling

Possible interactions:
- If you develop diarrhea while on this drug, don't take any anti-diarrheal medication without talking with your doctor first. You could make your diarrhea worse.

Other important information:
- This drug may be absorbed through your skin into your bloodstream and cause severe or fatal colitis, inflammation of the colon. Call your doctor immediately if you develop bloody diarrhea, stomach cramps, or fever.
- Talk to your doctor before taking this medication if you've ever had ulcerative colitis, antibiotic-associated colitis, or an intestinal inflammation.
- Be careful using this drug if you have eczema, asthma, or hay fever.

CLOMIPRAMINE HYDROCHLORIDE

Pregnancy category: C
No driving   MAO warning

Brand:
Anafranil

Clomipramine is a tricyclic antidepressant used to treat obsessive-compulsive disorder (OCD).

How to take this drug:
- Take your medicine with meals so it won't upset your stomach.

Possible side effects:

Sexual dysfunction in men	Dry mouth
Constipation	Nausea
Upset stomach	Sleepiness
Shakiness	Muscle spasms
Dizziness	Nervousness
Tiredness	Sweating
Urination problems	Weight gain
Vision changes	

Possible interactions:
- The antipsychotic drug haloperidol; the attention-deficit disorder drug methylphenidate; the ulcer drug cimetidine; and certain antidepressants, such as fluoxetine, may increase levels of clomipramine in your body.
- Clomipramine may increase levels of phenobarbital and the heart drugs warfarin and digoxin in your body.
- Smoking may reduce the effectiveness of clomipramine.
- People taking antipsychotics, other antidepressants, or people who have suddenly quit taking a benzodiazepine (a drug for anxiety) are at greater risk of seizures if they also take clomipramine.
- If you take clomipramine along with tranquilizers, alcohol, antihistamines, or muscle relaxers, the combination may dangerously depress your nervous system.
- Some blood-pressure-lowering drugs may not work as well if you also take clomipramine.
- Your doctor should supervise you closely for side effects if you take clomipramine along with any anticholinergic drugs, such as some antihistamines and muscle relaxants or along with any sympathomimetic drugs, such as some decongestants.
- The seizure drug phenytoin and various barbiturates may decrease levels of clomipramine in your body.

Other important information:
- Don't use this drug if you are recovering from a heart attack.
- Use clomipramine cautiously if you have a history of seizures, alcoholism, or brain damage.
- Quit taking clomipramine before surgery with general anesthetics if possible.
- If you have any of the following conditions, use clomipramine with caution: an overactive thyroid, increased pressure in the eye, urinary retention, poor liver function, or tumors of the adrenal medulla.
- You may experience some withdrawal symptoms, such as dizziness, nausea, sleep disturbances, or irritability, if you stop taking the drug suddenly.

CLONAZEPAM

Pregnancy category: NR
No driving

Brand:
Klonopin

Clonazepam treats certain types of seizures.

Possible side effects:

Drowsiness	Dizziness
Lack of coordination	Upper respiratory infection
Sinusitis	Depression
Fatigue	Flu-like symptoms

Possible interactions:
- If you take clonazepam along with tranquilizers, alcohol, antihistamines, muscle relaxers, monoamine oxidase (MAO) inhibitors and the tricyclic antidepressants, and other anticonvulsant drugs, the combination may dangerously depress your nervous system.

Other important information:
- People with a certain type of glaucoma (ask your doctor) and people with severe liver disease shouldn't use clonazepam.
- People with poor kidney function and people with chronic respiratory diseases should use clonazepam cautiously.
- You can become dependent on clonazepam. To avoid seizures and other less severe withdrawal symptoms, quit taking the drug gradually under your doctor's supervision.
- Have regular blood counts and liver function tests while you're taking clonazepam.

CLONIDINE HYDROCHLORIDE

Pregnancy category: C
No driving

Brand:
Catapres

Clonidine controls high blood pressure.

Possible side effects:
Dry mouth	Drowsiness
Dizziness	Constipation

Possible interactions:
- Some antidepressants may decrease the effectiveness of clonidine.
- If you take clonidine along with tranquilizers, alcohol, antihistamines, or muscle relaxers, the combination may dangerously depress your nervous system.
- This drug may increase your sensitivity to alcohol.

Other important information:
- People with severe heart problems, recent heart attack, disease of blood vessels in the brain, or kidney failure should take this drug with caution.
- Don't stop taking this drug without consulting your doctor. Quitting suddenly could cause dangerous withdrawal symptoms.
- This drug can cause very low blood pressure, especially when you first begin to take it. Be careful when you stand up quickly — you may feel lightheaded and dizzy.

CLORAZEPATE DIPOTASSIUM

Pregnancy category: D
No driving   MAO warning

Brand:
Gen-XENE	*Tranxene-SD*
Tranxene-SD Half Strength	*Tranxene T-Tab*

This benzodiazepine treats anxiety, helps manage seizures, and treats alcohol withdrawal by slowing down your nervous system. It acts as a sedative, stimulates your appetite, and works as a mild pain reliever.

Possible side effects:
Drowsiness	Dizziness
Stomach problems	Nervousness
Blurred vision	Dry mouth
Headache	Confusion

Possible interactions:
- If you take clorazepate along with other tranquilizers, alcohol, antihistamines, or muscle relaxers, the combination may dangerously depress your nervous system.
- If possible, don't take clorazepate when you are taking other drugs for mental disorders, such as phenothiazines.

Other important information:
- People with some kinds of glaucoma (ask your doctor) shouldn't use this drug.
- You can become dependent on clorazepate. To avoid seizures and other less severe withdrawal symptoms, quit taking the drug gradually under your doctor's supervision.
- People with poor liver, kidney, or lung function should use clorazepate cautiously. The drug may stay in your body longer and increase your risk of side effects.
- Have regular blood and urine tests if you are taking clorazepate for a long time.
- Older people should begin with a low dosage to reduce the chances of becoming oversedated.

CLOTRIMAZOLE AND BETAMETHASONE DIPROPIONATE

Pregnancy category: C

Brand:
Lotrisone

This drug combines an antifungal with a corticosteroid to treat skin infections caused by athlete's foot, fungus of the genital and anal areas, and whole body fungus.

How to take this drug:
- With clean hands, gently massage this cream into the affected and surrounding area.
- Apply this cream twice a day, in the morning and evening.
- Do not wrap or bandage the area after you apply the medicine (unless your doctor tells you to).

Possible side effects:

Itching	Blisters
Hives	Irritated skin
Peeling skin	Redness
Swelling	

Other important information:
- Don't use this drug if you are sensitive to clotrimazole, betamethasone dipropionate, other corticosteroids, or imidazoles.

- Use the full course of treatment even if symptoms improve.
- When you're treating a fungus in the groin area, wear loose-fitting clothing and apply the cream sparingly for two weeks only. Let your doctor know if the fungus hasn't disappeared after two weeks.
- For athlete's foot, let your doctor know if the fungus hasn't improved in two weeks.

COLESTIPOL HYDROCHLORIDE

Pregnancy category: NR

Brand:
Colestid

Colestipol is used to reduce blood cholesterol levels.

How to take this drug:
- Increase your fluid and fiber intake to help avoid constipation.
- Take other drugs one to two hours before or four to six hours after taking colestipol. Ask your doctor about dosing schedules.

Possible side effects:
Constipation	Irritated hemorrhoids
Stomach pain and bloating	Belching
Gas	Nausea
Diarrhea	

Possible interactions:
- Colestipol may decrease the absorption of other drugs, such as the beta blocker propranolol, the diuretics furosemide and chlorothiazide, the antibiotics tetracycline and penicillin G, the heart drugs digitoxin and digoxin, and the antilipemic gemfibrozil.

Other important information:
- Colestipol may reduce your body's absorption of folic acid and the fat-soluble vitamins A, D, E, and K. A shortage of vitamin K can cause bruising and longer bleeding times.

CROMOLYN SODIUM

Pregnancy category: B

Brand:
Gastrocrom   *Intal*

Cromolyn sodium helps prevent spasms of the bronchi (the air passages that lead to the lungs) caused by exercise, certain toxins, pollutants, and cold air.

How to take this drug:
- This drug is available as an aerosol, capsules, and an inhalation solution.

- Open the ampule and pour the contents into a half glass of hot water. Stir until completely dissolved, adding cold water while you are stirring. Don't mix with fruit juice, milk, or foods.
- Don't swallow the inhalation capsules. Try rinsing your mouth or taking a drink of water before and after inhaling to prevent coughing and throat irritation.
- Don't exceed the prescribed dose for the inhalation solution.
- For the nasal solution form, clear your nose before spraying. Inhale through your nose while you use the spray.

Possible side effects:
Oral concentrate:

Headache	Diarrhea
Itching	Nausea
Muscle pain	

Inhaled forms:

Coughing	Stuffy nose
Sneezing	Mild wheezing
Nausea	

Other important information:
- People with poor liver or kidney function may need a lower dose.
- Don't use cromolyn sodium to treat severe asthma attacks.
- People allergic to lactose should not take the inhalation capsule form.
- People with coronary artery disease or heart arrhythmias should use inhalers cautiously because of the propellants they contain.
- To prevent bronchospasm caused by exercise, cold air, etc., use the inhaler or nebulizing solution 10 to 15 minutes before exposure to whatever causes your asthma attack.
- You may need to take the drug for several weeks before you notice any improvement. Don't stop taking this drug or reduce the dose without talking to your doctor. Asthma symptoms may get worse.
- You usually begin taking cromolyn in addition to your regular asthma medicine, such as a bronchodilator. You may be able to gradually decrease your other medication under your doctor's supervision.

CYCLOBENZAPRINE HYDROCHLORIDE

Pregnancy category: B
No driving   MAO warning

Brand:
Flexeril

Cyclobenzaprine relieves muscle spasms and the associated pain, tenderness, and tightness.

Possible side effects:

Drowsiness   Dry mouth
Dizziness

Possible interactions:

- Cyclobenzaprine may decrease the effectiveness of some high blood pressure drugs, such as guanethidine.
- If you take cyclobenzaprine along with alcohol or tranquilizers, antihistamines, or muscle relaxants, the combination may dangerously depress your nervous system.

Other important information:

- Don't use this drug if you have an overactive thyroid, heart arrhythmias, congestive heart failure, heart block, or are recovering from a heart attack.
- Use with caution if you have a history of urinary retention or certain kinds of glaucoma (ask your doctor).
- If you suddenly stop taking this drug, you may have nausea, headache, and a tired, weak feeling.

CYCLOPHOSPHAMIDE

Pregnancy category: D

Brand:

Cytoxan

This drug treats various types of cancer.

How to take this drug:

- Take cyclophosphamide on an empty stomach. If stomach upset occurs, you may take it with food.

Possible side effects:

Loss of appetite   Nausea or vomiting

Possible interactions:

- Cyclophosphamide may change the effects of phenobarbital and the anticancer drug doxorubicin hydrochloride.

Other important information:

- Be on the lookout for signs that this drug is depressing your immune system: fever, sore throat, tiredness, weakness, bruising, unusual bleeding. Have your blood tested regularly.
- Cyclophosphamide can cause new cancerous growths, sometimes several years after treatment has stopped.
- Cyclophosphamide can also cause liver and kidney damage. Have regular liver and kidney tests while you're taking this drug.
- Your dose may need to be reduced if you've had one or both adrenal glands removed.

- This drug can cause sterility in men and women.

CYCLOSPORINE

Pregnancy category: C

Brand:
Neoral   *Sandimmune*
Sangcya

Cyclosporine is used to suppress the immune system and protect against rejection in heart, bone marrow, liver, and kidney transplants. Doctors may prescribe this drug for other illnesses including Crohn's disease, severe psoriasis, aplastic anemia, multiple sclerosis, alopecia areata, pemphigus and pemphigoid, Behçet's disease, myasthenia gravis, and atopic dermatitis.

How to take this drug:
- Stir the oral solution well and drink it all at once. Don't allow it to stand.
- The oral solution may be mixed with orange juice, milk, or chocolate milk to improve the taste.
- Take at room temperature.
- Use a glass container when taking the solution.

Possible side effects:
Excessive hair growth   Tremors
Acne   Enlarged gums
Cramps   Diarrhea
Nausea   Tingling
Convulsions

Possible interactions:
- This drug interacts dangerously with the anticonvulsant Dilantin.
- Don't take cyclosporine with other immunosuppressive drugs.
- Taking any of the following drugs while taking cyclosporine may increase your risk of kidney toxicity: gentamicin, tobramycin, vancomycin, cimetidine, ranitidine, diclofenac, amphotericin B, ketoconazole, melphalan, trimethoprim with sulfamethoxazole, and azapropazone.
- Drugs that decrease liver enzymes may increase levels of cyclosporine, and, conversely, drugs that increase liver enzymes may decrease levels of cyclosporine.
- Taking any of the following drugs may increase levels of cyclosporine in your body: diltiazem, nicardipine, verapamil, ketoconazole, fluconazole, itraconazole, danazol, bromocriptine, metoclopramide, erythromycin, and methylprednisolone.
- Taking any of the following may decrease levels of cyclosporine in your body: rifampin, phenobarbital, phenytoin, and carbamazepine.

- Talk to your doctor before drinking grapefruit juice while taking this drug.

Other important information:
- Be on the lookout for signs that this drug is depressing your immune system: fever, sore throat, tiredness, weakness, bruising, unusual bleeding. Have your blood tested regularly.
- Have your liver and kidney functions checked often while you take this drug.
- Don't take this drug if you are allergic to castor oil.
- This drug may increase your risk of skin cancer and cancer of the lymph system.

CYPROHEPTADINE HYDROCHLORIDE

Pregnancy category: B
No driving   MAO warning

Brand:
Periactin

This antihistamine relieves symptoms of food allergies, hay fever, allergy to cold temperatures, and other allergies. It helps relieve sneezing, runny nose, itching, rashes, hives, swelling, and difficulty breathing. Cyproheptadine can be used along with epinephrine to treat severe allergic reactions.

Possible side effects:

Sleepiness	Dry mouth
Dizziness	Lack of coordination
Stomach pain	Thickened mucus in your airways

Possible interactions:
- While taking cyproheptadine, avoid alcohol and other depressants, such as sleeping pills and tranquilizers.

Other important information:
- Don't use this drug if you have some kinds of glaucoma (ask your doctor), bladder neck obstruction, obstruction of the pylorus (opening from the stomach to the intestine), stomach ulcer, or an enlarged prostate.
- Don't use cyproheptadine if you have a lower respiratory disease, such as asthma, bronchitis, or pneumonia.
- Use cyproheptadine cautiously if you have increased pressure in the eye, an overactive thyroid, heart disease, or high blood pressure.
- If you are over 60, you're more likely to feel dizzy and sedated and have low blood pressure while taking cyproheptadine.

DESIPRAMINE HYDROCHLORIDE

Pregnancy category: NR
No driving   MAO warning

Brand:
Norpramin

Desipramine treats the symptoms of depression.

Possible side effects:

Dizziness	Drowsiness
Dry mouth	Headache
Increased appetite	Nausea
Unpleasant taste	Black tongue

Possible interactions:
- The ulcer drug cimetidine, the phenothiazine tranquilizers, and the heart drugs propafenone and flecainide can increase the levels of desipramine in your body.
- Cigarette smoking, barbiturates, and alcohol may decrease the effectiveness of this drug.
- Some blood-pressure-lowering drugs may not work as well if you also take desipramine.
- If you take desipramine along with tranquilizers, alcohol, antihistamines, or muscle relaxers, the combination may dangerously depress your nervous system.
- Your doctor should supervise you closely for side effects if you take desipramine along with any anticholinergic drugs, such as some antihistamines and muscle relaxants, or along with any sympathomimetic drugs, such as some decongestants.
- Any of the type of antidepressants called selective serotonin reuptake inhibitors (fluoxetine, sertraline, and paroxetine) can cause desipramine to reach dangerously high levels in your body.

Other important information:
- Don't take this drug if you are recovering from a heart attack.
- Take this drug very cautiously if you have heart disease, urinary retention, glaucoma, thyroid disease, or a history of seizures.
- When possible, quit taking desipramine several days before surgery.
- If you quit taking this drug suddenly, you could experience nausea, headache, and a general feeling of fatigue. If you gradually quit taking the drug, you may still experience irritability, restlessness, and dream and sleep disturbances.

DESONIDE

Pregnancy category: C

Brand:

DesOwen
Tridesilon

This drug is used to relieve and heal inflamed or irritated skin conditions including eczema, dermatitis, psoriasis, severe diaper rash, insect bites, minor burns, and sunburn.

How to take this drug:

- Don't wrap or bandage the area after you apply the medicine unless your doctor tells you to. For diaper rash, don't use tight-fitting diapers or plastic pants after applying this medicine.
- Avoid contact with your eyes.
- Don't use this drug for longer than prescribed.
- Apply a thin film and rub in gently and completely.

Possible side effects:

Stinging	Burning
Itching	Peeling
Irritation	Dryness

Other important information:

- Don't use this drug if you are allergic to other steroid creams.
- If your skin becomes irritated, contact your doctor.
- If you are covering a very large area of your skin and, therefore, using lots of medicine, have regular tests for hypothalamic-pituitary-adrenal axis suppression.
- If your skin is infected, you'll also need an antifungal or antibacterial medicine.

DESOXIMETASONE

Pregnancy category: C

Brand:

Topicort
Topicort LP

Desoximetasone is used to relieve and heal inflamed or irritated skin conditions, including eczema, dermatitis, psoriasis, severe diaper rash, insect bites, minor burns, and sunburn.

How to take this drug:

- Don't wrap or bandage the area after you apply the medicine unless your doctor tells you to. For diaper rash, don't use tight-fitting diapers or plastic pants after applying this medicine.
- Avoid contact with your eyes.
- Don't use this drug for longer than prescribed.
- Apply a thin film and rub in gently and completely.

Possible side effects:

Stinging	Burning
Itching	Peeling
Irritation	Dryness

Other important information:

- Don't use this drug if you are allergic to other steroid creams.
- If you are covering a very large area of your skin and, therefore, using lots of medicine, have regular tests for hypothalamic-pituitary-adrenal axis suppression.
- If your skin is infected, you'll also need an antifungal or antibacterial medicine.

DEXAMETHASONE AND TOBRAMYCIN

Pregnancy category: C

Brand:

TobraDex

This combination of tobramycin (an antibiotic) and dexamethasone (a steroid) is used to treat a bacterial infection with inflammation in the eye. It is also used to treat eye injuries from chemical or radiation burns or from foreign bodies.

How to take this drug:

- This medication comes as an ointment or as drops.
- Don't touch the dropper or tube to any surface.
- Your prescription should not be refilled without having your eye rechecked first.
- Shake well before use.

Possible side effects:

Eye irritation

Other important information:

- Don't use this drug if you have a viral disease, a mycobacterial infection, or a fungal disease of the eye.
- Using this drug for a long period of time could result in glaucoma, cataracts, or other eye damage.

DIAZEPAM

Pregnancy category: D
No driving   MAO warning

Brand:
Valium

This benzodiazepine treats anxiety, relieves muscle spasms, helps manage seizures, and treats alcohol withdrawal by slowing down your nervous system. It acts as a sedative, stimulates your appetite, and works as a mild pain reliever.

Possible side effects:
Drowsiness   Fatigue
Lack of coordination

Possible interactions:
- If you take diazepam along with other tranquilizers, alcohol, antihistamines, or muscle relaxers, the combination may dangerously depress your nervous system.
- Don't take diazepam when you are taking other drugs for mental disorders, such as phenothiazines.
- Effects of this drug may be increased by the ulcer drug cimetidine.

Other important information:
- People with some kinds of glaucoma (ask your doctor) shouldn't use this drug.
- You can become dependent on diazepam. To avoid seizures and other less severe withdrawal symptoms, quit taking the drug gradually under your doctor's supervision.
- People with poor liver, kidney, or lung function should use diazepam cautiously. The drug may stay in your body longer and increase your risk of side effects.
- Have regular blood and urine tests if you are taking diazepam for a long time.

DICLOFENAC POTASSIUM

Pregnancy category: B

Brand:
Cataflam

This drug is an NSAID used to relieve the symptoms of rheumatoid arthritis, osteoarthritis, and ankylosing spondylitis (arthritis of the spine). It is also used to relieve menstrual pain.

How to take this drug:
- If you take this drug with food, it will be absorbed more slowly, but you may avoid some of the digestive side effects it can cause.

- Never double a missed dose. Instead take it as soon as you remember or skip it and go on with your regular schedule.

Possible side effects:

Abdominal pain	Headache
Dizziness	Diarrhea
Indigestion	Nausea
Constipation	Fluid retention and swelling
Vision changes	

Possible interactions:

- Don't use with aspirin, other NSAIDs, or with other medications containing diclofenac.
- Diclofenac may interact with digoxin, insulin, oral hypoglycemic drugs, and phenobarbital.
- Diclofenac may prolong bleeding time if used with anticoagulants.
- Diclofenac may increase the levels or effects of the immunosuppressant cyclosporine, the psychosis drug lithium, the seizure drug phenytoin, and the anti-inflammatory methotrexate, possibly increasing toxicity of some of these drugs.
- Diclofenac may reduce the effects of beta blockers and loop diuretics.
- The gout drug probenecid may increase levels of NSAIDs.
- The ulcer drug cimetidine may increase or decrease blood levels of diclofenac.

Other important information:

- This formula of diclofenac is designed to dissolve immediately in the stomach. If you haven't eaten, it can be absorbed within 10 minutes.
- Don't take this drug if you are at risk of ulcers, kidney or liver disease, have a low body weight, are elderly, or are sensitive to aspirin or NSAIDs.
- Have your doctor monitor you closely for intestinal ulcers or bleeding.
- Tell your doctor immediately if you develop these signs of liver problems: nausea, fatigue, jaundice, abdominal pain, flu-like symptoms, or severe itching.
- Since this drug can cause fluid retention, be careful if you suffer from high blood pressure or poor blood circulation.
- Be on the lookout for signs that this drug is depressing your immune system: fever, sore throat, tiredness, weakness, bruising, or unusual bleeding. Have your blood tested regularly.

DICLOFENAC SODIUM

Pregnancy category: B

Brand:

Voltaren   *Voltaren-XR*

This drug is an NSAID used to relieve the symptoms of rheumatoid arthritis, osteoarthritis, and ankylosing spondylitis (arthritis of the spine).

How to take this drug:
- If you take this drug with food, it will be absorbed more slowly, but you may avoid some of the digestive side effects it can cause.
- Never double a missed dose. Instead take it as soon as you remember or skip it and go on with your regular schedule.

Possible side effects:
Abdominal pain
Dizziness
Indigestion
Constipation
Vision changes

Headache
Diarrhea
Nausea
Fluid retention and swelling

Possible interactions:
- Don't use with aspirin, other NSAIDs, or with other medications containing diclofenac.
- Diclofenac may interact with digoxin, insulin, oral hypoglycemic drugs, and phenobarbital.
- Diclofenac may prolong bleeding time if used with anticoagulants.
- Diclofenac may increase the levels or effects of the immunosuppressant cyclosporine, the psychosis drug lithium, the seizure drug phenytoin, and the anti-inflammatory drug methotrexate, possibly increasing toxicity of some of these drugs.
- Diclofenac may reduce the effects of beta blockers and loop diuretics.
- The gout drug probenecid may increase levels of diclofenac.
- The ulcer drug cimetidine may increase or decrease blood levels of diclofenac.

Other important information:
- The delayed-release formula is designed to resist dissolving in the stomach but release diclofenac quickly in the small intestines. The extended-release formula dissolves slowly over a longer period of time.
- Don't take this drug if you are at risk of ulcers, kidney or liver disease, have a low body weight, are elderly, or are sensitive to aspirin or NSAIDs.
- Have your doctor monitor you closely for intestinal ulcers or bleeding.
- Tell your doctor immediately if you develop these signs of liver problems: nausea, fatigue, jaundice, abdominal pain, flu-like symptoms, or severe itching.
- Since this drug can cause fluid retention, be careful if you suffer from high blood pressure or poor blood circulation.
- Be on the lookout for signs that this drug is depressing your immune system: fever, sore throat, tiredness, weakness, bruising, or unusual bleeding. Have your blood tested regularly.

DICLOFENAC WITH MISOPROSTOL

Pregnancy category: X

Brand:
Arthrotec

This drug combines diclofenac, an NSAID, and misoprostol, a synthetic prostaglandin that protects the stomach from ulcers. It is used to treat the symptoms of osteoarthritis and rheumatoid arthritis.

How to take this drug:
- Don't chew, crush, or dissolve the tablets.
- Never double a missed dose. Instead take it as soon as you remember or skip it and go on with your regular schedule.

Possible side effects:
Abdominal pain	Diarrhea
Indigestion	Nausea
Gas	Swelling

Possible interactions:
- Don't use with aspirin.
- If you take digoxin or lithium, have your doctor monitor you for possible toxic levels.
- This drug can interact with blood pressure medications, including ACE inhibitors.
- If you take this drug with warfarin, your risk of serious bleeding increases.
- Talk to your doctor about a possible interaction with insulin or oral hypoglycemic agents.
- Don't take with magnesium-containing antacids.

Other important information:
- This drug has severe consequences for women who are, or plan to become, pregnant.
- Don't take this drug if you have had allergic reactions to aspirin or other NSAIDs or if you have advanced kidney disease.
- Talk to your doctor if you have a history of asthma, kidney or liver problems, ulcer disease, GI bleeding, inflammatory bowel disease, cardiac decompensation, or high blood pressure.
- Your risk of bleeding is greater if you are taking oral corticosteroids, anticoagulants, or long-term NSAID therapy; if you are elderly or smoke; are an alcoholic; are in poor general health; or test positive for *Helicobacter pylori*.
- Make sure you are not dehydrated when taking this drug.
- Have your blood checked routinely for signs of anemia.
- Watch out for the signs of liver toxicity: nausea, fatigue, lethargy, itching, jaundice, abdominal pain, and flu-like symptoms. If you develop these, see your doctor immediately.

DICLOXACILLIN SODIUM

Pregnancy category: B

Brand:
Dycill   *Pathocil*

This penicillin antibiotic is used to treat a wide variety of infections by killing the bacteria that cause the infections.

How to take this drug:
- To improve absorption of this drug, take it on an empty stomach at least one hour before or two hours after a meal.

Possible side effects:
Nausea   Stomach pain
Gas   Loose stools

Possible interactions:
- The antibiotics neomycin and tetracycline may reduce the effects of this drug.
- This drug may interact with beta blockers and the antibiotics chloramphenicol and erythromycin.
- The effects of oral contraceptives and some other penicillins may be reduced.
- This drug can cause a false-positive urine glucose test, a false-positive Coombs' test, and a false-positive protein test.

Other important information:
- Don't use this drug if you are allergic to penicillin or other antibiotics. It may cause a dangerous allergic reaction, which can be fatal. Notify your doctor if you develop nausea, vomiting, severe diarrhea, fever, rash, hives, itching, wheezing, shortness of breath, sore throat, black tongue, swollen joints, or any unusual bleeding or bruising.
- Take all of the prescription, even after the infection goes away.

DICYCLOMINE

Pregnancy category: B
No driving

Brand:
Bentyl

Dicyclomine treats stomach disorders, such as irritable bowel syndrome (IBS), by relieving cramps or spasms of the stomach, intestines, and bladder.

How to take this drug:
- Don't take antacids within several hours of taking your dose of dicyclomine.

Possible side effects:

Dry mouth   Nausea or vomiting
Dizziness   Lightheadedness
Drowsiness   Weakness
Nervousness or excitement   Vision or eye problems

Possible interactions:

- The following drugs may increase the effects of dicyclomine: the antiparkinson drug amantadine, antihistamines, the antipsychosis drug phenothiazine, the antianxiety benzodiazepines, the antidepressant drugs called monoamine oxidase (MAO) inhibitors, narcotic painkillers, and other drugs with anticholinergic qualities.
- Dicyclomine may interact with glaucoma medication and the anti-nausea drug metoclopramide.
- This drug may increase the levels of the heart drug digoxin in the blood.
- Antacids may decrease levels of this drug in the blood.

Other important information:

- People with the following conditions should not use this drug: allergy to anticholinergic drugs; kidney disease; any obstructive disease of the stomach, intestines, or urinary tract; severe ulcerative colitis or ulcerative colitis complicated by dilation of the colon; a disease of the muscles called myasthenia gravis; reflux esophagitis; unstable heart problems; and glaucoma.
- People with the following conditions should use this drug very cautiously: disease of the autonomic nervous system; liver or kidney disease; ulcerative colitis; overactive thyroid; high blood pressure; coronary heart disease; congestive heart failure; irregular, rapid heartbeat; hiatal hernia; and prostate disease.
- This drug can make you become overheated if you are exposed to hot weather. Watch for signs of heatstroke or fever.

DIFLUNISAL

Pregnancy category: C

Brand:

Dolobid

Diflunisal relieves mild to moderate pain and treats the inflammation of osteoarthritis and rheumatoid arthritis.

How to take this drug:

- Swallow the tablets whole.
- Take your medicine with food or a full glass of milk or water to help prevent stomach irritation.

Possible side effects:

Nausea	Indigestion
Stomach pain	Diarrhea
Rash	Headache

Possible interactions:

- Don't use diflunisal with the NSAID indomethacin. The combination can cause dangerous stomach bleeding.
- Diflunisal may increase the effects of anticoagulants, such as warfarin. Your doctor may need to adjust the dose of your anticoagulant.
- Diflunisal may increase the levels of the diuretic hydrochlorothiazide in the blood but decrease its effects.
- It may increase levels of the analgesic acetaminophen, the anti-inflammatory drug methotrexate, and the immunosuppressant cyclosporine.
- It may decrease levels of the NSAID sulindac.
- Antacids may decrease levels of this drug in the blood.

Other important information:

- Take diflunisal with caution if you have active gastrointestinal bleeding or active peptic ulcer, a history of gastrointestinal disease, poor heart function, high blood pressure, a low blood platelet count, or other conditions that may cause fluid retention.
- Bleeding stomach ulcers and liver damage are the most common serious reactions to diflunisal. Warning signs of liver damage include nausea, tiredness, red and itchy skin, yellow eyes and skin (jaundice), and flu-like symptoms.
- Be on the lookout for signs that this drug is depressing your immune system: fever, sore throat, tiredness, weakness, bruising, unusual bleeding. Have your blood tested regularly.
- People allergic to aspirin or other NSAIDs should not use diflunisal.
- Don't use diflunisal to treat fever.

Digoxin

Pregnancy category: C

Brand:

Lanoxicaps
Lanoxin

Digoxin treats congestive heart failure and certain heart rhythm irregularities.

Possible side effects:

Nausea or vomiting	Loss of appetite
Diarrhea	Headache
Visual disturbances	Hallucinations
Breast enlargement in	Confusion
men and women	Depression

| Drowsiness | Weakness |
| Seizures | Irregular heartbeat |

Possible interactions:
- Antacids, the anti-inflammatory drug sulfasalazine, the cholesterol-lowering drugs colestipol and cholestyramine, the anti-nausea drug metoclopramide, and the antibiotic neomycin may decrease the effects of digoxin.
- The ulcer drug propantheline; the angina drug verapamil; the antispasmodic drug diphenoxylate; the antibiotics erythromycin, clarithromycin, and tetracycline; and the heartbeat regulators amiodarone and propafenone may increase the effects of digoxin.
- If you take digoxin along with drugs that decrease potassium levels in the blood, such as diuretics and the steroid prednisone, the combination may cause a dangerous loss of potassium.

Other important information:
- People with cardiovascular disease or thyroid problems should take digoxin with caution.
- If you have kidney problems, your doctor may need to carefully adjust your dose of digoxin.
- Digoxin can quickly reach toxic levels. Watch carefully for any side effects.
- Digoxin should not be used to treat obesity. It can cause dangerous irregular heartbeats, which can be fatal.
- It is important to maintain correct levels of potassium, calcium, and magnesium as these minerals also affect the heart. Talk to your doctor about a proper diet.

DILTIAZEM HYDROCHLORIDE

Pregnancy category: C
Brand:
Cardizem SR   *Dilacor XR*

Diltiazem is a calcium channel blocker. It lowers blood pressure and treats some forms of angina.

Possible side effects:
Weakness	Swollen hands or feet
Headache	Dizziness
Slow or irregular heartbeat	Flushing
Nausea	Rash

Possible interactions:
- Diltiazem may increase the effects of anesthetics and the immunosuppressant cyclosporine.
- The ulcer drug cimetidine may increase the effects of diltiazem.

- Using diltiazem with the beta blocker propranolol may result in various heartbeat irregularities. Don't suddenly stop taking beta blockers before or during treatment with this drug.
- Taking diltiazem and the heart drug digoxin could increase your blood level of digoxin to dangerous levels.

Other important information:
- Diltiazem should not be used by people with various heart conditions, including sick sinus syndrome, very low blood pressure, and some forms of irregular heartbeat.
- Use diltiazem cautiously if you have liver disease, kidney disease, congestive heart failure, or are already taking beta blockers.
- Be on the lookout for signs that this drug is depressing your immune system: fever, sore throat, tiredness, weakness, bruising, unusual bleeding. Have your blood tested regularly.

DIPHENHYDRAMINE HYDROCHLORIDE

Pregnancy category: B
No driving   MAO warning

Brand:
Benadryl

This sedating antihistamine relieves symptoms of food allergies, hay fever, and other allergies. It helps relieve sneezing, runny nose, itching, rashes, hives, swelling, and difficulty breathing. Diphenhydramine can be used to treat severe allergic reactions, motion sickness, and mild cases of parkinsonism.

How to take this drug:
- To ease motion sickness, take 30 minutes before traveling. While traveling, take the medicine before meals and when you go to bed.

Possible side effects:

Sleepiness	Dry mouth
Dizziness	Lack of coordination
Stomach pain	Thickened mucus in your airways

Possible interactions:
- While taking diphenhydramine, avoid alcohol and other depressants, such as sleeping pills and tranquilizers.

Other important information:
- Don't take this drug if you have certain kinds of glaucoma (ask your doctor), bladder neck obstruction, obstruction of the pylorus (opening from the stomach to the intestine), stomach ulcer, or an enlarged prostate.

- Don't use diphenhydramine if you have a lower respiratory disease, such as asthma, bronchitis, or pneumonia. It can dry out and thicken the mucus in your airways, making it more difficult to remove.
- Use diphenhydramine cautiously if you have increased pressure in the eye, an overactive thyroid, heart disease, or high blood pressure.
- If you're over 60, you're more likely to feel dizzy and sedated and have low blood pressure while taking diphenhydramine.

DIPHENOXYLATE HYDROCHLORIDE WITH ATROPINE SULFATE

Pregnancy category: C
No driving   MAO warning

Brand:
Lomotil
Lonox

This diphenoxylate/atropine combination medicine relieves diarrhea by slowing down the movements of the intestines.

Possible side effects:

Tiredness	Confusion
Dizziness	Numbness of fingers or toes
Drowsiness	Restlessness
Itching	Swelling
Rash	Headache
Stomach pain	Nausea
Fever	Rapid heartbeat
Difficulty urinating	Flushing
Dry skin and mouth	

Possible interactions:
- If you take this drug along with tranquilizers, alcohol, antihistamines, or muscle relaxers, the combination may dangerously depress your nervous system.

Other important information:
- People with some types of jaundice or some types of colitis (ask your doctor) should not use this drug.
- If you have liver or kidney problems, talk to your doctor about your condition before taking this drug.
- When you have diarrhea, you are losing water along with minerals, such as salt and potassium. This drug can put you at greater risk for dehydration. Make sure you drink extra fluids and eat a balanced diet.

DIPYRIDAMOLE

Pregnancy category: B

Brand:
Persantine

Dipyridamole is used to prevent clotting after heart valve replacement surgery. It is often used along with warfarin.

Possible side effects:
Dizziness	Headache
Rash	Upset stomach
Vomiting	Diarrhea
Flushing	Itching

Other important information:
* Be careful using dipyridamole if you have low blood pressure.

DIRITHROMYCIN

Pregnancy category: C

Brand:
Dynabac

Dirithromycin is an antibiotic used to treat specific strains of bacteria that cause acute and chronic bronchitis, pneumonia, strep throat, tonsillitis, and some skin infections.

How to take this drug:
* You must take this drug either with food or within an hour of eating.
* Don't cut, chew, or crush the tablets.
* Never double a missed dose. Instead take it as soon as you remember or skip it and go on with your regular schedule.

Possible side effects:
Abdominal pain	Headache
Nausea or vomiting	Diarrhea
Indigestion	Dizziness
Weakness	

Possible interactions:
* Dirithromycin may interact with theophylline, antacids, triazolam, digoxin, anticoagulants, ergotamine, cyclosporine, hexobarbital, carbamazepine, alfentanil, disopyramide, phenytoin, bromocriptine, valproate, astemizole, and lovastatin.

Other important information:
* Don't use dirithromycin if you have bacteria in your blood, commonly called blood poisoning.

- Many antibiotics kill the beneficial bacteria in your colon and allow the development of "antibiotic-associated colitis." The most common symptom is diarrhea. If you develop diarrhea after taking a round of dirithromycin, see your doctor.

DISOPYRAMIDE PHOSPHATE

Pregnancy category: C
No driving

Brand:

Norpace   *Norpace CR*

Disopyramide is an antiarrhythmic used to correct irregular heartbeats to a normal rhythm.

How to take this drug:
- Take your medicine on time and exactly as your doctor prescribes.
- Eat a high-fiber diet and drink plenty of liquids to relieve constipation, one of disopyramide's side effects.

Possible side effects:

Dry mouth	Constipation
Blurred vision	Gas or bloating
Frequent urination	Weakness
Headache	Impotence
Dizziness when standing suddenly	Fluid retention
Weight gain	Chest pain
Loss of appetite	Vomiting
Diarrhea	Itching
Nervousness	Rash
Dry nose, eyes, and throat	

Possible interactions:
- Other antiarrhythmic drugs, such as procainamide and lidocaine, may increase levels or effects of this drug.
- The seizure drug phenytoin may decrease levels of this drug.

Other important information:
- People with some types of heart rhythm disorders should not use this drug, including people with second- or third-degree AV block not being treated with a pacemaker.
- People with the following conditions should take this drug very cautiously: congestive heart failure, low blood pressure, urinary retention, the nerve/muscle disorder called myasthenia gravis, or glaucoma.
- You may need a lower dose if you have poor liver or kidney function.

- Have your blood sugar levels tested regularly if you have liver disease or congestive heart failure or if you are taking any other drugs that may affect your blood sugar levels.
- Men with enlarged prostates have an increased risk of urinary retention while taking disopyramide.
- Disopyramide may stimulate uterine contractions in pregnant women.

DISULFIRAM

Pregnancy category: C
No driving

Brand:
Antabuse

This drug is used to treat certain chronic alcoholics who want to remain sober.

How to take this drug:
- Take disulfiram at bedtime if it makes you drowsy.

Possible side effects:

Drowsiness	Restlessness
Weakness	Headache
Impotence	Joint disease
Metallic or garlic-like aftertaste	Psychotic reaction
Skin eruptions	

Possible interactions:
- You should not take disulfiram with the antibiotic metronidazole because a dangerous psychotic reaction can occur.
- If you take disulfiram with the seizure drug phenytoin, toxic levels of phenytoin may accumulate in your blood.
- Disulfiram may increase levels of some tranquilizers, including chlordiazepoxide and diazepam.
- It may increase the actions or effects of the anticoagulant warfarin.
- Difficulty walking or changes in behavior may occur if you use the tuberculosis drug isoniazid while taking disulfiram.

Other important information:
- Don't use alcohol in any form while you are taking this drug. Even in small amounts, it may produce a severe reaction that can cause slowed breathing, irregular heart rhythms, heart attack, unconsciousness, convulsions, and death. Ask your pharmacist about the alcohol content of any medications you intend to buy, including over-the-counter products. Also avoid vinegar, some sauces, after-shave lotions, colognes, and ointments.

- Don't use this drug if you are allergic to any thiuram derivatives, which are used in the production of rubber and pesticides. Also, don't take it if you suffer from psychoses, severe heart disease, or coronary thrombosis.
- People with brain damage, epilepsy, diabetes, kidney or liver disease, or underactive thyroid should use this drug with caution.

DIVALPROEX SODIUM

Pregnancy category: D
No driving

Brand:
Depakote

Divalproex sodium is used alone or along with other anticonvulsant drugs to treat certain types of seizures.

How to take this drug:
- If your medicine upsets your stomach, take it with food.
- You can swallow the capsules whole or open them and sprinkle the contents on a teaspoonful of soft food, such as applesauce. Swallow the mixture immediately. Don't chew it or store the mixture to use later.

Possible side effects:
Sleepiness   Nausea
Indigestion

Possible interactions:
- If you take divalproex sodium along with tranquilizers, alcohol, antihistamines, muscle relaxers, and other anticonvulsant drugs, the combination may dangerously depress your nervous system. Barbiturates combined with divalproex sodium can be especially dangerous. Your doctor should carefully monitor the levels of these drugs in your body.
- Taking divalproex sodium and aspirin, carbamazepine, dicumarol, or phenytoin at the same time can increase or decrease the levels of any of these drugs in your body.
- Drugs that affect blood clotting (aspirin and warfarin, for instance) should be used cautiously with divalproex sodium.
- Divalproex sodium may make birth control pills less effective.

Other important information:
- In rare cases, this drug can cause liver failure, which can be fatal. Have regular liver tests and look for side effects, such as fatigue, weakness, swelling of the face, loss of appetite, and vomiting. Usually, liver failure occurs in the first six months that you take divalproex sodium.
- This drug may cause a low blood platelet count. This means your blood may not clot properly. Look for unusual bruising and have regular blood tests.

DOLASETRON MESYLATE MONOHYDRATE

Pregnancy category: B

Brand:
Anzemet

Dolasetron mesylate is a selective serotonin receptor antagonist that prevents the nausea and vomiting that is a common side effect of surgery and chemotherapy.

Possible side effects:

Headache	Blood pressure changes
Tiredness	Diarrhea
Fever	Itching
Irregular heartbeat	Dizziness
Indigestion	Chills

Possible interactions:
- This drug may interact with cimetidine, rifampin, and drugs that change your heart rhythm, such as anti-arrhythmias.

Other important information:
- Be careful taking this drug if you suffer from hypokalemia (low blood levels of potassium), hypomagnesemia (low blood levels of magnesium), if you are on diuretics, anti-arrhythmic drugs, or anthracycline therapy.

DORZOLAMIDE HYDROCHLORIDE

Pregnancy category: C

Brand:
Trusopt

This ophthalmic solution is a sulfonamide used to reduce pressure within the eye caused by glaucoma or ocular hypertension.

How to take this drug:
- If you are using this medication with any other medication in your eye, take them at least 10 minutes apart.
- Remove contact lenses before using this medication. Wait 15 minutes, then reinsert them.
- Don't contaminate the solution or the tip of the bottle by allowing it to touch anything, including your eye.

Possible side effects:

Burning or stinging eyes	Bitter taste
Gray spots in the cornea (superficial punctate keratitis)	Blurred vision
	Red eyes
Watery eyes	Dryness
Light sensitivity	

Possible interactions:
- Don't use these drops if you are also taking an oral carbonic anhydrase inhibitor.

Other important information:
- Allergic reactions to sulfonamides can be serious, even fatal.
- This drug is not recommended if you have severe kidney or liver problems.
- If you use this drug over a long period of time, you could develop allergic eye and eyelid irritations, such as conjunctivitis. If this happens, stop using the solution immediately and see your doctor.

DORZOLAMIDE HYDROCHLORIDE – TIMOLOL MALEATE
Pregnancy category: C

Brand:
Cosopt

This ophthalmic solution combines a topical sulfonamide and a topical beta-adrenergic receptor blocking agent. It is used to lower the pressure in your eye caused by glaucoma or ocular hypertension.

How to take this drug:
- If you are using this drug with any other eye medication, use them at least 10 minutes apart.
- Remove contact lenses before using this medication. Wait 15 minutes, then reinsert them.
- Don't contaminate the solution or the tip of the bottle by allowing it to touch anything, including your eye.

Possible side effects:
Unpleasant taste	Burning, stinging, itching eyes
Conjunctivitis	Eyelid irritation
Muscle weakness	Gray spots in the cornea (superficial
Blurred vision	punctate keratitis)
Blood spot on the eye	

Possible interactions:
- Don't use this drug with oral carbonic anhydrase inhibitors or other topical beta-adrenergic blocking agents.
- Be careful taking this drug with digitalis; catecholamine-depleting drugs, like reserpine; or oral or IV calcium antagonists, especially if you have heart problems.

Other important information:
- Don't use this medication if you have bronchial asthma, kidney disease, liver disease, chronic lung disease (severe chronic obstructive pulmonary

disease), or certain heart conditions (sinus bradycardia, atrioventricular block, overt cardiac failure, or cardiogenic shock).

- Allergic reactions to sulfonamides can be serious, even fatal. Report any unusual effects.
- You may need to stop this medication if you are scheduled for surgery. Talk to your doctor.
- If you are diabetic or subject to hypoglycemia or hyperthyroidism, use this medication cautiously.
- While on this medication, you may be more susceptible to any allergic reactions.

DOXAZOSIN

Pregnancy category: C
No driving

Brand:
Cardura

Doxazosin controls high blood pressure by relaxing and expanding blood vessel walls.

How to take this drug:
- Taking the first dose at bedtime may help reduce the "first-dose" effect.

Possible side effects:
Dizziness when standing suddenly   Lightheadedness
Fainting

Possible interactions:
- If you take doxazosin with other blood pressure drugs, you're more likely to experience very low blood pressure and fainting.
- Alcohol can make your blood pressure drop even further while you're taking this drug.

Other important information:
- Take this drug cautiously if you are taking other blood pressure-lowering drugs or if you have poor liver function.
- Doxazosin may cause you to have very low blood pressure when you first start taking it. Your blood pressure can drop so low that you faint or lose consciousness. This is known as the "first-dose" effect. It can also occur if your dose is increased quickly, if your treatment is restarted after you've missed several doses, or if you begin taking another high blood pressure drug.
- Move slowly and carefully when you get up from a sitting or lying position.

DOXEPIN HYDROCHLORIDE

Pregnancy category: NR
No driving   MAO warning

Brand:
Sinequan

Doxepin treats the symptoms of depression and anxiety.

Possible side effects:

Drowsiness	Dizziness
Dry mouth	Headache
Increased appetite	Nausea
Unpleasant taste	Black tongue

Possible interactions:
- Avoid alcohol while taking this drug. It could dangerously increase your normal response to the alcohol.
- The ulcer drug cimetidine, the phenothiazine tranquilizers, the heart drugs propafenone and flecainide, and any of the type of antidepressants called selective serotonin reuptake inhibitors (fluoxetine, sertraline, and paroxetine) can increase the levels of doxepin in your body. If you are taking doxepin and any of these other drugs at the same time, you may need lower than normal doses of both drugs.
- Your doctor should supervise you closely for side effects if you take doxepin along with any anticholinergic drugs, such as some antihistamines and muscle relaxers.
- For diabetics, taking tolazamide and doxepin at the same time can cause severe hypoglycemia.

Other important information:
- People with glaucoma or urinary retention should not use doxepin.
- You may need to take doxepin for two to three weeks before your depression is relieved.
- If you suddenly quit taking this drug, you could have nausea, headache, and a general feeling of fatigue. If you gradually quit taking the drug, you may still experience irritability, restlessness, and dream and sleep disturbances.

DOXYCYCLINE HYCLATE

Pregnancy category: D

Brand:

Doryx	*Doxychel Hyclate*
Doxy-Lemmon	*Doxy-Tabs*
Vibramycin	*Vibra-Tabs*
Periostat	

This antibiotic is used to treat a variety of infections. Periostat is prescribed specifically to treat adult periodontitis.

How to take this drug:
- Take with food or milk to avoid irritation of the stomach. Make sure you wash down the drug with plenty of liquid to help prevent ulcers and irritation of the esophagus and throat, especially if you will be lying down afterward.
- If you miss a dose, take it as soon as possible. If several hours have passed or it is nearing time for the next dose, don't try to catch up by doubling your dose unless your doctor tells you to.

Possible side effects:
Headache
Diarrhea
Sore throat or hoarseness
Difficulty swallowing
Sensitivity to light
Hives
Fluid retention
Joint pain

Nausea
Loss of appetite
Inflamed mouth or tongue
Rash
Blue-gray discoloration of the
   skin and mucous membranes
Fever

Possible interactions:
- This drug may reduce the effectiveness of birth control pills, resulting in unplanned pregnancy.
- This drug may increase the levels or effects of anticoagulants, and it may interfere with the actions of penicillin antibiotics.
- Antacids and iron-containing products may reduce absorption of this drug.

Other important information:
- Don't use if you are allergic to tetracycline antibiotics.
- Discontinue use if an allergic skin reaction appears after exposure to sunlight.
- If you have kidney problems, tetracyclines can accumulate to toxic levels in your body.
- Be on the lookout for signs that this drug is depressing your immune system: fever, sore throat, tiredness, weakness, bruising, unusual bleeding. Have your blood tested regularly.
- Taking an antibiotic for a long time can cause bacteria or fungus to overgrow, leading to another infection, such as fungal infections of the mouth, anus, or vagina. If you get one of these "superinfections," you may need to quit taking doxycycline and start taking another antibiotic for the second infection.
- Doxycycline may cause increased pressure on the brain in adults. Let your doctor know immediately if you develop headache, nausea, or visual disturbances.

- This drug may cause colitis, an inflammation of the colon. Symptoms include bloody diarrhea, stomach cramps, and fever.
- It may make your skin extra-sensitive to sunlight, so protect your skin if you'll be outdoors.

DYPHYLLINE

Pregnancy category: C

Brand:
Dilor   *Lufyllin*

Dyphylline is a bronchodilator. It relieves acute asthma and the wheezing and bronchial spasms that accompany bronchitis and emphysema.

Possible side effects:
Nausea or vomiting   Headache
Irritability   Restlessness
Sleeplessness   Irregular heartbeat

Possible interactions:
- If you take the gout drug probenecid, your blood levels of dyphylline may increase.
- If you take another bronchodilator, such as theophylline, and ephedrine along with dyphylline, the effects of all three drugs may be increased, and your central nervous system may be overstimulated. Some over-the-counter drugs contain theophylline and ephedrine.

Other important information:
- Don't use if you are allergic or hypersensitive to caffeine or any of the other bronchodilators that are "xanthine derivatives."
- Use with caution if you have heart disease, overactive thyroid, high blood pressure, damage to the heart, or stomach ulcer.

ENALAPRIL MALEATE

Pregnancy category: C/D

Brand:
Vasotec

This angiotensin converting enzyme (ACE) inhibitor treats high blood pressure.

Possible side effects:
Dizziness   Headache
Tiredness   Cough

Possible interactions:
- If this drug is taken with the antipsychotic drug lithium, it may cause lithium to accumulate to toxic levels.

- Nonsteroidal anti-inflammatory drugs (NSAIDs) may decrease the blood-pressure-lowering effects of enalapril.
- You could have a dangerous drop in blood pressure if you drink alcohol or take barbiturates or narcotics with enalapril.

Other important information:
- Take this drug very cautiously if you have kidney problems, heart failure, or collagen vascular diseases.
- Enalapril may cause a severe drop in blood pressure after the first dose, particularly in people taking diuretics, on dialysis, or with congestive heart failure. Be careful when you stand quickly. You may feel lightheaded and dizzy.
- Be on the lookout for signs that this drug is depressing your immune system: fever, sore throat, tiredness, weakness, bruising, unusual bleeding. Have your blood tested regularly.
- Mild swelling can occur in the throat, face, lips, tongue, mucous membranes, hands, or feet, but swelling of the throat can be extremely dangerous. If this happens, call for emergency help immediately.
- If you develop jaundice (yellow eyes or skin), contact your doctor immediately.
- Enalapril may cause dangerously high levels of potassium in the blood, which can be fatal. Don't use potassium-sparing diuretics or take potassium supplements without talking to your doctor.
- Be careful in hot weather and during exercise. Sweating can cause loss of fluid, low blood pressure, and, therefore, lightheadedness.

ERGOTAMINE TARTRATE

Pregnancy category: X

Brand:
Ercaf   *Ercatab*
Ergomar   *Wigraine*

This drug is used to prevent or relieve throbbing migraine and cluster headaches.

How to take this drug:
- Take medicine at the first sign of headache. If necessary, take another tablet in a half-hour, but don't take more than three tablets in 24 hours. You shouldn't take more than five tablets in one week.
- Don't take more than the recommended dose. Prolonged or excessive use can lead to ergotism (ergot poisoning).

Possible side effects:
Nausea or vomiting	Weakness in the legs
Numbness and tingling in fingers and toes	Muscle pain in extremities
	Irregular heartbeat
Itching	Swelling

Possible interactions:
- Taking ergotamine with other drugs that constrict blood vessels may result in dangerously high blood pressure.

Other important information:
- Don't use this drug if you have coronary artery disease, high blood pressure, poor liver or kidney function, severe itching, peripheral vascular disease (such as arteriosclerosis or Raynaud's disease), blood poisoning, or hypersensitivity to ergot alkaloids.
- You can become dependent on ergotamine if you take it for a long time. You may need increasingly larger amounts to relieve your headache. And, once you stop taking it, you may have "rebound headache" that is even more severe than your original headache.
- Ercatab and Wigraine contain caffeine.

ERYTHROMYCIN, TOPICAL

Pregnancy category: B

Brand:
A/T/S	*Emgel*
Erycette	*Erygel*
Erymax	*Erythra-Derm*
Theramycin	

These antibiotic gels and ointments are used to treat acne.

How to take this drug:
- For the gel and ointment forms, wash with soap and warm water, rinse well, and pat dry before applying the drug. Apply in the morning and evening and wash your hands after applying.

Possible side effects:
Peeling	Dryness
Itching	Burning
Redness	Oily skin
Eye irritation	

Possible interactions:
- Talk to your doctor before combining this product with any other topical medications. You could badly irritate your skin.

Other important information:
- You may not see improvement for several weeks. Continue to use it regularly. However, if you still don't notice any improvement after eight weeks, call your doctor.

ERYTHROMYCIN, ORAL

Pregnancy category: B

Brand:
Ery-Tab   *E-Mycin*

This antibiotic is used to treat various respiratory illnesses and skin and soft tissue infections.

How to take this drug:
- The effectiveness of erythromycin is decreased in some people when they take it with food. Take it with food if it upsets your stomach, but if it doesn't, take it on an empty stomach — one hour before or two hours after meals.
- Take each dose at evenly spaced intervals throughout the day with at least 6 ounces of fluids.

Possible side effects:

Nausea	Loss of appetite
Diarrhea	Stomach cramps and discomfort
Itching	Skin eruptions (such as hives)
Irregular heartbeat	

Possible interactions:
- This drug may cause rhabdomyolysis (a disease that destroys muscle tissue) in people who are taking the cholesterol-reducer lovastatin.
- This drug may increase the levels or effects of anticoagulants, the seizure drug carbamazepine (Tegretol), the heart drug digoxin, the migraine drug ergotamine, the asthma drug theophylline, and the insomnia drug triazolam.
- Taking terfenadine and erythromycin together can cause life-threatening heart rhythm disturbances.

Other important information:
- People with liver disease should not take this drug.
- Abnormal liver function, including jaundice, is a rare side effect. If you develop yellow eyes and skin, dark urine, or feel unusually tired, contact your doctor.
- Taking an antibiotic for a long time can cause bacteria or fungus to overgrow, leading to another infection, such as fungal infections of the mouth, anus, or vagina. If you get one of these "superinfections," you may need to quit taking erythromycin and start taking another antibiotic for the second infection.
- Take all of the prescription, even after you begin to feel better.

ESTERIFIED ESTROGENS

Pregnancy category: X

Brand:

Estratab   *Menest*

This drug is used to treat symptoms of menopause, such as vaginal dryness and hot flashes. It also helps prevent osteoporosis (loss of bone mass).

How to take this drug:
- Take this drug after meals or with a snack if you experience nausea.
- Never double a missed dose. Instead take it as soon as you remember or skip it and go on with your regular schedule.
- Try to take your medicine at the same time every day to reduce side effects and help it work better.

Possible side effects:

Nausea or vomiting
Menstrual changes
Cramps or bloating
Dizziness
Changes in skin tone

Changes in sex drive
Breast tenderness or enlargement
Headache
Weight changes

Possible interactions:
- Carbamazepine, phenobarbital, and rifampin may decrease this estrogen's effectiveness.
- Corticosteroids may increase estrogen's effectiveness.
- Taking estrogen with cyclosporine or dentrolene could produce toxic levels of these drugs.
- Your dose of oral anticoagulants may have to be adjusted.
- Estrogen may make tamoxifen less effective.

Other important information:
- Smoking increases your chances of developing serious side effects, such as strokes, heart attacks, and blood clots.
- If you experience any signs of a blood clot — shortness of breath, pain in your chest or legs, a severe headache, dizziness, or faintness — call your doctor immediately.
- Taking estrogen for a number of years may increase your risk of endometrial cancer (cancer of the lining of the uterus). Adding progestin (another female hormone) to your estrogen dose reduces that increased risk.
- Drugs containing estrogen cause some people's gums to bleed, swell, and become tender. You can help prevent this side effect by brushing and flossing your teeth regularly and massaging your gums.
- Use this drug cautiously if you have high blood pressure; depression; heart, liver, or kidney problems; bone diseases; migraine; seizures; or diabetes.

ESTRADIOL

Pregnancy category: X

Brand:

Estrace   *Gynodiol*

Estradiol is used to treat symptoms of menopause, such as vaginal dryness and hot flashes. It also helps prevent osteoporosis (loss of bone mass).

How to take this drug:
- Take this drug after meals or with a snack if you experience nausea.
- Never double a missed dose. Instead take it as soon as you remember or skip it and go on with your regular schedule.
- Try to take your medicine at the same time every day to reduce side effects and help it work better.

Possible side effects:

Nausea	Change in appetite or weight
Breast tenderness	Headache
Eye problems	Diarrhea
Fluid retention	Dizziness
Depression	Vaginal discharge or bleeding
Breast lumps	Nipple discharge
Rash	Joint pain
A spotty darkening of the skin	

Possible interactions:
- Check with your doctor if you are also taking phenobarbital, warfarin, phenytoin, rifampin, amitriptyline, or imipramine.

Other important information:
- Smoking increases your chances of developing serious side effects, such as strokes, heart attacks, and blood clots.
- If you experience any signs of a blood clot — shortness of breath, pain in your chest or legs, a severe headache, dizziness, or faintness — call your doctor immediately.
- Taking estrogen for a number of years may increase your risk of endometrial cancer (cancer of the lining of the uterus). Adding progestin (another female hormone) to your estrogen dose reduces that increased risk.
- Drugs containing estrogen cause some people's gums to bleed, swell, and become tender. You can help prevent this side effect by brushing and flossing your teeth regularly and massaging your gums.
- This drug will increase your skin's sensitivity to the sun. Always use a sunscreen and wear protective clothes when you will be exposed to the sun.

ESTRADIOL TRANSDERMAL SYSTEM

Pregnancy category: X

Brand:

Vivelle   Estraderm

Climara

The estradiol patch is worn on your skin to treat symptoms of menopause, such as vaginal dryness and hot flashes. It also helps prevent osteoporosis (loss of bone mass).

How to take this drug:

- Place adhesive side of patch on clean, dry skin of the buttocks or stomach. Avoid the waistline area since clothing may rub off the patch. Change the site of the patch weekly to help prevent skin irritation. If the patch falls off, reapply the same patch or use a new one.

Possible side effects:

Nausea

Breast tenderness

Eye problems

Fluid retention

Depression

Breast lumps

Rash

A spotty darkening of the skin

Change in appetite or weight

Headache

Diarrhea

Dizziness

Vaginal discharge or bleeding

Nipple discharge

Joint pain

Possible interactions:

- Check with your doctor if you are also taking phenobarbital, warfarin, phenytoin, rifampin, amitriptyline, or imipramine.

Other important information:

- Smoking increases your chances of developing serious side effects, such as strokes, heart attacks, and blood clots.
- If you experience any signs of a blood clot — shortness of breath, pain in your chest or legs, a severe headache, dizziness, or faintness — call your doctor immediately.
- Taking estrogen for a number of years may increase your risk of endometrial cancer (cancer of the lining of the uterus). Adding progestin (another female hormone) to your estrogen dose reduces that increased risk.
- Drugs containing estrogen cause some people's gums to bleed, swell, and become tender. You can help prevent this side effect by brushing and flossing your teeth regularly and massaging your gums.
- This drug will increase your skin's sensitivity to the sun. Always use a sunscreen and wear protective clothes when you will be exposed to the sun.

ESTROGENS, CONJUGATED

Pregnancy category: X

Brand:
Premarin

This female hormone is used to treat symptoms of menopause, such as vaginal dryness and hot flashes. It also helps prevent osteoporosis (loss of bone mass).

How to take this drug:
- Take this drug after meals or with a snack if you experience nausea.
- Never double a missed dose. Instead take it as soon as you remember or skip it and go on with your regular schedule.
- Try to take your medicine at the same time every day to reduce side effects and help it work better.

Possible side effects:

Nausea	Change in appetite or weight
Breast tenderness	Headache
Eye problems	Diarrhea
Fluid retention	Dizziness
Depression	Vaginal discharge or bleeding
Breast lumps	Nipple discharge
Rash	Joint pain
A spotty darkening of the skin	

Possible interactions:
- Talk to your doctor if you are also taking phenobarbital, warfarin, phenytoin, rifampin, amitriptyline, imipramine, carbamazepine, corticosteroids, cyclosporine, dantrolene, oral anticoagulants, or tamoxifen.

Other important information:
- Smoking increases your chances of developing serious side effects, such as strokes, heart attacks, and blood clots.
- If you experience any signs of a blood clot — shortness of breath, pain in your chest or legs, a severe headache, dizziness, or faintness — call your doctor immediately.
- Taking estrogen for a number of years may increase your risk of endometrial cancer (cancer of the lining of the uterus). Adding progestin (another female hormone) to your estrogen dose reduces that increased risk.
- If you suffer from nearsightedness or astigmatism, your condition could get worse. You may also find you have less tolerance for contact lenses.
- Your menstrual flow could change.
- Drugs containing estrogen cause some people's gums to bleed, swell, and become tender. You can help prevent this side effect by brushing and flossing your teeth regularly and massaging your gums.

- This drug will increase your skin's sensitivity to the sun. Always use a sunscreen and wear protective clothes when you will be exposed to the sun.

ESTROGENS, CONJUGATED AND MEDROXYPROGESTERONE ACETATE

Pregnancy category: X

Brand:
Premphase   *Prempro*

This female hormone is used to treat symptoms of menopause, such as vaginal dryness and hot flashes. It also helps prevent osteoporosis (loss of bone mass).

How to take this drug:
- Take this drug after meals or with a snack if you experience nausea.
- Never double a missed dose. Instead take it as soon as you remember or skip it and go on with your regular schedule.
- Try to take your medicine at the same time every day to reduce side effects and help it work better.

Possible side effects:
Nausea	Change in appetite or weight
Breast tenderness	Headache
Eye problems	Diarrhea
Fluid retention	Dizziness
Depression	Vaginal discharge or bleeding
Breast lumps	Nipple discharge
Rash	Joint pain
A spotty darkening of the skin	

Possible interactions:
- Talk to your doctor if you are also taking phenobarbital, warfarin, phenytoin, rifampin, amitriptyline, imipramine, carbamazepine, corticosteroids, cyclosporine, dantrolene, oral anticoagulants, or tamoxifen.

Other important information:
- Smoking increases your chances of developing serious side effects, such as strokes, heart attacks, and blood clots.
- If you experience any signs of a blood clot — shortness of breath, pain in your chest or legs, a severe headache, dizziness, or faintness — call your doctor immediately.
- Taking estrogen for a number of years may increase your risk of endometrial cancer (cancer of the lining of the uterus). Adding progestin (another female hormone) to your estrogen dose reduces that increased risk.
- If you suffer from nearsightedness or astigmatism, your condition could get worse. You may also find you have less tolerance for contact lenses.

- Your menstrual flow could change.
- Drugs containing estrogen cause some people's gums to bleed, swell, and become tender. You can help prevent this side effect by brushing and flossing your teeth regularly and massaging your gums.
- This drug will increase your skin's sensitivity to the sun. Always use a sunscreen and wear protective clothes when you will be exposed to the sun.

ESTROPIPATE

Pregnancy category: X

Brand:
Ogen

This female hormone is used to treat symptoms of menopause, such as vaginal dryness and hot flashes. It also helps prevent osteoporosis (loss of bone mass).

How to take this drug:
- Take this drug after meals or with a snack if you experience nausea.
- Never double a missed dose. Instead take it as soon as you remember or skip it and go on with your regular schedule.
- Try to take your medicine at the same time every day to reduce side effects and help it work better.

Possible side effects:

Nausea	Change in appetite or weight
Breast tenderness	Headache
Eye problems	Diarrhea
Fluid retention	Dizziness
Depression	Vaginal discharge or bleeding
Breast lumps	Nipple discharge
Rash	Joint pain
A spotty darkening of the skin	

Possible interactions:
- Talk to your doctor if you are also taking phenobarbital, warfarin, phenytoin, rifampin, amitriptyline, or imipramine.

Other important information:
- Smoking increases your chances of developing serious side effects, such as strokes, heart attacks, and blood clots.
- If you experience any signs of a blood clot — shortness of breath, pain in your chest or legs, a severe headache, dizziness, or faintness — call your doctor immediately.
- Taking estrogen for a number of years may increase your risk of endometrial cancer (cancer of the lining of the uterus). Adding progestin (another female hormone) to your estrogen dose reduces that increased risk.

- Drugs containing estrogen cause some people's gums to bleed, swell, and become tender. You can help prevent this side effect by brushing and flossing your teeth regularly and massaging your gums.
- This drug will increase your skin's sensitivity to the sun. Always use a sunscreen and wear protective clothes when you will be exposed to the sun.

ETANERCEPT

Pregnancy category: B
Refrigerate

Brand:
Enbrel

Etanercept is an injectable drug used to relieve the symptoms of rheumatoid arthritis.

How to take this drug:
- You usually give yourself injections of this drug. The first time, do it while your doctor is watching.
- Dispose of needles and syringes properly and never reuse them.
- Carefully follow all instructions for mixing, injecting, and storing this drug.
- Don't add other medications to the solution.
- Change injection sites: thigh, abdomen, upper arm.
- Inject at least an inch from an earlier injection site.
- Never inject into areas of skin that are bruised, tender, red, or hard.
- Never double a missed dose. Instead take it as soon as you remember or skip it and go on with your regular schedule.

Possible side effects:

Injection site reactions (redness, itching, pain, swelling)	Dizziness
	Cough
Colds	Weakness
Sinusitis	Abdominal pain
Infection	Rash
Headache	Upset stomach

Other important information:
- This drug can be used along with methotrexate.
- Don't take it if you have bacteria in the blood, commonly called blood poisoning or sepsis.
- It's possible that this drug will suppress your immune system, so stop taking it if you develop a serious infection.
- Don't get a vaccination containing live vaccines while on this medication.

ETHAMBUTOL HYDROCHLORIDE

Pregnancy category: C
No driving

Brand:
Myambutol

Ethambutol hydrochloride is used to treat pulmonary tuberculosis in combination with other anti-tuberculous drugs. Ethambutol prevents growth of the bacteria that causes tuberculosis.

How to take this drug:
- If you miss a dose, take it as soon as possible. If several hours have passed or it is nearing time for the next dose, don't try to catch up by doubling your dose unless your doctor tells you to.

Possible side effects:

Nausea	Stomach upset or pain
Loss of appetite	Visual disturbances
Hallucinations	Disorientation
Dizziness	Confusion
Headache	Fever
Numbness and tingling in the hands and feet	Joint pain
	Itching
Dermatitis	Gout

Possible interactions:
- Antacids may delay and reduce absorption of this drug.

Other important information:
- People with poor kidney function may need smaller doses. Periodically check your kidney and liver functions and blood levels if you take this drug for a long time.
- This drug may cause vision problems, which can be irreversible in some cases. Have regular eye exams. Use with extreme caution if you have cataracts, optic neuritis, disorder of the retina of the eye caused by diabetes, or recurring eye inflammation. These conditions make it more difficult to determine changes in vision. Report any changes in vision in one or both eyes to your doctor.

ETHOSUXIMIDE

Pregnancy category: NR
No driving

Brand:
Zarontin

Ethosuximide controls petit mal seizures for people with epilepsy.

Possible side effects:

Upset stomach	Nausea
Cramps	Diarrhea
Loss of appetite	

Possible interactions:

- Ethosuximide may increase levels of the seizure drug phenytoin.

Other important information:

- Use this drug very cautiously if you have liver or kidney problems.
- Ethosuximide can also cause liver and kidney damage. Have regular liver and kidney tests while you're taking this drug.
- Be on the lookout for signs that this drug is depressing your immune system: fever, sore throat, tiredness, weakness, bruising, unusual bleeding. Have your blood tested regularly.
- Never stop taking your medicine or change your dose without talking to your doctor. Any sudden change could cause a seizure.

ETIDRONATE DISODIUM

Pregnancy category: C

Brand:

Didronel

This hormone is used to treat the symptoms of bone loss in Paget's disease and to aid in proper bone healing after hip replacement surgery.

How to take this drug:

- Take this drug two hours before meals, especially before eating foods high in calcium, such as milk or other dairy products.
- Avoid taking vitamin and mineral supplements or antacids high in calcium, iron, magnesium, or aluminum within two hours of taking this drug.

Possible side effects:

Nausea	Diarrhea
Bone pain	Mouth ulcers
Rash, hives, or itching	Fluid retention
Memory loss	Confusion
Mental depression	

Possible interactions:

- Vitamin and mineral supplements, food (especially milk and other dairy products), and antacids that contain calcium, iron, magnesium, or aluminum may decrease levels of etidronate.

Other important information:

- People with kidney disease should take etidronate with caution.

- Have your doctor monitor your kidney function if you are being treated for hypercalcemia.
- Taking high doses of etidronate or taking it for a long time may increase the risk of fractures. If you experience a fracture, your doctor may stop your drug treatment for a while.

ETODOLAC

Pregnancy category: C

Brand:
Lodine

This nonsteroidal anti-inflammatory drug (NSAID) is used to control the symptoms of osteoarthritis and to relieve pain.

Possible side effects:

Nausea	Diarrhea
Dizziness	Stomach pain or cramps
Indigestion	Constipation
Black and tarry feces	Mental depression
Weakness	Nervousness
Blurred vision	Ringing in the ears
Itching	Rash
Frequent urination	

Possible interactions:
- Avoid aspirin while taking NSAIDs, such as etodolac.
- Etodolac may decrease the effectiveness of anticoagulants such as warfarin.
- Etodolac may increase the levels or effects of the heart drug digoxin, the immunosuppressant cyclosporine, the antipsychotic drug lithium, and the cancer drug methotrexate, possibly increasing the toxicity of some of these drugs.

Other important information:
- Don't use etodolac if you are allergic to aspirin or other NSAIDs.
- Taking etodolac is more likely to cause kidney problems if you are elderly; if you take diuretics; or if you have lupus, heart failure, or poor liver or kidney function.
- Take etodolac with caution if you have heart failure, high blood pressure, or clotting disorders.
- Bleeding stomach ulcers and liver or kidney damage are the most common serious reactions to using etodolac for long periods. Warning signs of liver damage include nausea, tiredness, red and itchy skin, yellow eyes and skin (jaundice), and flu-like symptoms.
- Be on the lookout for signs that this drug is depressing your immune system: fever, sore throat, tiredness, weakness, bruising, unusual bleeding. Have your blood tested regularly.

ETRETINATE

Pregnancy category: X
No driving

Brand:
Tegison

Etretinate is used to treat severe psoriasis in people who cannot use other drugs.

How to take this drug:
* Take etretinate with food or milk to increase absorption of the drug.
* Use a moisturizer to help relieve dry skin. Apply one hour after using etretinate.

Possible side effects:

Dry nose	Chapped lips
Hair loss	Peeling hands and feet
Thirst	Sore mouth
Dry and fragile skin	Itching
Rash	Red and scaly face
Bone or joint pain	Tiredness

Possible interactions:
* Don't take vitamin supplements containing vitamin A while you are taking this drug.
* Alcohol combined with etretinate may cause very high triglyceride levels.

Other important information:
* Don't use this drug if you are allergic to vitamin A.
* Have a liver function test before you begin taking etretinate.
* If you are diabetic, obese, or drink alcohol, or have a family history of these conditions, use this drug with caution.
* Etretinate commonly raises triglyceride and cholesterol levels.
* This drug may cause eye and vision disorders, often making contact lenses difficult to wear and decreasing night vision.
* Two common risks of taking etretinate for long periods of time are liver damage (including hepatitis and cirrhosis) and increased pressure on the brain. Let your doctor know immediately if you develop headache, nausea, fluid retention, or visual disturbances.
* Even if etretinate makes your psoriasis worse at first, don't stop taking it.
* This drug may make your skin extra-sensitive to sunlight.

FAMOTIDINE

Pregnancy category: B

Brand:
Pepcid

Famotidine decreases the amount of acid your stomach produces. It helps stomach ulcers heal, treats gastroesophageal reflux disease (severe heartburn), controls bleeding in the stomach or intestines, and treats Zollinger-Ellison disease, a condition in which your stomach produces too much acid.

Possible side effects:

Headache	Diarrhea
Constipation	Dizziness
Confusion	Hallucinations
Depression	Anxiety

Possible interactions:
* You can take antacids along with famotidine.

Other important information:
* Don't take famotidine if you are allergic to any anti-ulcer drug.
* Your doctor may need to adjust your dose if you have liver or kidney problems.
* Be on the lookout for signs that this drug is depressing your immune system: fever, sore throat, tiredness, weakness, bruising, unusual bleeding. Have your blood tested regularly.

FELODIPINE

Pregnancy category: C
No driving

Brand:
Plendil

Felodipine is a calcium channel blocker used to lower blood pressure.

How to take this drug:
* Tablets should be swallowed whole. Don't crush or chew.

Possible side effects:

Headache	Flushing
Swollen feet, ankles, and hands	Dizziness
Common cold symptoms	Weakness
Prickling or tingling sensation	Upset stomach
Chest pain	Nausea
Muscle cramps	Rapid heartbeat
Constipation	Diarrhea
Back pain	Swollen gums
Rash	

Possible interactions:
* Talk to your doctor before drinking grapefruit juice while taking this drug.

- If you take felodipine with beta blockers, the combination may cause very low blood pressure or heart irregularities. Don't suddenly stop taking beta blockers before or during treatment with calcium-channel blockers.
- If you take felodipine with the pain drug fentanyl, the combination may cause dangerously low blood pressure.
- Felodipine may increase the effects of the heart drug digitalis.
- Felodipine may decrease the effects of the asthma drug theophylline.
- The ulcer drugs cimetidine and ranitidine and the antibiotic erythromycin may increase the levels or effects of felodipine.
- Barbiturates and the seizure drug carbamazepine may decrease levels or effects of felodipine.

Other important information:
- Use this drug cautiously if you have heart failure or liver disease or are older than 65.
- Felodipine can cause your gums to swell and bleed. Brushing, flossing, and visiting your dentist regularly will make this side effect less severe.
- Don't stop taking this drug suddenly. It can cause chest pain.

FENOFIBRATE

Pregnancy category: C

Brand:
TriCor

Fenofibrate is used to lower triglyceride levels, especially in people at risk of pancreatitis.

How to take this drug:
- Take with meals.

Possible side effects:

Infection	Body pain
Fatigue	Flu-like symptoms
Headache	Indigestion
Nausea or vomiting	Decreased sex drive
Rash	Stuffy nose
Intestinal problems	

Possible interactions:
- Because fenofibrate can interact with bile acid binding resins, take them several hours apart.
- Use this drug cautiously if you are also taking anticoagulants. You may need to adjust doses.
- Combining fenofibrate with drugs like lovastatin, pravastatin, or simvastatin may cause severe muscle problems (myopathy, rhabdomyolysis, or myositis) or kidney damage.

- This drug may interact with cyclosporine.

Other important information:
- If you suffer from severe kidney problems, you may need an adjusted dose of this drug.
- Follow a healthy, low-cholesterol diet in addition to this medication.
- Weight and alcohol problems should be addressed before beginning drug treatment.
- Fenofibrate does not claim to prevent heart disease.
- Fenofibrate may increase your likelihood of developing gallstones. Have your gallbladder checked periodically and don't use fenofibrate if you already have gallbladder disease.
- Have your liver monitored regularly while on this drug.
- If you experience muscle pain, see your doctor immediately.

FENOPROFEN CALCIUM

Pregnancy category: NR
No driving

Brand:
Nalfon   *Nalfon 200*

This nonsteroidal anti-inflammatory drug (NSAID) relieves mild to moderate pain associated with conditions such as rheumatoid arthritis and osteoarthritis.

How to take this drug:
- Take your medicine with food or a full glass of milk or water to help prevent stomach irritation.

Possible side effects:

Nausea	Constipation
Stomach pain or cramps	Indigestion
Gas	Loss of appetite
Diarrhea	Headache
Sleepiness	Dizziness
Confusion	Itching or rash
Sweating	Hearing problems
Blurred vision	Rapid heartbeat
Nervousness	Difficulty breathing
Swollen hands or feet	

Possible interactions:
- Avoid alcohol and aspirin while taking NSAIDs, such as fenoprofen.
- Fenoprofen may increase the effects of anticoagulants.
- Levels or effects of fenoprofen may be decreased by the sedative phenobarbital.

Other important information:
- Don't use fenoprofen if you are allergic to aspirin or any NSAID.
- Take fenoprofen with caution if you have stomach ulcers, poor heart function, high blood pressure, or blood-clotting disorders.
- Taking fenoprofen is more likely to cause kidney problems if you are elderly; if you take diuretics; or if you have lupus, heart failure, or poor liver or kidney function.
- Be on the lookout for signs that this drug is depressing your immune system: fever, sore throat, tiredness, weakness, bruising, unusual bleeding. Have your blood tested regularly.
- Bleeding stomach ulcers and liver or kidney damage are the most common serious reactions to using fenoprofen for long periods of time. Warning signs of liver damage include nausea, tiredness, red and itchy skin, yellow eyes and skin (jaundice), and flu-like symptoms.

FERROUS SULFATE

Pregnancy category: A

Brand:
Feosol   *Fero-Folic*
Iberet-Folic

This drug is used to treat iron-deficiency anemia and to prevent iron deficiency.

How to take this drug:
- Take this drug on an empty stomach. However, if it causes an upset stomach, you can take it with or after food.
- Mix liquid formulas with water or juice and drink through a straw to help prevent stained teeth.
- Do not chew or crush sustained-release tablets or capsules.
- If you miss a dose, take it as soon as you remember. But if it is nearing time for your next dose, don't double up your doses (unless your doctor tells you to).
- Certain foods, such as eggs, milk, yogurt, whole-grain breads and cereals, coffee, and tea, may decrease iron absorption.

Possible side effects:
Constipation   Nausea
Diarrhea

Possible interactions:
- Iron may decrease the effectiveness of the antibiotic tetracycline. Don't take antibiotics within two hours of taking iron.
- Antacids may decrease levels or effects of this drug. Don't take antacids within two hours of taking iron.

Other important information:
- Discuss any plans for pregnancy with your doctor.
- Liquid forms may temporarily stain teeth.

FEXOFENADINE HYDROCHLORIDE

Pregnancy category: C
No driving

Brand:
Allegra

Fexofenadine hydrochloride is an antihistamine used to relieve the symptoms of seasonal allergies, like sneezing, runny nose, and itchy, watering eyes.

How to take this drug:
- Never double a missed dose. Instead take it as soon as you remember or skip it and go on with your regular schedule.

Possible side effects:
Colds   Nausea
Menstrual pain   Drowsiness
Upset stomach   Fatigue

Other important information:
- If you have kidney problems, you may need to adjust your dose of fexofenadine hydrochloride.

FEXOFENADINE HYDROCHLORIDE AND PSEUDOEPHEDRINE HYDROCHLORIDE

Pregnancy category: C
MAO warning

Brand:
Allegra-D

This drug is a combination antihistamine and decongestant used to relieve the symptoms of seasonal allergies, like sneezing, stuffy nose, and itchy, watering eyes.

How to take this drug:
- Don't take this drug with food.
- Don't take more than the prescribed amount.
- Don't break or chew the tablet. Swallow it whole.

Possible side effects:
Headache   Sleeplessness
Nausea   Dry mouth
Upset stomach   Sore throat

Dizziness

Nervousness or anxiety

Back pain

Rapid heartbeat

Upper respiratory infection

Abdominal pain

Possible interactions:
- Don't take this drug with other over-the-counter antihistamines and decongestants or if you have a pacemaker and take digoxin.
- Talk to your doctor before taking it with mecamylamine (Inversine), methyldopa (Aldomet), or reserpine (Diupress or Hydropres).

Other important information:
- If you have kidney problems, you may need your dose of this drug adjusted.
- Don't take it if you have narrow-angle glaucoma, urinary retention, high blood pressure, or severe heart disease.
- Take this drug cautiously if you have diabetes, hyperthyroidism, or enlarged prostate.

FINASTERIDE

Pregnancy category: X

Brand:

Proscar   *Propecia*

Proscar helps shrink an enlarged prostate, a symptom of benign prostatic hyperplasia (BPH). By doing this, it reduces the risk of acute urinary retention and the need for prostate surgery, including transurethral resection of the prostate (TURP) and prostatectomy. Propecia, which comes in a lower dose, is prescribed to treat male pattern hair loss.

How to take this drug:
- You can take finasteride with or without food.
- Never double a missed dose. Instead take it as soon as you remember or skip it and go on with your regular schedule.

Possible side effects:

Impotence

Decreased sex drive

Ejaculation changes

Breast enlargement

Skin rash

Swollen lips

Other important information:
- Talk to your doctor before taking this drug if you have liver problems.
- If you are taking Propecia for baldness, let your doctor know this before having a PSA screening test for prostate cancer.
- This drug is not for use in children or women.
- Women who are pregnant should not handle crushed or broken finasteride tablets because of the risk of damage to male babies.

- Before taking Proscar make sure you don't have another condition that could be mistaken for BPH, like an infection, prostate cancer, stricture disease, hypotonic bladder, or other neurogenic disorders.
- You may need to take this drug for several months before you see any improvement.
- Propecia works only as long as you are taking it. If you stop, you will continue to lose hair.

FLECAINIDE ACETATE

Pregnancy category: C
No driving

Brand:
Tambocor

Flecainide is an antiarrhythmic used to correct irregular heartbeats to a normal rhythm.

Possible side effects:

Dizziness	Difficulty breathing
Headache	Nausea
Fatigue	Blurred vision
Rapid heartbeat	Chest pain
Loss of strength	Tremors
Constipation	Fluid retention
Stomach pain	

Possible interactions:
- Flecainide may increase levels of the heart drug digoxin.
- Taking flecainide along with the beta-blocker propranolol may increase the effects of both drugs.
- Levels of flecainide may be increased by the ulcer drug cimetidine, the seizure drugs carbamazepine and phenytoin, the sedative phenobarbital, and the heart drug amiodarone.

Other important information:
- If you've had a heart attack, don't use this drug because of the possibility of fatal cardiac arrest.
- People with some types of heart rhythm disorders should not use this drug. This includes people with second- or third-degree AV block not being treated with a pacemaker. People with cardiogenic shock should not take this drug either.
- Take flecainide acetate with extreme caution if you have poor liver function, the heart condition called sick sinus syndrome, a history of congestive heart failure, severe kidney disease, or use a pacemaker. This drug may worsen irregular heartbeats or cause heart failure in people with poor heart function.

- Any potassium imbalance should be corrected before beginning treatment because high or low potassium levels can alter the effects of this drug on the heart.
- Be on the lookout for signs that this drug is depressing your immune system: fever, sore throat, tiredness, weakness, bruising, unusual bleeding. Have your blood tested regularly.
- Take your medicine on time and exactly as your doctor prescribes.

FLUCONAZOLE

Pregnancy category: C

Brand:
Diflucan

Fluconazole is used to treat certain yeast infections of the vagina, mouth, throat, and esophagus. It also treats other fungal infections, including pneumonia, peritonitis, urinary tract infections, and meningitis.

Possible side effects:
Nausea   Diarrhea
Stomach pain   Headache
Rash   Seizures

Possible interactions:
- This drug may increase levels or effects of the immunosuppressant cyclosporine; the seizure drug phenytoin; the anticoagulant warfarin; and the diabetes drugs tolbutamide, glyburide, and glipizide.
- The tuberculosis drug rifampin may decrease effects or levels of this drug.

Other important information:
- If you are allergic to any other anti-fungal drugs, use this drug with caution.
- If you have an impaired immune system and develop a rash, see your doctor. You may need to stop treatment.
- People with poor kidney function may need a reduced dose.
- Have regular liver function tests while you're taking this drug. Liver damage is rare but serious.
- Take all of your medicine, even after you begin to feel better.

FLUCYTOSINE

Pregnancy category: C

Brand:
Ancobon

This drug is used to treat serious fungal infections caused by specific yeast and bacteria.

How to take this drug:
* If your dose is more than one capsule, you may want to take them over a 15-minute period to help prevent stomach irritation.

Possible side effects:
Nausea	Diarrhea
Stomach pain	Headache
Fever	Confusion
Dizziness	Rash

Possible interactions:
* The herpes virus drug cytosine arabinoside may decrease the effectiveness of this drug.
* The antibiotic amphotericin B increases the action and toxicity of this drug.

Other important information:
* Have regular blood, kidney, and liver tests while you're taking this drug.
* Monitor your blood levels of flucytosine to prevent accumulation and toxicity.
* If you have poor kidney function, take this drug with extreme caution.
* Flucytosine may cause liver damage, with or without jaundice (yellow eyes and skin, dark urine, and light-colored stools).
* Flucytosine may damage nerve tissues. Symptoms include numbness or tingling in your hands or feet, lack of muscle coordination, and weakness.
* Be on the lookout for signs that this drug is depressing your immune system: fever, sore throat, tiredness, weakness, bruising, unusual bleeding. Have your blood tested regularly.
* Your infection may not begin clearing up for weeks or months. Keep taking the drug as prescribed.

FLUNISOLIDE

Pregnancy category: C

Brand:
AeroBid   *AeroBid-M*

Flunisolide is an anti-inflammatory steroid that you inhale through your mouth to treat and control asthma.

How to take this drug:
* You can avoid fungal infections in your mouth and throat by rinsing your mouth and gargling with warm water after using your inhaler. Don't swallow the water.
* You should do your best to take your medicine at regular time intervals.
* For people with asthma, if you use a bronchodilator, use it several minutes before the flunisolide. This will help you get the full effect of your medicine.

Possible side effects:

Hoarseness

Yeast infections in the mouth
and throat (oral thrush)

Dry mouth

Nausea or vomiting

Headache

Other important information:

- This drug won't stop a severe asthma attack. If you do have an asthma attack and you don't get relief from a bronchodilator, call 911 or go to the nearest emergency room. You may need steroid pills or shots.
- If you are switching to flunisolide from steroid pills or shots, make sure you get off the other drug slowly. People have died after switching quickly from steroid pills to inhaled steroids. Report to your doctor any signs of corticosteroid withdrawal, including fatigue, weakness, painful joints or muscles, low blood pressure when you stand up, and difficulty breathing.
- If you were taking steroid pills and you are now taking flunisolide, you may need to get back on the former drug during a severe asthma attack or during times of stress, such as surgery, infection, or an injury. It can take your body several months to begin producing enough steroid hormones on its own after you have been taking steroid pills. In case of an emergency, carry a card that says you have used cortisone-related drugs in the past year.
- Take extra care to avoid exposure to people with chickenpox or measles because corticosteroid drugs can weaken your immune system. If you are exposed, let your doctor know right away.
- People with tuberculosis, herpes simplex of the eye, or an untreated infection (fungal, viral, or bacterial) shouldn't use flunisolide.
- Don't use inhaled steroids more often than your doctor recommends or you may suffer some serious side effects. Your adrenal glands may also quit producing natural steroids.

FLUOCINOLONE ACETONIDE

Pregnancy category: C

Brand:

Derma-Smoothe/FS

FS Shampoo

Synemol

Fluonid

Synalar

Fluocinolone acetonide is used to relieve and heal inflamed or irritated skin conditions, including eczema, dermatitis, psoriasis, severe diaper rash, insect bites, minor burns, and sunburn.

How to take this drug:

- Do not wrap or bandage the area after you apply the medicine unless your doctor tells you to. For diaper rash, you should not use tight-fitting diapers or plastic pants after applying this medicine.

- Avoid contact with your eyes.
- Apply a thin film and rub in gently and completely.

Other important information:
- Don't use this drug if you are allergic to other steroid creams.
- If you are covering a very large area of your skin and, therefore, using lots of medicine, have regular tests for hypothalamic-pituitary-adrenal axis suppression.
- If your skin is infected, you'll also need an antifungal or antibacterial medicine.

FLUOCINONIDE

Pregnancy category: C

Brand:
Lidex   *Lidex-E*

This drug is used to relieve and heal inflamed or irritated skin conditions, including eczema, dermatitis, psoriasis, severe diaper rash, insect bites, minor burns, and sunburn.

How to take this drug:
- Do not wrap or bandage the area after you apply the medicine unless your doctor tells you to. For diaper rash, don't use tight-fitting diapers or plastic pants after applying this medicine.
- Avoid contact with your eyes.
- Apply a thin film and rub in gently and completely.

Other important information:
- Don't use this drug if you are allergic to other steroid creams.
- If you are covering a very large area of your skin and, therefore, using lots of medicine, have regular tests for hypothalamic-pituitary-adrenal axis suppression.
- If your skin is infected, you'll also need an antifungal or antibacterial medicine.

FLUOXETINE

Pregnancy category: B
No driving   MAO warning

Brand:
Prozac

Fluoxetine treats the symptoms of depression and obsessive-compulsive disorder by increasing the amount of serotonin in your central nervous system.

How to take this drug:
- You can take fluoxetine with or without food. However, avoid foods high in tryptophan.

Possible side effects:

Anxiety	Sleeplessness
Weight loss	Drowsiness
Fatigue	Shakiness
Sweating	Upset stomach
Nausea	Diarrhea
Dizziness	Lightheadedness

Possible interactions:

- This drug interacts dangerously with MAO inhibitors like Eldepryl, Marplan, Nardil, and Parnate.
- Taking fluoxetine while you are also taking other antidepressants can increase the levels of both drugs in your body.
- If you are taking flecainide, vinblastine, carbamazepine, or any tricyclic antidepressant, you may need to decrease your dosage of the drug once you start taking fluoxetine. Consult your doctor.
- Tryptophan and paroxetine together can cause agitation, restlessness, and upset stomach. You may want to avoid foods high in tryptophan, such as meats, poultry, fish, liver, kidney, eggs, nuts, peanut butter, broad beans, and wheat germ.
- Fluoxetine may increase or decrease levels of the antipsychotic drug lithium, which means lithium levels should be monitored while using this drug.
- Fluoxetine may cause diazepam to stay in your body longer than usual.
- Fluoxetine may increase levels of phenytoin in your body.
- Digoxin and coumadin may interact with fluoxetine.

Other important information:

- Fluoxetine can stay in your body for up to five weeks after you stop taking it. You may need to wait five weeks before you take any drug that may interact with fluoxetine.
- You may need a lower than normal dose of fluoxetine if you have liver or kidney disease. Your doctor should monitor you closely for side effects.
- Take this drug with caution if you have a history of seizures.
- For people with diabetes, fluoxetine can affect your blood sugar control.

FLUPHENAZINE

Pregnancy category: NR
No driving

Brand:

Prolixin

This phenothiazine is a tranquilizer used to treat symptoms of various mental illnesses, such as schizophrenia and mania.

Possible side effects:

Sleepiness   Dry mouth
Urine retention   Confusion

Possible interactions:

- If you take any phenothiazine along with other tranquilizers, alcohol, antihistamines, or muscle relaxers, the combination may dangerously depress your nervous system.
- This drug may increase the effects of atropine.

Other important information:

- People with brain damage, severely depressed people, and people taking large doses of sleep-inducing drugs shouldn't take fluphenazine.
- Take this drug very cautiously if you have a history of epilepsy, heart disease, or liver disease. Be careful with this drug if you work in extreme heat or around phosphorus insecticides.
- This drug can cause pregnancy test results to be unreliable.
- Don't quit taking this drug suddenly or you may experience stomach pain, nausea, dizziness, and shakiness.

FLURANDRENOLIDE

Pregnancy category: C

Brand:

Cordran

This drug is used to relieve and heal inflamed or irritated skin conditions including eczema, dermatitis, psoriasis, insect bites, and minor burns.

How to take this drug:

- Avoid contact with your eyes.
- Do not wrap or bandage the area after you apply the medicine unless your doctor tells you to. For diaper rash, you should not use tight-fitting diapers or plastic pants after applying this medicine.
- If you have psoriasis or a similar skin condition and your doctor has told you to wrap or bandage the area, you may want to follow these steps: 1) Soak in a bath and remove as much of the scaling skin as possible. 2) Rub in the lotion thoroughly. 3) Place moist gauze or a dampened cloth over the area and cover with a plastic wrap. 4) Seal the edges with tape.

Possible side effects:

Irritation   Acne
Dryness   Itching
Burning   Skin discoloration
Mild infection   Excessive hair growth
Dry and itching skin   Inflamed hair follicles
around the mouth   Blocked sweat glands
Skin wasting   Streaks on the skin

Other important information:
- Don't use this drug if you are allergic to other steroid creams.
- If you are covering a very large area of your skin and, therefore, using lots of medicine, have regular tests for hypothalamic-pituitary-adrenal axis suppression.
- If your skin is infected, you'll also need an antifungal or antibacterial medicine.

FLURAZEPAM HYDROCHLORIDE

Pregnancy category: NR
No driving

Brand:
Dalmane

Flurazepam is a sleep-inducing drug used to treat insomnia.

Possible side effects:
Dizziness	Drowsiness
Lightheadedness	Lack of coordination

Possible interactions:
- If you take flurazepam along with tranquilizers, alcohol, antihistamines, or muscle relaxants, the combination may dangerously depress your nervous system.

Other important information:
- You can become dependent on flurazepam. To avoid seizures and other less-severe withdrawal symptoms, quit taking the drug gradually under your doctor's supervision.
- People with poor liver, kidney, or lung functions should use flurazepam cautiously. The drug may stay in your body longer and increase your risk of side effects.
- You may have trouble sleeping for the first couple of nights after you stop taking this drug.

FLURBIPROFEN

Pregnancy category: B
No driving

Brand:
Ansaid

This nonsteroidal anti-inflammatory drug (NSAID) is used to relieve the symptoms of arthritis.

Possible side effects:
Water retention	Nausea

Diarrhea	Constipation
Stomach pain or cramps	Indigestion
Gas	

Possible interactions:
- Avoid alcohol and aspirin while taking flurbiprofen.
- Flurbiprofen may prolong bleeding time if used at the same time as anticoagulants.
- Flurbiprofen may decrease the effects of beta blockers and diuretics.

Other important information:
- Don't use flurbiprofen if you are allergic to aspirin or any NSAID.
- Take flurbiprofen with caution if you have stomach ulcers, poor heart function, high blood pressure, or blood-clotting disorders.
- Taking flurbiprofen is more likely to cause kidney problems if you are elderly; if you take diuretics; or if you have lupus, heart failure, or poor liver or kidney function.
- Bleeding stomach ulcers and liver or kidney damage are the most common serious reactions to using flurbiprofen for long periods of time. Warning signs of liver damage include nausea, tiredness, red and itchy skin, yellow eyes and skin (jaundice), and flu-like symptoms.
- Be on the lookout for signs that this drug is depressing your immune system: fever, sore throat, tiredness, weakness, bruising, unusual bleeding. Have your blood tested regularly.

FLUTAMIDE

Pregnancy category: D

Brand:
Eulexin

This drug treats cancer of the prostate that has spread to other parts of the body.

Possible side effects:

Vomiting	Nausea
Diarrhea	Hot flashes
Impotence	Breast enlargement in men
Decreased sex drive	Depression
Nervousness	Anxiety
Confusion	Loss of appetite
Fluid retention	

Other important information:
- Don't stop treatment without consulting your doctor.
- Have periodic liver function tests.

FLUTICASONE PROPIONATE

Pregnancy category: C
Refrigerate

Brand:

Flonase   *Flovent*

Flonase is a nasal spray for relief from the symptoms of allergies. Flovent is an inhalation aerosol used to prevent asthma attacks.

How to take this drug:
- Use regularly as your doctor instructs.
- Never double a missed dose. Instead take it as soon as you remember or skip it and go on with your regular schedule.

Possible side effects:
Sinusitis   Runny or stuffy nose
Upper respiratory infection Headache

Possible interactions:
- Have your doctor monitor you if you take fluticasone along with keto-conazole.

Other important information:
- Be especially careful if you are changing from steroid tablets for asthma to Flovent. The change should be gradual so your body has time to adjust.
- Flovent is not for emergency treatment of asthma attacks.
- Contact your doctor if you are exposed to chickenpox or measles.

FLUVASTATIN SODIUM

Pregnancy category: X

Brand:

Lescol

Fluvastatin sodium is used to lower cholesterol, especially in those at risk of atherosclerosis.

How to take this drug:
- Take with or without food.
- Never double a missed dose. Instead take it as soon as you remember or skip it and go on with your regular schedule.
- If you are combining this drug with another cholesterol medication, take them at least two hours apart.

Possible side effects:
Upper respiratory infection Back pain
Upset stomach   Headache
Muscle or joint pain   Diarrhea

Stuffy nose	Sore throat
Abdominal pain	Constipation

Possible interactions:

- Fluvastatin sodium can interact with cyclosporine, gemfibrozil, erythromycin, or niacin to increase your risk of developing muscle problems.
- It can also interact with cholestyramine, digoxin, cimetidine, ranitidine, omeprazole, rifampicin, and anticoagulants.

Other important information:

- Be careful taking this drug if you have a history of liver disease or alcohol abuse.
- Have your liver tested throughout treatment with this drug.
- In addition to taking this drug, eat a low-fat, low-cholesterol diet and exercise.
- Make sure your doctor tests you for these conditions before prescribing fluvastatin sodium: diabetes, hypothyroidism, and nephrotic syndrome.
- Tell your doctor immediately if you develop muscle pain or weakness.

FLUVOXAMINE MALEATE

Pregnancy category: C
No driving   MAO warning

Brand:

Luvox

Fluvoxamine maleate treats the symptoms of Obsessive Compulsive Disorder (OCD).

Possible side effects:

Nausea	Sleeplessness
Sleepiness	Headache
Muscle weakness	Vomiting
Nervousness	Dizziness

Possible interactions:

- Don't take this drug with terfenadine or cisapride since it can cause an interaction resulting in heart problems.
- This drug can affect your body's levels of clozapine; carbamazepine; theophylline; and benzodiazepines, like alprazolam, midazolam, and triazolam. You may need to adjust your dose.
- Don't take it with diazepam.
- If you take this drug with an anticoagulant, like warfarin, have your clotting time checked regularly.
- Be careful combining fluvoxamine maleate with lithium. You may experience seizures.

- Be careful taking tricyclic antidepressants (amitriptyline, clomipramine, or imipramine) with this drug. You may need to adjust your dose.
- Taking fluvoxamine maleate with tryptophan has resulted in cases of severe vomiting.
- If you take a beta blocker, you may have to adjust your dose while on this drug.

Other important information:
- This drug has not been tested for longer than 10 weeks. Have your doctor evaluate you periodically if you'll be taking it for an extended period of time.
- Be careful using this drug if you have any type of liver, circulatory, or metabolic disorder.
- Use it cautiously if you have a history of seizures and stop using it immediately if you develop seizures.

FOSINOPRIL

Pregnancy category: C/D

Brand:
Monopril

This angiotensin converting enzyme (ACE) inhibitor treats high blood pressure.

Possible side effects:
Tiredness   Dizziness
Headache   Cough
Sexual dysfunction   Diarrhea
Nausea

Possible interactions:
- This drug may increase levels or effects of the anti-psychotic drug lithium, so lithium levels should be monitored while using this drug.
- Antacids can keep fosinopril from being absorbed properly. Don't take antacids within two hours of taking fosinopril.

Other important information:
- People with poor kidney and liver functions should take this drug very cautiously.
- Fosinopril may cause a severe drop in blood pressure after the first dose, particularly in people taking diuretics, on dialysis, or with congestive heart failure. Be careful when you stand up quickly — you may feel lightheaded and dizzy. If you faint, stop taking the drug and immediately contact your doctor.

- Mild swelling can occur in the throat, face, lips, tongue, mucous membranes, hands, or feet, but swelling of the throat can be extremely dangerous. Contact your doctor immediately.
- If you develop jaundice (yellow eyes or skin), contact your doctor immediately.
- Fosinopril may cause dangerously high levels of potassium in the blood. Don't use potassium-sparing diuretics or take potassium supplements without talking to your doctor. Very high levels of potassium can be fatal.
- Make sure you drink plenty of fluids to help prevent a drop in blood pressure.
- Be careful in hot weather and during exercise. Sweating can cause loss of fluid, low blood pressure, and, therefore, lightheadedness.
- Be on the lookout for signs that this drug is depressing your immune system: fever, sore throat, tiredness, weakness, bruising, unusual bleeding. Have your blood tested regularly.

FURAZOLIDONE

Pregnancy category: NR

Brand:
Furoxone

Furazolidone is a broad spectrum antibiotic that treats the symptoms of diarrhea and inflamed intestines (enteritis) caused by a variety of bacteria, such as *E. coli*, *staphylococci*, *Salmonella*, *Shigella*, etc.

How to take this drug:
- Furazolidone comes in either tablet or liquid form.

Possible side effects:

Hives	Fever
Joint pain	Rash
Nausea or vomiting	Headache
General discomfort	

Possible interactions:
- Be careful taking this drug with other MAO inhibitors.
- Don't take with foods containing tyramine, such as broad beans; avocado; banana; chocolate; colas; mushrooms; raisins; sour cream; aged cheeses and meats; beer; wine; salted, smoked, or pickled fish; chicken livers; soy sauce; and yeast extracts, like Marmite or brewer's yeast.
- Don't take with indirectly acting sympathomimetic amines, like those found in nasal decongestants (phenylephrine, ephedrine) and anorectics (amphetamines).

- Talk to your doctor before combining furazolidone with sedatives, anti-histamines, tranquilizers, or narcotics.

Other important information:
- Don't drink alcohol within four days of taking this medication.
- This drug blocks the enzyme monoamine oxidase and, therefore, can interact with certain foods to raise your blood pressure. If you develop symptoms of hypertensive crisis, such as headache, chest pain, nausea, or vomiting, or any other unusual symptoms, contact your doctor immediately.

FUROSEMIDE

Pregnancy category: C

Brand:
Lasix

This diuretic is used to reduce fluid retention associated with congestive heart failure, liver or kidney disease, and to reduce high blood pressure.

Possible side effects:

Muscle cramps or spasms	Dizziness when standing suddenly
Bladder spasms	Weakness
Restlessness	Dizziness
Headache	Nausea
Loss of appetite	Stomach or mouth irritation
Cramping	Diarrhea
Constipation	Yellow skin or eyes
Tingling	Vision problems
Hearing loss	Rash
Increased sensitivity to light	

Possible interactions:
- Don't use furosemide with antibiotics called aminoglycosides or the diuretic ethacrynic acid because of potential damage to hearing.
- Furosemide may increase levels of the anti-psychotic drug lithium and blood pressure drugs called beta blockers.
- Furosemide may decrease effects of norepinephrine.
- The anti-inflammatory indomethacin may decrease effects of furosemide.

Other important information:
- Diabetics should use this drug with caution because it can raise your blood sugar levels.
- Use furosemide with caution if you have kidney disease.
- Be on the lookout for signs that this drug is depressing your immune system: fever, sore throat, tiredness, weakness, bruising, unusual bleeding. Have your blood tested regularly.

- Furosemide may increase levels of uric acid in the blood (this puts you at risk for gout, a form of arthritis) and may worsen symptoms of lupus.
- This diuretic may cause dangerously low levels of potassium and other electrolytes. Eat extra potassium-rich foods, like bananas. Contact your doctor if you experience any of the symptoms of potassium loss: unusual thirst, tiredness, drowsiness, restlessness, muscle pains or cramps, nausea, or rapid heart rate.
- Weigh daily so you'll know if you're losing too much fluid, which can cause dehydration and possibly blood clots. Warning signs include dry mouth, thirst, drowsiness, and weakness. Contact your doctor immediately if you stop urinating.
- If you have high blood pressure, avoid using over-the-counter cold remedies or diet pills, which can increase blood pressure.

GABAPENTIN

Pregnancy category: C
No driving

Brand:
Neurontin

Gabapentin is used along with other medication to treat epileptic seizures.

How to take this drug:
- Take this drug with or without food.

Possible side effects:

Tiredness	Weight gain
Indigestion	Muscle pain
Dizziness	Loss of muscle control
Involuntary eye movement	Tremors
Nervousness	Speech difficulties
Vision problems	Amnesia
Stuffy nose	Sore throat
Sleepiness	

Possible interactions:
- Gabapentin can interact with antacids such as Maalox. Take these two medications at least two hours apart.
- This drug could affect the results of urine protein tests.

Other important information:
- If you have kidney problems, you may need to adjust your dose of this drug.
- If you are taking this drug along with other anti-epileptic medications, your side effects may be different.

GEMFIBROZIL

Pregnancy category: C

Brand:
Lopid

Gemfibrozil decreases "bad" LDL cholesterol levels and increases "good" HDL cholesterol levels in people who haven't been able to lower their cholesterol through diet, exercise, and weight loss.

How to take this drug:
- If you take two doses a day, take one tablet a half-hour before you eat breakfast and one tablet a half-hour before your evening meal.

Possible side effects:

Indigestion	Stomach pain
Diarrhea	Nausea
Irregular heartbeat	Itchy and inflamed skin
Rash	Dizziness
Constipation	Headache

Possible interactions:
- Using gemfibrozil with the lipid-lowering drug lovastatin can cause severe kidney damage.
- Gemfibrozil may increase the effects of anticoagulants, so your dose of the anticoagulant may need to be reduced.

Other important information:
- People with gallbladder disease, poor liver function, or poor kidney function should not use gemfibrozil. If you develop gallstones, follow your doctor's advice about using this drug.
- This drug may cause the dangerous and sometimes fatal disease that destroys muscle tissue called rhabdomyolysis. Notify your doctor immediately if you develop any pain, tenderness, or weakness in your muscles.
- It is very important to try to improve your cholesterol levels with a low-fat diet and exercise while you are taking gemfibrozil.
- Check your blood counts, kidney function, and liver function regularly while you're taking gemfibrozil.

GLIMEPIRIDE

Pregnancy category: C

Brand:
Amaryl

This sulfonylurea is used to lower the blood sugar levels in type II diabetics.

How to take this drug:
- Take this drug with food.

Possible interactions:

- This drug may interact with nonsteroidal anti-inflammatory drugs (NSAIDs), such as aspirin and ibuprofen; salicylates, such as aspirin; sulfonamides; chloramphenicol; coumarin; probenecid; MAO inhibitors; and beta adrenergic blocking agents.
- You may become hyperglycemic if you take glimepiride with diuretics, corticosteroids, phenothiazines, thyroid products, estrogens, oral contraceptives, phenytoin, nicotinic acid, sympathomimetics, or isoniazid.

Other important information:

- Don't take glimepiride if you have diabetic ketoacidosis.
- While taking this drug, you are at a higher risk of developing fatal heart problems.
- You are at risk of developing hypoglycemia while taking glimepiride, especially if you have kidney problems.
- Before taking this drug, talk to your doctor if you have liver or kidney problems.
- Use along with a controlled diet and plenty of exercise to control diabetes.

GLIPIZIDE

Pregnancy category: C

Brand:

Glucotrol   *Glucotrol XL*

This drug is used to treat noninsulin dependent (type II) diabetes by lowering blood sugar.

How to take this drug:

- Take this drug 30 minutes before eating a meal.

Possible side effects:

Nausea	Diarrhea
Constipation	Dizziness
Drowsiness	Headache
Allergic skin reactions, such as itching or hives	Increased sensitivity to light

Possible interactions:

- Glipizide is more likely to cause low blood sugar if you are also taking antidepressant drugs called monoamine oxidase (MAO) inhibitors, blood pressure drugs called beta blockers, anticoagulants, sulfonamides, the gout drug probenecid, nonsteroidal anti-inflammatory drugs (NSAIDs), the antifungal miconazole, or the antibiotic chloramphenicol.
- Glipizide may cause high blood sugar if you take it with calcium channel blockers, diuretics, the seizure drug phenytoin, corticosteroids, sympathomimetics, estrogen, or the tuberculosis drug isoniazid.

Other important information:

- While taking this drug, you are at a higher risk of developing fatal heart problems.
- Don't use this drug if you have diabetes complicated by ketoacidosis.
- If you have liver or kidney problems or congestive heart failure, use glipizide with caution.
- Check your blood and urine periodically for abnormal sugar levels while taking this drug.
- Wear identification that states you are diabetic.
- Use along with a controlled diet and plenty of exercise to control diabetes.
- Since this drug can cause low blood sugar, especially when you haven't eaten enough, when you've exercised, or when you've consumed alcohol, learn to recognize the signs of hypoglycemia and know how to treat it.
- This drug can lose its effectiveness after you've taken it for a long time.
- Tell your doctor about any stressful events you experience, such as surgery, trauma, infection, or fever. You may need insulin or some other special treatment.

GLYBURIDE

Pregnancy category: C

Brand:

DiaBeta   Glynase
Micronase

This drug is used to treat noninsulin dependent (type II) diabetes by encouraging the pancreas to release insulin. It also has some diuretic effect (it helps your kidneys get rid of water) and lowers blood sugar.

Possible side effects:

Nausea   Heartburn
Allergic skin reactions,   Increased sensitivity to light
such as itching or hives

Possible interactions:

- Glyburide is more likely to cause low blood sugar if you are also taking antidepressant drugs called monoamine oxidase (MAO) inhibitors, blood pressure drugs called beta blockers, anticoagulants, sulfonamides, the gout drug probenecid, nonsteroidal anti-inflammatory drugs (NSAIDs), the antifungal miconazole, the antibiotic chloramphenicol, or the fluoroquinolone antibiotics.
- Glyburide may cause high blood sugar if you take it with calcium channel blockers, diuretics, the seizure drug phenytoin, corticosteroids, nicotinic acid, sympathomimetics, estrogen, or the tuberculosis drug isoniazid.

Other important information:
- While taking this drug, you are at a higher risk of developing fatal heart problems.
- Don't use this drug if you have diabetes complicated by ketoacidosis.
- If you have liver or kidney problems or congestive heart failure, use this drug with caution.
- Check your blood and urine periodically for abnormal sugar levels while taking this drug.
- Wear identification that states you are diabetic.
- Use along with a controlled diet and plenty of exercise to control diabetes.
- Since this drug can cause low blood sugar, especially when you haven't eaten enough, when you've exercised, or when you've consumed alcohol, learn to recognize the signs of hypoglycemia and know how to treat it.
- This drug can lose its effectiveness after taking it for a long period of time.
- Tell your doctor about any stressful events you experience, such as surgery, trauma, infection, or fever. You may need insulin or some other special treatment.

GRISEOFULVIN

Pregnancy category: X

Brand:
Fulvicin P/G	*Grifulvin V*
Grisactin	*Gris-PEG*

Griseofulvin is an antibiotic used to treat fungal infections, such as ringworm and athlete's foot.

Possible side effects:
Hives or rash	Nausea
Diarrhea	Upset stomach
Oral thrush (yeast infection	Headache
in the mouth)	Fatigue
Confusion	Dizziness
Sleeplessness	

Possible interactions:
- Griseofulvin may increase the effects of alcohol and cause rapid heartbeat and flushing.
- This drug may decrease the effects of oral contraceptives and anticoagulants.
- Barbiturates may decrease the effectiveness of griseofulvin.

Other important information:
- Don't use this drug if you have liver disease.

- If you are allergic to penicillin, you may be allergic to this drug also.
- Good hygiene and skin care are important during treatment.
- This drug may make your skin extra-sensitive to sunlight, so protect your skin if you'll be outdoors.
- If you will be taking this drug for a long period of time, be sure your doctor orders regular liver, kidney, and bone marrow tests.
- You may need an ointment or cream in addition to griseofulvin, especially for athlete's foot.

GUANFACINE HYDROCHLORIDE

Pregnancy category: B
No driving

Brand:
Tenex

Guanfacine lowers your blood pressure and heart rate.

How to take this drug:
- Take this medicine at bedtime since it may cause sleepiness.

Possible side effects:
Dry mouth	Constipation
Sleepiness	Weakness
Dizziness	Sleeplessness
Headache	Impotence

Possible interactions:
- Taking guanfacine with alcohol or other depressants, such as tranquilizers or sleeping pills, may cause dangerous depressant effects.
- Phenobarbital and phenytoin reduce the effectiveness of guanfacine.

Other important information:
- People with severe heart disease, a recent heart attack, chronic liver or kidney failure, or cerebrovascular disease should use this drug cautiously.
- If you develop a skin rash or "rebound hypertension" (a rise in your blood pressure after two to four days on the drug), quit taking guanfacine under your doctor's supervision.
- You may experience nausea and dizziness when you stand up.
- Don't stop taking guanfacine suddenly. You may feel nervous and anxious, and your blood pressure may suddenly increase.

HALCINONIDE

Pregnancy category: C

Brand:
Halog   *Halog-E*

Halcinonide is a corticosteroid used to relieve and heal inflamed or irritated skin conditions, including eczema, dermatitis, psoriasis, severe diaper rash, insect bites, minor burns, and sunburn.

How to take this drug:
- Halcinonide is available as an ointment, cream, and solution.
- Avoid contact with your eyes.
- Don't wrap or bandage the area after you apply the medicine unless your doctor tells you to. For diaper rash, you should not use tight-fitting diapers or plastic pants after applying this medicine.
- If you have psoriasis or a similar skin condition and your doctor has told you to wrap or bandage the area, you may want to follow these steps: 1) Rub in a small amount of cream thoroughly. Then add a thin coating of cream. 2) Wet the area or place a dampened cloth over it and cover with a plastic wrap. 3) Seal the edges with tape.

Possible side effects:
Irritation	Burning
Itching	Dryness
Acne	Skin discoloration
Infection	Weakening and wasting of the skin
Excessive hair growth	Dermatitis around the mouth
Streaks on the skin	

Other important information:
- Don't use this drug if you are allergic to other steroid creams.
- If your skin is infected, you'll also need an antifungal or antibacterial medicine.
- If you are covering a very large area of your skin and, therefore, using lots of medicine, be tested regularly for hypothalamic-pituitary-adrenal axis suppression.

HALOPERIDOL

Pregnancy category: C
No driving

Brand:
Haldol

This tranquilizer treats schizophrenia and other mental illnesses, severe hyperactivity and other behavior problems in children, and the tics and offensive language of Tourette's syndrome.

Possible side effects:
Sleepiness	Dry mouth
Urine retention	Blurred vision
Confusion	Lightheadedness

Possible interactions:

- Taking haloperidol with lithium may cause toxic effects on the brain and nervous system. Your doctor should monitor you closely.
- If you take haloperidol along with other tranquilizers, alcohol, antihistamines, or muscle relaxers, the combination may dangerously depress your nervous system. Alcohol and haloperidol combined can also cause very low blood pressure.
- Be very careful when taking haloperidol and an antiparkinson drug at the same time.

Other important information:

- People with Parkinson's disease should not use this drug.
- If you have a history of heart problems or seizures or if you take anticoagulants, take this drug with extreme caution.
- You may get dehydrated while on this drug. Drink lots of fluids even if you don't feel thirsty.
- Don't quit taking haloperidol suddenly or you may experience stomach pain, nausea, dizziness, and shakiness.

HYDRALAZINE HYDROCHLORIDE

Pregnancy category: C
MAO warning

Brand:

Apresoline

Hydralazine dilates blood vessels and quickly reduces very high blood pressure.

How to take this drug:

- Take the oral form with meals to increase absorption.

Possible side effects:

Nausea or vomiting	Diarrhea
Constipation	Difficulty urinating
Difficulty breathing	Numbness or tingling
Chest pain	Irregular heartbeat
Flushing	Fluid retention
Dizziness	Tremors
Depression	Anxiety
Disorientation	Headache
Conjunctivitis	Watery eyes
Stuffy nose	Hoarseness
Loss of appetite	Muscle cramps
Lightheadedness	

Possible interactions:

- If you take hydralazine with other high blood pressure drugs, you may develop very low blood pressure.

Other important information:
- Don't take this drug if you have coronary artery disease or rheumatic heart disease.
- Use this drug with caution if you have kidney damage or cerebral vascular problems.
- Have regular liver function tests while you are taking this drug.
- Be on the lookout for signs that this drug is depressing your immune system: fever, sore throat, tiredness, weakness, bruising, or unusual bleeding. Have your blood tested regularly.
- This drug can cause very low blood pressure, especially when you first begin to take it. Be careful when you stand up — you may feel lightheaded and dizzy.

HYDROCHLOROTHIAZIDE

Pregnancy category: B

Brand:
Esidrix   *HydroDIURIL*
Oretic   *Microzide*

This diuretic is used to reduce blood pressure and to treat fluid retention associated with kidney disease, congestive heart failure, cirrhosis of the liver, estrogen therapy, and corticosteroid therapy.

Possible side effects:
Lightheadedness	Loss of appetite
Sensitivity to light	Nausea
Stomach pain or cramps	Diarrhea
Constipation	Tingling
Blurred vision	Yellow skin or eyes
Hives or rash	Dizziness
Headache	Weakness
Restlessness	Muscle cramps or spasms

Possible interactions:
- Hydrochlorothiazide may increase the effects of the heart drug digitalis and the muscle relaxer tubocurarine.
- It may increase blood levels of the anti-psychotic drug lithium to toxic levels.
- It may increase the effects of other blood pressure drugs.
- Nonsteroidal anti-inflammatory drugs (NSAIDs) may decrease the effectiveness of this drug.

Other important information:
- Take hydrochlorothiazide with caution if you have poor kidney function or liver disease.

- This diuretic may cause dangerously low levels of potassium and other electrolytes. Eat extra potassium-rich foods, like bananas. Contact your doctor if you experience any of the symptoms of potassium loss: unusual thirst, tiredness, drowsiness, restlessness, muscle pains or cramps, nausea, or rapid heart rate.
- Weigh daily so you'll know if you're losing too much fluid, which can cause dehydration and possibly blood clots. Warning signs of dehydration include dry mouth, thirst, drowsiness, and weakness. Contact your doctor immediately if you stop urinating.
- Hydrochlorothiazide may increase levels of uric acid in the blood (this puts you at risk for gout), may worsen symptoms of lupus, and may raise blood sugar levels.
- Be on the lookout for signs that this drug is depressing your immune system: fever, sore throat, tiredness, weakness, bruising, or unusual bleeding. Have your blood tested regularly.

HYDROQUINONE

Pregnancy category: C

Brand:

Lustra Cream	*Eldopaque Forte 4% Cream*
Eldoquin Forte 4% Cream	*Solaquin Forte 4% Cream/Gel*
Melanex Topical Solution	

These creams are used to gradually bleach skin that has become discolored from various conditions, including the use of oral contraceptives or hormone replacement therapy, or from skin trauma, freckling, aging, or pregnancy.

How to take this drug:

- Apply these products only to small areas of your body at a time.

Possible interactions:

- Avoid using products containing peroxide since these may cause staining on your skin treated with hydroquinone.

Other important information:

- Check for skin sensitivity on a small area. If your skin becomes inflamed, itches, or develops blisters, do not use.
- You must use sunscreen along with hydroquinone treatment. Some of these products already contain sunscreen. If not, apply your own and avoid sun exposure.
- Some people have serious allergic reactions to a sulfite in these products. Contact your doctor if you experience hives, itching, wheezing, or difficulty breathing.
- Hydroquinone can make your lips go numb. It also tastes bitter.
- It will irritate the skin near your nostrils and eyes.

HYDROXYCHLOROQUINE SULFATE

Pregnancy category: C

Brand:
Plaquenil

This drug is used to treat severe attacks of malaria, rheumatoid arthritis, and lupus.

How to take this drug:
- If this drug upsets your stomach, take it with food.

Possible side effects:

Ringing in the ears	Skin problems
Itching	Stomach cramps
Nausea	Diarrhea
Loss of appetite	Headache
Psychotic episodes	

Other important information:
- Hydroxychloroquine sulfate may worsen the skin disease psoriasis.
- People with liver disease, alcoholism, or G6PD deficiency should use this drug with caution.
- Be on the lookout for signs that this drug is depressing your immune system: fever, sore throat, tiredness, weakness, bruising, or unusual bleeding. Have your blood tested regularly.
- This drug may cause irreversible damage to the retina of your eye. See your doctor immediately if any vision changes occur. Have regular eye exams.
- It may take several weeks before you get any relief from your rheumatoid arthritis symptoms. If you don't improve in six months, your doctor may stop your drug treatment.

HYDROXYUREA

Pregnancy category: D

Brand:
Droxia   *Hydrea*

Hydroxyurea is used to treat tumors associated with melanoma, leukemia, and ovarian cancer. It is also used to treat sickle cell anemia, and, with radiation therapy, treats squamous cell carcinomas of the head and neck.

How to take this drug:
- You can take this drug by emptying the capsule into a glass of water. But don't let the powder touch your skin and don't inhale it.

Possible side effects:

Loss of appetite	Nausea or vomiting
Diarrhea	Constipation

Inflamed mouth	Rash
Redness	Hair loss
Fever	Weight gain

Other important information:

- Be careful using hydroxyurea if you have received radiotherapy or cytotoxic cancer chemotherapeutic drugs, if your immune system is suppressed, or if you have kidney problems.
- You may need a lower dose if you are elderly.
- This drug can suppress your immune system. Have your doctor monitor your blood regularly.
- Your doctor should monitor your kidneys and liver throughout treatment with hydroxyurea.
- Keep in mind that side effects may be more severe if you are receiving hydroxyurea and radiation therapy together.
- Hydroxyurea can have cancerous side effects. Talk to your doctor about this risk.

HYDROXYZINE HYDROCHLORIDE

Pregnancy category: NR
No driving

Brand:

Atarax

This drug is used as a sedative before surgery and to relieve anxiety, tension, pain, and the itching caused by allergies. It also relieves nausea and works as a bronchodilator.

Possible side effects:

| Dry mouth | Drowsiness |

Possible interactions:

- Hydroxyzine may increase the action of drugs that depress the nervous system, such as meperidine, barbiturates, narcotics, and non-narcotic pain relievers. These drugs are sometimes used together before surgery.
- When you're taking hydroxyzine, avoid alcohol and other depressants, such as tranquilizers and sleeping pills.

Other important information:

- Check with your doctor before taking hydroxyzine if you have an enlarged prostate, urination problems, glaucoma, or heart rhythm problems.

HYOSCYAMINE SULFATE

Pregnancy category: C
No driving

Brand:
Cystospaz

Levbid

Levsin

Levsinex

Hyoscyamine sulfate relieves the spasms of many stomach and intestinal disorders, including diverticulitis, peptic ulcer, pancreatitis, colitis, and irritable bowel syndrome (IBS). It treats bladder spasms, certain cases of heart block, and helps dry out a runny nose. This drug also controls tremors and muscle rigidity in Parkinson's disease.

Possible side effects:
Dry mouth

Difficulty urinating

Nervousness

Irregular heartbeat

Abnormal dilation of pupils

Impotence

Headache

Blurred vision

Hives

Drowsiness

Possible interactions:
- You have an added risk of negative side effects if you take hyoscyamine along with any of the following drugs: the psychosis drug haloperidol, the antiparkinson drug amantadine, tranquilizers called phenothiazines, antidepressant drugs called monoamine oxidase (MAO) inhibitors, and tricyclic antidepressants.
- Antacids may reduce the effectiveness of this drug. Take the hyoscyamine before meals and antacids after meals.

Other important information:
- People with the following conditions should not take this drug: kidney disease; obstructive diseases of the stomach, intestines, or bladder; severe ulcerative colitis or ulcerative colitis complicated by dilation of the colon; liver disease; paralysis of the intestines; the elderly or debilitated with reduced muscle tone in the intestines; the nerve/muscle disease called myasthenia gravis; rapid heartbeat; angina; and some kinds of glaucoma (ask your doctor).
- People with the following conditions should take this drug very cautiously: overactive thyroid, diseases of the autonomic nervous system, congestive heart failure, coronary heart disease, high blood pressure, irregular heartbeat, enlarged prostate, chronic lung disease, asthma, allergies, hiatal hernia with stomach acid that washes back up into the esophagus, obstruction of the intestines, and glaucoma.
- This drug can make you become overheated if you are exposed to hot weather. Watch for signs of heatstroke or fever.

IMIPRAMINE HYDROCHLORIDE

Pregnancy category: NR
No driving   MAO warning

Brand:
Tofranil   *Tofranil PM*

Imipramine is a tricyclic antidepressant that treats the symptoms of depression.

How to take this drug:
* Since imipramine has a sedative effect, you may want to take the largest dose in the late afternoon or at bedtime.

Possible side effects:

Drowsiness	Dizziness
Dry mouth	Headache
Increased appetite	Nausea
Unpleasant taste	Black tongue

Possible interactions:
* If you take imipramine along with tranquilizers, alcohol, antihistamines, or muscle relaxers, the combination may dangerously depress your nervous system.
* Your doctor should supervise you closely for side effects if you take imipramine along with any anticholinergic drugs, such as some antihistamines and muscle relaxants, or along with any sympathomimetic drugs, such as some decongestants.
* Cimetidine, an ulcer drug, methylphenidate, and fluoxetine can increase the levels of imipramine in your body.
* Some blood-pressure-lowering drugs, such as guanethidine and clonidine, may not work as well if you also take imipramine.
* Barbiturates and phenytoin can decrease levels of imipramine in your body.

Other important information:
* Don't use this drug if you are recovering from a heart attack.
* If you have a history of seizures, liver or kidney problems, urinary retention, thyroid problems, increased pressure in the eye, or heart problems, talk with your doctor about your condition before you take imipramine.
* When possible, quit taking imipramine several days before surgery.
* If you suddenly quit taking this drug, you could have nausea, headache, and a general feeling of fatigue. If you gradually quit taking the drug, you may still experience irritability, restlessness, and dream and sleep disturbances.

- If you develop a fever and a sore throat while taking this drug, you need to have certain blood tests done.
- This drug will increase your skin's sensitivity to the sun. Always use sunscreen and wear protective clothes when you will be exposed to the sun.

INDAPAMIDE

Pregnancy category: B

Brand:
Lozol

This diuretic is used to reduce blood pressure and fluid retention associated with congestive heart failure.

Possible side effects:

Anxiety	Nervousness
Weakness	Headache
Dizziness	Blurred vision
Drowsiness	Depression
Stomach pain	Diarrhea
Vomiting	Constipation
Frequent urination	Impotence
Dry mouth	Rash, itching, or hives

Possible interactions:
- Taking indapamide with the antipsychotic drug lithium may cause lithium to accumulate to toxic levels.
- Indapamide may increase the effects of other high blood pressure drugs.
- Indapamide may decrease the effects of the heart drug norepinephrine.
- Since indapamide may raise blood sugar levels, people with diabetes may need adjustments to their doses of insulin or other glucose-lowering agents if they begin taking it.

Other important information:
- People with poor kidney function or liver disease should use this drug with caution.
- Indapamide may increase levels of uric acid in the blood (this puts you at risk for gout), may worsen symptoms of lupus, and may raise blood sugar levels.
- This diuretic may cause dangerously low levels of potassium and other electrolytes. Contact your doctor if you experience any of the symptoms of potassium loss: unusual thirst, tiredness, drowsiness, restlessness, muscle pains or cramps, nausea, or rapid heart rate. Your electrolyte balances should also be watched carefully if you get sick and are vomiting or have diarrhea.

- Weigh daily so you'll know if you're losing too much fluid, which can cause dehydration and possibly blood clots. Warning signs include dry mouth, thirst, drowsiness, and weakness. Contact your doctor immediately if you stop urinating.

INDOMETHACIN

Pregnancy category: NR

Brand:

Indocin   *Indocin SR*

This nonsteroidal anti-inflammatory drug (NSAID) relieves the pain and inflammation of arthritis, gout, ankylosing spondylitis, and bursitis or tendinitis in the shoulder.

How to take this drug:

- Take with food, after meals, or with antacids to help prevent stomach irritation.

Possible side effects:

Nausea	Indigestion
Diarrhea	Constipation
Heartburn	Ringing in the ears
Dizziness	Depression
Tiredness	Headache

Possible interactions:

- Avoid alcohol and aspirin while taking NSAIDs, such as indomethacin.
- Taking indomethacin and the arthritis drug diflunisal together could cause dangerous intestinal bleeding.

Other important information:

- Don't use indomethacin if you are allergic to aspirin or any NSAID.
- Take indomethacin with caution if you have stomach ulcers, poor liver or kidney function, heart problems, high blood pressure, or blood-clotting disorders.
- Indomethacin may cause gastrointestinal bleeding.
- Taking this drug is more likely to cause kidney problems if you are elderly; if you take diuretics; or if you have lupus, heart failure, or poor liver or kidney function.
- Indomethacin may cause or worsen Parkinson's disease, epilepsy, and depression.
- Be on the lookout for signs that this drug is depressing your immune system: fever, sore throat, tiredness, weakness, bruising, or unusual bleeding. Have your blood tested regularly.

IODOQUINOL

Pregnancy category: C

Brand:
Yodoxin

This drug is used to treat amoeba infestation of the intestines.

How to take this drug:
- You can crush the tablets and mix them with a soft food, such as applesauce.

Possible side effects:

Rash, itching, or hives	Enlarged thyroid
Fever	Chills
Headache	Eye problems
Stomach cramps	Nausea
Vomiting	Diarrhea
Itching around the anus	Dizziness

Possible interactions:
- This drug may alter the results of some thyroid function tests.

Other important information:
- Don't use this drug if you have liver damage.
- Long-term treatment can cause damage to the optic nerve.
- People with thyroid disease should use this drug with caution.
- Don't prepare food for others until the infection is completely cleared up.

IPRATROPIUM

Pregnancy category: B

Brand:
Atrovent

Ipratropium is a bronchodilator that treats the bronchial spasms associated with emphysema and chronic bronchitis.

How to take this drug:
- Don't skip a dose. You need to use ipratropium consistently to get the full effect.

Possible side effects:

Coughing	Dry mouth
Nervousness	Dizziness
Headache	Nausea
Stomach pain	Blurred vision

Other important information:
- Don't use ipratropium if you are allergic to atropine or its derivatives or if you are allergic to food products, such as soybean or lecithin (found in milk, egg yolks, corn, etc.).

- Use ipratropium cautiously if you have some kinds of glaucoma (ask your doctor), bladder neck obstruction, or enlarged prostate.
- Avoid accidentally spraying ipratropium in your eyes. Your vision may be blurred temporarily.

IRBESARTAN

Pregnancy category: C/D

Brand:
Avapro

Irbesartan is an angiotensin II blocker used to treat high blood pressure.

How to take this drug:
- You can take this drug with or without food.
- Never double a missed dose. Instead take it as soon as you remember or skip it and go on with your regular schedule.

Possible side effects:

Diarrhea	Indigestion
Muscle pain	Tiredness
Upper respiratory infection	

Other important information:
- You can combine this drug with other blood pressure medications, including diuretics.
- If you are taking high doses of diuretics or are on hemodialysis, your sodium levels may need to be adjusted before taking irbesartan.
- Certain people will develop excessively low blood pressure (hypotension). Warning signs include dizziness and lightheadedness.
- Use cautiously if you have kidney problems or congestive heart failure.
- You must take irbesartan regularly, even though you may not see results for a couple of weeks.

ISOCARBOXAZID

Pregnancy category: C
No driving   MAO warning

Brand:
Marplan

Isocarboxazid is an MAO inhibitor used to treat depression.

Possible side effects:

Dizziness	Headache
Nausea	Dry mouth
Sleeplessness	Tremors
Constipation	

Possible interactions:
- Don't take this drug with other MAO inhibitors; SSRIs (Prozac, Zoloft, Paxil); dibenzazepine derivatives; sympathomimetics; metrizamide (Amipaque); meperidine; amphetamines; over-the-counter drugs for colds, hay fever, or weight loss; narcotics; alcohol; drugs for high blood pressure, including diuretics; antihistamines; sedatives; anesthetics; the antidepressant bupropion (Wellbutrin, Zyban); the antianxiety bus-pirone (BuSpar); or the cough suppressant dextromethorphan.
- Avoid these foods while taking isocarboxazid: caffeine; broad beans; avocado; banana; chocolate; colas; mushrooms; raisins; sour cream; aged cheeses and meats; beer; wine; liqueurs; salted, smoked, or pick-led fish; chicken livers; sauerkraut; yogurt; soy sauce; and yeast extracts, like Marmite or brewer's yeast.
- Isocarboxazid can interact with disulfiram (Antabuse).

Other important information:
- Don't take isocarboxazid if you have heart disease, liver or kidney problems, high blood pressure, or severe or frequent headaches.
- Avoid surgery requiring a general anesthesia. Certain local anesthesias must be avoided, too. Talk to your doctor.
- Watch out for signs of drastic increases in your blood pressure: headaches, heart palpitations, stiff neck, nausea or vomiting, tightness in the chest, sweating, and sensitivity to light.
- Tell your dentist you are using this drug.
- Some people on this medication experience sudden dizziness when they stand up. Be careful to avoid falls.
- If you are epileptic or suffer other kinds of seizures, this drug can increase the number of seizures you have.
- Have your liver tested regularly while taking this medication.
- Use this drug cautiously if you are diabetic or have thyroid problems.
- You may not see improvement for several weeks. Continue to take the drug regularly.

ISONIAZID

Pregnancy category: C

Brand:
Laniazid

Isoniazid treats all forms of tuberculosis.

How to take this drug:
- You can take your medicine with food to help prevent stomach irritation.
- If you miss a dose, take it as soon as possible. If several hours have passed or it is nearing time for the next dose, don't try to catch up by doubling your dose unless your doctor tells you to.

Possible side effects:

Nausea	Upset stomach
Fever	Rashes
Breast enlargement in men	

Possible interactions:

- This drug may increase the effects of the seizure drug phenytoin.
- Avoid alcohol, which increases the risk of liver damage from isoniazid.
- Taking this drug with large doses of acetaminophen increases your risk of liver damage.

Other important information:

- Don't use this drug if you have had a severe reaction to isoniazid, including liver damage.
- Some people, particularly alcoholics and diabetics, may need vitamin B supplements. Ask your doctor.
- Hepatitis is a rare but sometimes fatal side effect. Call your doctor if you experience weakness, loss of appetite, or vomiting.
- If you have chronic liver disease or poor kidney function, use this drug with caution.
- Be on the lookout for signs that this drug is depressing your immune system: fever, sore throat, tiredness, weakness, bruising, or unusual bleeding. Have your blood tested regularly.

ISOSORBIDE DINITRATE

Pregnancy category: C

Brand:

Isordil   *Sorbitrate*

Isosorbide dinitrate prevents angina (chest pain).

How to take this drug:

- Take your medicine regularly, as prescribed, and keep it easily available at all times.
- You can take an additional dose before a stressful time or at bedtime if you have angina at night. Discuss these options with your doctor.

Possible side effects:

Headache	Flushing
Weakness	Dizziness

Possible interactions:

- Don't drink alcohol while you take this drug. The combination may cause very low blood pressure.

Other important information:
- If you have low blood pressure, have had a recent heart attack, or are sensitive to nitrates or nitrites, take this drug very cautiously.
- Don't stop taking this drug suddenly — you could experience chest pain or even a heart attack. Instead, withdraw from the medication gradually under your doctor's supervision.
- Since this drug can cause very low blood pressure and dizziness, sit or stand up slowly and be careful on stairs.

ISOSORBIDE MONONITRATE

Pregnancy category: B/C
No driving

Brand:
Imdur   *Ismo*
Monoket

Isosorbide mononitrate helps prevent angina attacks due to coronary artery disease. However, it cannot stop an angina attack once it has started.

How to take this drug:
- Follow the dosing instructions carefully.
- Imdur is an extended release dose and is taken on a different schedule.
- Don't chew or crush the Imdur Extended Release Tablets, and take with plenty of liquid.
- Never double a missed dose. Instead take it as soon as you remember or skip it and go on with your regular schedule.

Possible side effects:
Daily headaches   Dizziness
Nausea or vomiting

Possible interactions:
- Taking calcium channel blockers or blood pressure medication, or drinking alcohol with this drug increases your risk of experiencing a drop in blood pressure. Be careful — you may feel lightheaded if you stand up suddenly.
- Taking Imdur with sildenafil can cause severely low blood pressure.
- You may have falsely low cholesterol readings while on isosorbide mononitrate.

Other important information:
- Don't use this drug if you are allergic to organic nitrates.
- Isosorbide mononitrate is not proven useful to treat myocardial infarction or congestive heart failure.

- Use this drug cautiously if you have low blood pressure since it can make the condition worse. Watch out for lightheadedness upon standing suddenly.
- If you are an industrial worker who has been exposed to high doses of organic nitrates over a long period of time, you may have built up a tolerance. Discuss with your doctor how this could affect treatment with isosorbide mononitrate.

ISOTRETINOIN

Pregnancy category: X

Brand:
Accutane

This form of vitamin A is used to treat severe acne that does not respond to other treatments.

How to take this drug:
- Take this drug with meals.
- Do not crush the capsules.
- If you miss a dose, take it as soon as possible. If several hours have passed or it's almost time for your next dose, don't try to catch up by doubling the dose (unless your doctor tells you to).

Possible side effects:
Swollen lips	Conjunctivitis (inflamed eyelids)
Muscle pain	Chest pain

Possible interactions:
- Don't take vitamin supplements containing vitamin A while you are taking this drug.
- Avoid alcohol while taking this drug because it may cause very high triglyceride levels.
- Taking this drug with the antibiotic tetracycline may cause increased pressure in the brain.

Other important information:
- Stop treatment with this drug if hepatitis, inflammatory bowel disease, or visual disorders develop.
- Isotretinoin may cause increased pressure on the brain in adults. Signs of this high pressure include headache, nausea, and visual disturbances. Let your doctor know immediately if you develop these symptoms.
- Isotretinoin may also raise your cholesterol and triglyceride levels and lower your red and white blood cell counts. A low red blood cell count could cause anemia and a low white blood cell count could lower your resistance to infection.
- Be extra careful when driving at night since this drug may cause a decrease in night vision.

- Your acne may get worse when you first begin taking isotretinoin. That doesn't mean you should stop taking the drug.
- This drug may make your skin extra-sensitive to sunlight, so protect your skin if you'll be outdoors.
- Do not donate blood while you are taking this drug or for 30 days after you quit taking this drug.

ISRADIPINE

Pregnancy category: C

Brand:
DynaCirc   *DynaCirc CR*

Isradipine is a calcium channel blocker used to lower blood pressure.

Possible side effects:

Headache	Fluid retention
Flushing	Dizziness
Nausea	Diarrhea
Rash	Fatigue
Rapid heartbeat	

Possible interactions:
- If you take isradipine along with blood pressure drugs called beta blockers, you may experience very low blood pressure or heart irregularities.
- You may also have severe low blood pressure if you take isradipine along with the pain drug fentanyl.

Other important information:
- Take isradipine with caution if you have congestive heart failure. Tell your doctor immediately if you have any signs of congestive heart failure, such as night cough; swelling and fluid retention in your legs, feet, or hands; or difficulty breathing, especially when lying down or after physical exertion.
- If you stop taking calcium channel blockers suddenly, you could have rebound angina. If you have to stop, do it gradually under your doctor's supervision.

KETOCONAZOLE

Pregnancy category: C
No driving

Brand:
Nizoral

Ketoconazole is used to treat fungal infections, including oral thrush and skin infections.

How to take this drug:
- This drug comes as a cream, shampoo, or tablets.
- Take your medicine with food to help prevent nausea. Nausea should go away after you've been taking the drug for a while.

Possible side effects:

Nausea	Itching
Stomach pain	

Possible interactions:
- Do not take ketoconazole with the allergy drug terfenadine because it may cause a dangerously rapid heartbeat.
- Taking this drug with the antihistamine astemizole may cause heartbeat irregularities.
- Take antacids two hours after this drug because they reduce absorption.
- Anticholinergics, histamine blockers, and the tuberculosis drug rifampin may decrease effects or levels of this drug.
- This drug may increase levels or effects of corticosteroids, anticoagulants, and the immunosuppressant cyclosporine.
- If taken with the antifungal drug miconazole, this drug may cause very low blood sugar.

Other important information:
- This drug can cause liver toxicity. Test liver functions before treatment begins and carefully monitor them during treatment, especially in people with a history of liver disease. Contact your doctor if you have severe diarrhea, stomach pain, or fever or if you develop any symptoms of possible liver damage, such as nausea, dark urine, light-colored stools, yellow eyes or skin, loss of appetite, or unusual fatigue.
- This drug should be used with caution by men with prostate cancer.
- Be on the lookout for signs that this drug is depressing your immune system: fever, sore throat, tiredness, weakness, bruising, or unusual bleeding. Have your blood tested regularly.
- This drug may make your skin extra-sensitive to sunlight, so protect your skin if you'll be outdoors.
- You may see improvement quickly, but continue to treat jock itch and ringworm for two weeks so the fungus won't come back.

KETOROLAC TROMETHAMINE

Pregnancy category: C

Brand:
Toradol

The tablet form of this nonsteroidal anti-inflammatory drug (NSAID) is used to relieve short-term pain.

Possible side effects:

Stomach or intestinal pain	Headache
Nausea	Indigestion
Gas	Constipation
Inflamed mouth	Stuffy nose
Hearing loss	Rash
Itching	Fluid retention
Dizziness	Drowsiness
Sweating	

Possible interactions:

- Ketorolac tablets may increase the levels or effects of the antipsychotic drug lithium and the cancer drug methotrexate, possibly increasing them to toxic levels.
- Ketorolac tablets may increase the effectiveness of diuretics and the anticoagulant warfarin.
- The gout drug probenecid may increase levels of ketorolac.

Other important information:

- Don't use ketorolac tablets if you have an allergy to aspirin or other NSAIDs.
- People with nasal polyps, fluid retention, an active stomach ulcer, or asthma should not use ketorolac tablets.
- Take the tablets with caution if you have poor liver or kidney function, poor heart function, high blood pressure, blood clotting disorders, are taking diuretics, or are over 65.
- Bleeding stomach ulcers and liver or kidney damage are rare but serious reactions to using ketorolac tablets for long periods of time. Warning signs of liver damage include nausea, tiredness, red and itchy skin, yellow eyes and skin (jaundice), and flu-like symptoms.
- Be on the lookout for signs that this drug is depressing your immune system: fever, sore throat, tiredness, weakness, bruising, or unusual bleeding. Have your blood tested regularly.

LABETALOL HYDROCHLORIDE

Pregnancy category: C
No driving

Brand:

Normodyne   *Trandate*

Labetalol is an alpha/beta blocker that controls high blood pressure and regulates heart rhythm.

Possible side effects:

Headache	Indigestion
Weakness	Dizziness
Stuffy nose	

Possible interactions:
- The ulcer drug cimetidine may increase levels of labetalol.
- Taking labetalol while you're taking the anesthesia drug halothane or the angina drug nitroglycerin may cause dangerously low blood pressure.

Other important information:
- People with severely slow heartbeat, greater than first-degree heart block, heart failure, or asthma should not use labetalol.
- Take labetalol with extreme caution if you have a history of heart failure, poor liver function, emphysema, or bronchitis.
- If you have diabetes, use this drug cautiously because beta blockers can mask the signs of low blood sugar. Labetalol may also reduce the effects of insulin. Diabetics may need to have their insulin dosages adjusted.
- Labetalol can also mask signs of an overactive thyroid.
- Discuss your medication with your doctor before having surgery. He may want to discontinue the drug before your surgery.
- Tell your doctor immediately if you have any signs of congestive heart failure, such as night cough; swelling of your legs, feet, or hands; or difficulty breathing, especially when lying down or after physical exertion.
- Never quit taking this drug without talking to your doctor. It could increase your risk of angina and heart attack.

LAMOTRIGINE

Pregnancy category: C
No driving

Brand:
Lamictal

Lamotrigine is used to treat seizures, usually from epilepsy or Lennox-Gastaut syndrome and usually in combination with other drugs.

How to take this drug:
- This drug is available as a pill or chewable tablet.
- Take with or without food.
- The chewable tablets may be swallowed whole, chewed, or dissolved in water or fruit juice.
- Don't take a higher dose than your doctor prescribes or increase your dose faster than prescribed.
- Never double a missed dose, instead take it as soon as you remember or skip it and go on with your regular schedule.

Possible side effects:

Rash	Dizziness
Headache	Sleepiness
Loss of muscle control	Vision problems
Nausea or vomiting	Stuffy nose
Sore throat	

Possible interactions:

- Although lamotrigine is often combined with acetaminophen, carbamazepine, phenobarbital, phenytoin, primidone, and valproic acid, they still can interact with each other. Talk with your doctor if you develop unusual symptoms.

Other important information:

- Although many develop a rash when taking lamotrigine, there is a rare chance of developing a serious, even life-threatening skin reaction. Show any rash to your doctor immediately, especially if you develop hives, fever, swollen lymph glands, mouth sores, or swollen lips or tongue.
- Lamotrigine should be given to patients younger than 16 only if they have seizures from the Lennox-Gastaut syndrome.
- Don't stop taking this drug abruptly.
- Be careful taking lamotrigine if you have kidney, liver, or heart problems. Your body may not be able to use or get rid of the drug properly.
- Taking lamotrigine over a long period of time may damage eye tissues.

LANSOPRAZOLE

Pregnancy category: B

Brand:

Prevacid

This delayed-release form of lansoprazole is prescribed to treat duodenal ulcers, benign gastric ulcers, the symptoms of gastroesophageal reflux disease (GERD), erosive esophagitis, or Zollinger-Ellison syndrome. It is often combined with amoxicillin and clarithromycin to treat *H. pylori* infection, which causes most duodenal ulcers.

How to take this drug:

- Take this drug either without food or before meals.
- If you have difficulty swallowing capsules, empty the contents onto a tablespoon of applesauce and swallow it immediately. You can also stir it into apple, cranberry, grape, orange, pineapple, prune, tomato, or V-8 juice and store it for up to 30 minutes.
- Never double a missed dose. Instead take it as soon as you remember or skip it and go on with your regular schedule.

Possible side effects:

Diarrhea   Abdominal pain
Nausea

Possible interactions:

- Lansoprazole may interact with theophylline, sucralfate, omeprazole, ketoconazole, ampicillin esters, iron salts, and digoxin.

Other important information:
- If you have severe liver problems, you may need an adjusted dose of lansoprazole.

LATANOPROST

Pregnancy category: C
Refrigerate   No driving

Brand:
Xalatan

This sterile ophthalmic solution is used to reduce pressure within the eyeball caused by glaucoma or ocular hypertension.

How to take this drug:
- Don't put this solution in your eyes while wearing contact lenses. Reinsert them 15 minutes after using the medication.
- Don't allow the bottle tip to touch your skin or eye. You could contaminate it or the solution.
- If you are using more than one medication in your eye, apply them at least five minutes apart.
- Never double a missed dose. Instead take it as soon as you remember or skip it and go on with your regular schedule.

Possible side effects:
Permanent eye color change   Permanent eyelid darkening
Permanent eyelash changes   Blurred vision
Burning, stinging, itching eyes

Possible interactions:
- Other eye medications containing thimerosal could interact with latanoprost. Use them at least five minutes apart.

Other important information:
- If you are receiving latanoprost treatment in only one eye, be aware that the drug can cause permanent changes in eye and eyelid color and number, length, and thickness of eyelashes. After several months of drug use, your eyes may look remarkably different.
- Use this drug cautiously if you have inflammation within your eye.
- Discuss latanoprost treatment with your doctor if you have kidney or liver problems.
- See your doctor immediately if you develop an eye infection, injure your eye, or have eye surgery.

LEFLUNOMIDE

Pregnancy category: X

Brand:
Arava

Leflunomide is used to reduce the symptoms of rheumatoid arthritis and to slow down joint damage.

How to take this drug:
- Never double a missed dose. Instead take it as soon as you remember or skip it and go on with your regular schedule.

Possible side effects:
Diarrhea	Hair loss
Rash	Nausea
Respiratory infection	Headache
Abdominal pain	

Possible interactions:
- Combining leflunomide with rifampin can increase levels of both these drugs in your body.
- Leflunomide can interact with cholestyramine, activated charcoal, and tolbutamide.
- Any substances that are toxic to the liver will increase the side effects of leflunomide.

Other important information:
- Use this drug cautiously if you have kidney problems.
- Don't take it if you have liver problems, including Hepatitis B or C. Your doctor may monitor your liver function throughout treatment.
- Since your body may not be able to fight infection while you are taking this drug, it is not recommended for people with a severely depressed immune system, or those who have cancer, bone marrow problems, or severe infections.
- You can continue to take aspirin, NSAIDs, or low-dose corticosteroids with leflunomide.
- Don't take vaccinations with live vaccines while taking this drug.

LEVALBUTEROL HYDROCHLORIDE

Pregnancy category: C

Brand:
Xopenex

Levalbuterol hydrochloride is an inhalant that treats and prevents bronchospasms from conditions like asthma.

How to take this drug:
- If you find that this drug is not working for you, don't increase the dose or frequency without talking with your doctor first.
- Carefully follow the dosing and storage instructions that come with this medication.
- Don't combine other drugs with levalbuterol hydrochloride in your inhaler.

Possible side effects:

Rapid heartbeat	Tremors
Nervousness	Chest pain
Headache	Dizziness

Possible interactions:
- These drugs may interact with levalbuterol hydrochloride: beta blockers, diuretics, digoxin, MAO inhibitors, or tricyclic antidepressants.

Other important information:
- Don't take this medication if you've had a reaction to albuterol.
- Levalbuterol hydrochloride can cause a negative reaction in some people where the airways narrow instead of open (paradoxical bronchospasm). This can be a life-threatening condition. Stop taking the drug and call your doctor immediately.
- Talk to your doctor about this drug if you have a heart condition, especially arrhythmias and high blood pressure, since it can cause heart-related side effects.
- Don't take more than the recommended amount. It can be fatal.
- You may not be able to take levalbuterol hydrochloride if you have seizures, high thyroid hormones, or diabetes.

LEVODOPA

Pregnancy category: NR
No driving   MAO warning

Brand:
Dopar   *Larodopa*

Levodopa treats the symptoms of Parkinson's disease.

How to take this drug:
- Take this drug with food.

Possible side effects:

Loss of appetite	Nausea
Dry mouth	Numbness
Dizziness	Confusion
Nightmares	Teeth grinding
Difficulty swallowing	

Possible interactions:
- Levodopa can increase the effects of blood-pressure-lowering drugs.
- Vitamin B6 may decrease levels or effects of this drug.

Other important information:
- Don't use this drug if you have certain kinds of glaucoma (ask your doctor), a history of skin cancer, or any undiagnosed skin lesions.
- If you have severe lung or heart disease; an irregular heartbeat; disease of the brain, liver, kidney, or endocrine system; or a history of heart attack, asthma, stomach ulcer, or mental disturbances, talk with your doctor about your condition before you take this drug.
- Be on the lookout for signs that this drug is depressing your immune system: fever, sore throat, tiredness, weakness, bruising, or unusual bleeding. Have your blood tested regularly.
- Have regular liver, blood, heart, and kidney tests while you're taking this drug.
- Since levodopa can cause low blood pressure and dizziness when you stand or sit up, be careful when you change positions.

LEVOFLOXACIN

Pregnancy category: C
No driving

Brand:
Levaquin

Levofloxacin is an antibiotic prescribed to treat various bacterial infections, including sinusitis, bacterial bronchitis, pneumonia, certain skin infections, urinary tract infections, and kidney infections caused by E. coli.

How to take this drug:
- Take this drug with or without food but with plenty of fluids.
- Never double a missed dose. Instead take it as soon as you remember or skip it and go on with your regular schedule.

Possible side effects:
Nausea	Diarrhea
Headache	Constipation

Possible interactions:
- Take these medications at least two hours before or after levofloxacin: antacids with magnesium or aluminum, sucralfate, iron, and multi-vitamins with zinc.
- Levofloxacin may interact with theophylline for asthma, the blood-thinning drug warfarin, and NSAIDs.

Other important information:
- This drug is not recommended for those under 18 years old.

- Watch out for serious drug reactions that might include tremors, restlessness, lightheadedness, confusion, hallucinations, paranoia, depression, nightmares, insomnia, seizures, difficulty breathing, severe drops in blood pressure, swelling, or skin reactions. Stop using levofloxacin and contact your doctor.
- Using an antibiotic can destroy the helpful bacteria in your digestive system, leading to a condition called antibiotic-associated colitis. If you develop diarrhea after taking this medication, see your doctor.
- Some people experience tendon inflammation or damage after taking this type of drug, especially in the shoulder, hand, and Achilles tendons. Avoid exercise and call your doctor.
- Be careful using this drug if you have kidney problems. You may need your dose adjusted and your kidneys monitored.
- Avoid excessive exposure to sunlight.
- Use this drug cautiously if you are subject to seizures.
- If you are diabetic, levofloxacin can affect your blood glucose levels.

LEVOTHYROXINE

Pregnancy category: A

Brand:

Levothroid   Levoxyl
Synthroid

This drug is used to replace thyroid hormones when the thyroid gland does not produce enough. It is also used to suppress the release of thyroid stimulating hormone from the pituitary gland for people with some forms of goiter and thyroid cancer.

Possible interactions:
- This drug may increase the effects of the anticoagulant warfarin and decrease the levels or effects of insulin in diabetics.
- The cholesterol reducers cholestyramine and colestipol may reduce levels of this drug.

Other important information:
- Don't use this drug if you have abnormal adrenal or thyroid glands.
- If you have heart or blood vessel abnormalities, such as angina, or if you have diabetes or adrenal gland abnormalities, use this drug with extreme caution.
- Diabetics may need their dosage of antidiabetic medication adjusted.
- Have periodic lab tests to reassess thyroid function and speed of blood clotting.
- Call your doctor if you have any signs of overdose, including diarrhea, nervousness, stomach cramps, rapid heartbeat, headache, weight loss, palpitations, fever, sweating, chest pain, insomnia, or irregular heartbeat.

LIOTHYRONINE SODIUM

Pregnancy category: A

Brand:
Cytomel   *Triostat*

Liothyronine sodium is used to replace thyroid hormones when the thyroid gland does not produce enough. It is also used to suppress the release of thyroid stimulating hormone from the pituitary gland for people with some forms of goiter and thyroid cancer.

Possible interactions:
- This drug may increase the effects of the anticoagulant warfarin and decrease the levels or effects of insulin in diabetics.
- Cholesterol reducers cholestyramine and colestipol may reduce levels of this drug.
- Taking this drug with the asthma drug epinephrine may cause heart problems.

Other important information:
- Don't use this drug if you have abnormal adrenal or thyroid gland function.
- If you have heart or blood vessel abnormalities, such as angina, diabetes, or adrenal gland abnormalities, use with extreme caution.
- Diabetics may need their dosage of antidiabetic medication adjusted.
- Have periodic lab tests to reassess thyroid function and speed of blood clotting.
- Call your doctor if you have any signs of overdose, including diarrhea, nervousness, stomach cramps, rapid heartbeat, headache, weight loss, palpitations, fever, sweating, chest pain, insomnia, or irregular heartbeat.

LISINOPRIL

Pregnancy category: C/D

Brand:
Prinivil   *Zestril*

This angiotensin converting enzyme (ACE) inhibitor treats high blood pressure and helps manage heart failure.

Possible side effects:

Fatigue	Headache
Cough	Vomiting
Diarrhea	Nausea

Possible interactions:
- This drug may increase levels or effects of the antipsychotic drug lithium. This means lithium levels should be monitored while using this drug.
- Nonsteroidal anti-inflammatory drugs (NSAIDs) may decrease the blood-pressure-lowering effects of lisinopril.

Other important information:
- People with poor kidney and liver functions should take this drug very cautiously.
- Lisinopril may cause a severe drop in blood pressure after the first dose, particularly in people taking diuretics, on dialysis, or with congestive heart failure. Be careful when you rise quickly — you may feel light-headed and dizzy. If you faint, stop taking the drug and immediately contact your doctor.
- Lisinopril may cause dangerously high levels of potassium in the blood. Don't use potassium-sparing diuretics or take potassium supplements without talking with your doctor. Very high levels of potassium can be fatal.
- Be careful in hot weather and during exercise. Sweating can cause loss of fluid, low blood pressure, and, therefore, lightheadedness. Drink plenty of fluids.
- Be on the lookout for signs that this drug is depressing your immune system: fever, sore throat, tiredness, weakness, bruising, or unusual bleeding. Have your blood tested regularly.
- This drug can cause swelling. Mild swelling can occur in the throat, face, lips, tongue, mucous membranes, hands, or feet, but swelling of the throat can be extremely dangerous. Contact your doctor immediately.

LISINOPRIL AND HYDROCHLOROTHIAZIDE

Pregnancy category: C/D

Brand:
Zestoretic   *Prinzide*

This medication combines an ACE inhibitor and a diuretic to control high blood pressure.

How to take this drug:
- You can take this medication with or without food.
- Never double a missed dose. Instead take it as soon as you remember or skip it and go on with your regular schedule.
- Don't allow yourself to become dehydrated while taking this medication. Drink lots of fluids.

Possible side effects:
Cough   Dizziness when standing suddenly
Tiredness   Headache

Possible interactions:
- This medication can interact with potassium-sparing diuretics, potassium supplements, and salt substitutes containing potassium.
- Lithium; barbiturates; narcotics; antidiabetic drugs, including insulin; other medications to lower blood pressure; cholestyramine and colestipol

resins; corticosteroids; pressor amines; muscle relaxants; and NSAIDs can all interact with this medication.

Other important information:
- It may be several weeks before you see any improvements, but you must continue to take the medication regularly.
- Watch out for potentially serious allergic reactions to this drug, including swelling or difficulty swallowing or breathing.
- Your blood pressure may drop severely while you are taking this medication. Watch out for dizziness, especially after you stand up suddenly.
- Be careful using this drug if you have diabetes, liver problems, congestive heart failure, allergies, bronchial asthma, or lupus erythematosus.
- Have your kidneys checked regularly if you have kidney problems.
- Don't take this drug if you are on dialysis.
- This drug can cause liver damage. Warning signs include nausea, tiredness, red and itchy skin, yellow eyes and skin (jaundice), and flu-like symptoms.
- Contact your doctor immediately if you develop any kind of infection, like sore throat, fever, etc.

LITHIUM CARBONATE

Pregnancy category: D
No driving

Brand:
Eskalith   *Eskalith CR*
Lithobid   *Lithonate*
Lithotabs

Lithium treats the manic stages of manic depression.

Possible side effects:
Shaky hands   Frequent urination
Thirst   Nausea
General discomfort

Possible interactions:
- Taking lithium and the anti-psychotic haloperidol at the same time may cause toxicity and brain damage. If you take lithium along with any anti-psychotic, you and your doctor should watch closely for side effects, such as shakiness, weakness, fever, and confusion.
- Lithium may increase the effects of neuromuscular blockers, such as metocurine iodide.
- Nonsteroidal anti-inflammatory drugs (NSAIDs), such as indomethacin and piroxicam, can increase lithium levels.
- Diuretics, calcium channel blockers, and ACE inhibitors, such as captopril, can increase lithium levels in your body. That increases your risk of lithium toxicity.

- The following may decrease the effects of lithium: acetazolamide, caffeine, and sodium bicarbonate.
- Taking carbamazepine and lithium at the same time can cause toxic side effects.
- Fluoxetine can increase or decrease your lithium levels.

Other important information:
- Use this drug with extreme caution if you have cardiovascular disease, kidney disease, dehydration, or low sodium levels, or if you take diuretics.
- Lithium can be toxic at low doses. Watch for early symptoms, such as tremors, lack of coordination, diarrhea, weakness, vomiting, and drowsiness. If you have these symptoms, don't take your next dose of lithium and call your doctor immediately. Later symptoms of toxicity are blurred vision, dizziness, and convulsions.
- Drink plenty of fluids and eat a balanced diet that includes salt. If you sweat a lot or have diarrhea, you need extra fluids, and you may need salt supplements.

LOMEFLOXACIN HYDROCHLORIDE

Pregnancy category: C
No driving

Brand:
Maxaquin

This fluoroquinolone antibiotic is used to treat adults with mild to moderate infections of the lower respiratory tract and urinary tract. It is also used before surgery to protect against urinary tract infections that may develop after surgery.

How to take this drug:
- Drink extra fluids while taking this drug.
- You may take this drug with or without meals.
- If you miss a dose, take it as soon as possible. If several hours have passed or it is nearing time for the next dose, don't try to catch up by doubling your dose unless your doctor tells you to.

Possible side effects:

Sensitivity to light	Headache
Nausea	Dizziness
Diarrhea	

Possible interactions:
- This drug may increase the effects of the anticoagulant warfarin, and it may increase levels of the immunosuppressant cyclosporine.
- Levels of lomefloxacin may be increased by the ulcer drug cimetidine and the drug probenecid, which is used to treat gout.

- Take antacids or any products containing iron or zinc four hours before or two hours after taking this drug.

Other important information:
- Don't use if you have any allergies to quinolone antibiotics. Serious, sometimes fatal, allergic reactions can occur.
- Taking an antibiotic for a long time can cause bacteria or fungus to overgrow, leading to another infection. If you get one of these "super-infections," you may need to quit taking lomefloxacin and start taking another antibiotic for the second infection.
- This drug may cause mild to severe colitis. Colitis is inflammation of the colon, and symptoms include bloody diarrhea, stomach cramps, and fever.
- Severe sensitivity to light may occur in some people exposed to sunlight or ultraviolet light.
- If you have any disorders of the central nervous system, such as epilepsy, or any other condition that increases your risk of seizures, use this drug with caution.

LOPERAMIDE

Pregnancy category: B
No driving

Brand:
Imodium

Loperamide relieves diarrhea by slowing down the movements of the intestines.

Possible side effects:

Nausea	Vomiting
Constipation	Stomach pain or bloating
Dry mouth	Tiredness
Drowsiness	Dizziness
Skin rash	

Other important information:
- Don't take loperamide if you have bloody diarrhea or a fever over 101 degrees Fahrenheit. Contact your doctor immediately if you develop a fever or severe stomach pain.
- If you are taking antibiotics or have poor liver function, talk with your doctor before taking loperamide.
- When you have diarrhea, you are losing water along with minerals, such as salt and potassium. This drug can put you at greater risk for dehydration. Make sure you drink extra fluids and eat a balanced diet.
- Don't use this drug for more than two days unless your doctor told you to do so. Tell your doctor if diarrhea has not improved within 48 hours.

LORACARBEF

Pregnancy category: B

Brand:
Lorabid

This cephalosporin antibiotic is used to combat infections of the respiratory tract, throat, tonsils, ears, urinary tract, and skin by killing the organisms that cause them.

How to take this drug:
- Take one hour before or two hours after food.
- Never double a missed dose. Instead take it as soon as you remember or skip it and go on with your regular schedule.

Possible side effects:

Skin rash	Diarrhea
Stomach pain	Nausea
Headache	Inflamed vagina (vaginitis)

Possible interactions:
- The effects of this drug may be increased by the drug probenecid, which is used to treat gout.

Other important information:
- Don't use this drug if you are allergic to cephalosporin antibiotics.
- If you are allergic to penicillin, use this drug with caution.
- People who have impaired kidney function or a history of intestinal disease, particularly colitis, should use this drug with caution. Tell your doctor if you have diarrhea, particularly if it is severe or contains blood, pus, or mucus.
- Be on the lookout for signs that this drug is depressing your immune system: fever, sore throat, tiredness, weakness, bruising, or unusual bleeding. Have your blood tested regularly.

LORATADINE

Pregnancy category: B

Brand:
Claritin

Loratadine is a long-acting, nonsedating antihistamine used to relieve seasonal allergy symptoms, such as sneezing, runny nose, itching, rashes, hives, swelling, and difficulty breathing.

How to take this drug:
- Take this drug on an empty stomach — at least two hours after or one hour before a meal. Food makes your body absorb the drug more slowly.

Possible side effects:

Headache	Sleepiness
Fatigue	Dry mouth

Possible interactions:

- The antifungal drug ketoconazole may increase the levels of loratadine in your blood.

Other important information:

- You may need to take the tablets every other day if you have cirrhosis or another liver disease.

LORATADINE AND PSEUDOEPHEDRINE SULFATE

Pregnancy category: B
MAO warning

Brand:

Claritin-D   *Claritin-D 24 hour*

This medication is a combination of an antihistamine and a nasal decongestant used to relieve the symptoms of seasonal allergies.

How to take this drug:

- Take this drug with a full glass of water.
- Don't break or chew this tablet.

Possible side effects:

Dry mouth	Sleepiness
Sleeplessness	Sore throat
Dizziness	Coughing
Fatigue	Nausea
Nervousness	Loss of appetite
Menstrual pain	

Possible interactions:

- Don't take any over-the-counter antihistamines or decongestants along with this medication.

Other important information:

- This medication comes in 12-hour and 24-hour extended release forms.
- Don't use this product if you suffer from glaucoma, urinary retention, high blood pressure, liver problems, or heart disease.
- Use this drug cautiously if you have diabetes, high levels of thyroid hormones, kidney problems, or enlarged prostate.
- If you are over age 60, you are more likely to have adverse reactions.
- Don't take this product if you have difficulty swallowing pills.

LORAZEPAM

Pregnancy category: D
No driving

Brand:
Ativan

This benzodiazepine treats anxiety and anxiety associated with depression by slowing down your nervous system.

Possible side effects:
Drowsiness   Dizziness

Possible interactions:
* If you take lorazepam along with other tranquilizers, alcohol, antihistamines, or muscle relaxers, the combination may dangerously depress your nervous system.

Other important information:
* People with some kinds of glaucoma (ask your doctor) shouldn't use this drug.
* You can become dependent on lorazepam. To avoid seizures and other less-severe withdrawal symptoms, quit taking the drug gradually under your doctor's supervision.
* People with poor liver, kidney, or lung functions should use lorazepam cautiously. The drug may stay in your body longer and increase your risk of side effects.
* Have regular blood and urine tests if you are taking lorazepam for a long time.

LOSARTAN POTASSIUM

Pregnancy category: C/D
No driving

Brand:
Cozaar

This angiotensin II receptor antagonist is prescribed to control high blood pressure.

How to take this drug:
* You can take this medication with or without food.

Possible side effects:
Dizziness   Back pain
Upper respiratory infection   Cough

Possible interactions:
- These drugs may interact with losartan potassium: ketoconazole and troleandomycin.
- Don't take potassium-sparing diuretics, potassium supplements, or salt substitutes containing potassium without talking to your doctor first.

Other important information:
- Watch out for severe drops in blood pressure. You may feel dizzy or faint when you stand up suddenly. Talk to your doctor if this becomes a problem.
- Be careful about becoming dehydrated. Some warning signs are dry mouth, fatigue, or confusion.
- It may be several weeks before you see any improvements, but you must continue to take the medication regularly.
- Talk to your doctor about any liver or kidney problems you have.

LOSARTAN POTASSIUM AND HYDROCHLOROTHIAZIDE

Pregnancy category: C/D

Brand:
Hyzaar

This medication, prescribed to control high blood pressure, is a combination of an angiotensin II receptor antagonist and a diuretic.

How to take this drug:
- You can take this medication with or without food.

Possible side effects:
Dizziness	Back pain
Upper respiratory infection	Cough

Possible interactions:
- This drug may interact with salt substitutes containing potassium, potassium supplements, or potassium-sparing diuretics to increase blood levels of potassium.
- These drugs may interact with losartan potassium hydrochlorothiazide: barbiturates, narcotics, anti-diabetic drugs, other medications to lower blood pressure, cholestyramine and colestipol resins, corticosteroids, pressor amines, muscle relaxants, lithium, and NSAIDs.

Other important information:
- Don't use this medication if you have liver problems, difficulty producing urine, or are especially sensitive to sulfa drugs.
- If you suffer from allergies or bronchial asthma, you are more likely to have a reaction to this drug.
- While taking this medication, systemic lupus erythematosus or diabetes can get worse.

- It may be several weeks before you see any improvements, but you must continue to take the medication regularly.
- Your doctor must monitor your kidneys while you are taking this drug if you have any type of kidney disease.
- Watch out for severe drops in blood pressure. You may feel dizzy or faint when you stand up suddenly. Talk to your doctor.
- Be careful about becoming dehydrated. Some warning signs are dry mouth, fatigue, or confusion.

LOTEPREDNOL ETABONATE

Pregnancy category: C

Brand:

Lotemax   *Alrex*

Loteprednol etabonate is a corticosteroid used to treat certain inflammatory conditions of the eye, like seasonal allergies. It gives temporary relief from itching and redness. Lotemax is also used to treat inflammation after cataract surgery.

How to take this drug:

- Don't allow the applicator tip to touch your eye or any other surface. If the tip or the medication becomes contaminated, you can develop an infection.
- Don't wear soft contact lenses when using this product.
- Shake vigorously before using.

Possible side effects:

Burning	Discharge
Dry eyes	Blurred vision
Watery eyes	Feeling of something in your eye
Itching	Red eyes
Headache	Runny nose
Increased sensitivity to light	Sore throat

Other important information:

- Don't use this drug to treat contact lens-related problems or if you have an eye infection caused by viruses, such as herpes or the chickenpox virus.
- Steroid eye drops used over a long period of time can cause glaucoma and increase your likelihood of developing a fungal infection. Use them carefully if you already have glaucoma.
- They can also lower your ability to fight infections.
- Using steroid eye drops after cataract surgery may delay healing time.
- If you don't see improvement after two days, see your doctor.
- Don't use longer than 10 days without having your doctor check the pressure in your eye.

LOVASTATIN

Pregnancy category: X

Brand:

Mevacor

Lovastatin is used to reduce total cholesterol and LDL cholesterol levels.

How to take this drug:

- Take lovastatin with your evening meal.

Possible side effects:

Nausea

Heartburn

Gas

Stomach ulcers

Joint pain

Rash

Weakness

Decreased sexual ability

Diarrhea

Constipation

Stomach pain or cramps

Headache

Itching

Blurred vision

Altered sense of taste

Possible interactions:

- Lovastatin may increase effects of the anticoagulant warfarin.
- The following drugs may increase the risk of rhabdomyolysis (a muscle-destroying disease) when you take them with lovastatin: the immuno-suppressant cyclosporine, the antibiotic erythromycin, the vitamin niacin, and the blood-fat reducer gemfibrozil.

Other important information:

- Lovastatin should not be used by people with liver disease or suspected liver problems.
- Use lovastatin with caution if you have a history of high alcohol consumption or poor kidney function.
- This drug may cause the dangerous and sometimes fatal disease that destroys muscle tissue called rhabdomyolysis. Notify your doctor immediately if you develop any pain, tenderness, or weakness in your muscles.
- This drug can also lead to kidney failure (caused by the rhabdomyolysis) in people with severe infections; uncontrolled seizures; low blood pressure; any kind of trauma, such as major surgery; or severe metabolic, electrolyte, or endocrine disorders.

MAFENIDE ACETATE

Pregnancy category: C

Brand:

Sulfamylon

Use mafenide acetate to control bacterial infection on second- and third-degree burns.

How to take this drug:
- Mafenide acetate is sold as a topical solution and a cream.

Possible side effects:

Rash	Itching
Redness	Swelling
Hives	Blisters
Metabolic acidosis (Excessive acidity in body fluids)	Hyperventilation
	Rapid breathing

Other important information:
- Be careful using this medication if you suffer from acute kidney failure or are sensitive to sulfites.

MAPROTILINE

Pregnancy category: B
No driving   MAO warning

Brand:
Ludiomil

Maprotiline treats the symptoms of depression and the anxiety that can accompany depression.

Possible side effects:

Drowsiness	Dry mouth
Nervousness	Anxiety
Sleeplessness	Agitation
Dizziness	Shakiness
Constipation	Blurred vision
Nausea	Weakness
Fatigue	Headache

Possible interactions:
- Taking maprotiline with phenothiazines (a type of tranquilizer) increases your risk of seizures.
- If you take maprotiline along with tranquilizers, alcohol, antihistamines, or muscle relaxers, the combination may dangerously depress your nervous system.
- Your doctor should supervise you closely for side effects if you take maprotiline along with any anticholinergic drugs, such as some antihistamines and muscle relaxants, or along with any sympathomimetic drugs, such as some decongestants.
- Some blood-pressure-lowering drugs such as guanethidine may not work as well if you also take maprotiline.
- Any of the type of antidepressants called selective serotonin reuptake inhibitors (fluoxetine, sertraline, and paroxetine) can cause maprotiline

to reach dangerously high levels in your body. You may need lower than normal doses of both drugs.

- Cimetidine, an ulcer drug, can increase the levels of maprotiline in your body.
- The seizure drug phenytoin and various barbiturates may lower the levels of maprotiline in your body.

Other important information:
- Don't use this drug when you are recovering from a heart attack.
- If you have a history of seizures, liver problems, urinary retention, thyroid problems, increased pressure in the eye, or heart problems, talk with your doctor about your condition before you take maprotiline.
- When possible, quit taking maprotiline several days before surgery.

MECLIZINE HYDROCHLORIDE

Pregnancy category: B
No driving

Brand:
Antivert   Antivert/25
Antivert/50   Bonine

Meclizine is an antihistamine that controls the nausea, vomiting, and dizziness associated with motion sickness.

Possible side effects:
Dry mouth   Drowsiness

Possible interactions:
- If you take meclizine along with tranquilizers, alcohol, antihistamines, or muscle relaxers, the combination may dangerously depress your nervous system.

Other important information:
- People with glaucoma, emphysema, asthma, chronic bronchitis, or an enlarged prostate should use this drug cautiously.

MECLOFENAMATE SODIUM

Pregnancy category: C/D

Brand:
Meclomen

This nonsteroidal anti-inflammatory drug (NSAID) relieves mild to moderate pain associated with arthritis and menstrual cramps.

How to take this drug:
- Take with food, after meals, or with antacids to help prevent stomach irritation.

Possible side effects:

Nausea	Diarrhea
Constipation	Stomach pain or cramps
Heartburn	Gas
Dizziness	Headache
Rash, hives, or itching	Loss of appetite
Constipation	Inflamed mouth
Ringing in the ears	Fluid retention and swelling

Possible interactions:

- Avoid alcohol and any products containing aspirin while taking meclofenamate.
- Meclofenamate may increase the effects of the anticoagulant warfarin.

Other important information:

- Don't use this drug if you are allergic to aspirin or other aspirin substitutes, such as NSAIDs.
- People with stomach ulcers should not take this drug.
- Liver and kidney damage are rare but serious reactions to using meclofenamate for long periods of time. Warning signs of liver damage include nausea, tiredness, red and itchy skin, yellow eyes and skin (jaundice), and flu-like symptoms.
- Taking meclofenamate is more likely to cause kidney problems if you are elderly; if you take diuretics; or if you have lupus, heart failure, or poor liver or kidney function.
- Be on the lookout for signs that this drug is depressing your immune system: fever, sore throat, tiredness, weakness, bruising, or unusual bleeding. Have your blood tested regularly.

MEDROXYPROGESTERONE ACETATE

Pregnancy category: X

Brand:

Cycrin   *Provera*

This female hormone is used to treat endometriosis, certain forms of endometrial or kidney cancers, abnormal uterine bleeding, and some menstrual disorders.

Possible side effects:

Rash, itching, or hives	Skin eruptions
Hair loss	Blood clots
Menstrual changes	Fluid retention and swelling
Nausea	Fever
Mental depression	Yellow eyes or skin
Dark urine	

Possible interactions:
- The effects of this drug may be decreased by the cancer drug amino-glutethimide.

Other important information:
- Don't use this drug if you have a history of any type of clotting disorder, brain hemorrhage, liver problems, breast cancer, or unexplained vaginal bleeding.
- Get a complete physical examination, including a pap smear, before treatment begins.
- Stop this drug if vision problems occur.
- Changes in menstruation may occur, and if treatment is prolonged, menstruation may stop.
- If you have heart or kidney problems, asthma, epilepsy or migraines, use with caution as water retention (a side effect of the drug) can adversely affect these conditions.

MEPERIDINE HYDROCHLORIDE

Pregnancy category: B
No driving   MAO warning

Brand:
Demerol

This drug is a narcotic pain reliever.

Possible side effects:
Dizziness or lightheadedness	Sleepiness
Nausea or vomiting	Sweating

Possible interactions:
- If you take meperidine along with alcohol or tranquilizers, antihistamines, or muscle relaxants, the combination may dangerously depress your nervous system.

Other important information:
- Take meperidine with extreme caution if you have head injuries, asthma, or other respiratory diseases.
- People with a history of convulsions, kidney or liver problems, Addison's disease, underactive thyroid, enlarged prostate, or irregular heartbeat should take meperidine with caution.
- The major risks of taking this drug are slowed or irregular breathing (some people have stopped breathing) and slowed circulation (some people have had cardiac arrest, which means their circulation has stopped).
- You may become physically and psychologically dependent on this drug if you take high doses for long periods of time. Never take more medicine than you are prescribed.

MEPHOBARBITAL

Pregnancy category: D
No driving

Brand:
Mebaral

Mephobarbital is a barbiturate used to treat seizures for people with epilepsy and to relieve apprehension, anxiety, and tension.

How to take this drug:
- Take your dose at bedtime if you usually have seizures during the night. If you usually have seizures during the day, then you should take your medicine during the day.

Possible side effects:
Daytime sleepiness

Possible interactions:
- If you take this drug along with tranquilizers, alcohol, antihistamines, or muscle relaxers, the combination may dangerously depress your nervous system.
- Mephobarbital may increase the effects of corticosteroids.
- It may decrease the effectiveness of anti-clotting drugs like warfarin, the antifungal drug griseofulvin, birth control pills, and doxycycline.
- If you take mephobarbital and phenytoin together, your doctor may need to adjust your dosages of both drugs. They can affect the levels of each other.
- Sodium valproate, valproic acid, and monoamine oxidase (MAO) inhibitors may increase the depressant effects of mephobarbital.

Other important information:
- You can become addicted to this drug. Don't increase your dose without talking to your doctor. Some symptoms of intoxication with barbiturates are walking unsteadily, slurred speech, confusion, and irritability.
- Withdraw from mephobarbital slowly, over four or five days. If you quit taking the drug suddenly, you may have nightmares, insomnia, anxiety, dizziness, or nausea. If you're addicted to the drug and you quit taking it suddenly, you may have delirium, seizures, or death.
- Your doctor should adjust your dosage carefully and watch you closely for side effects if you have poor kidney function, a heart disorder, respiratory problems, the nerve/muscle disorder called myasthenia gravis, poor thyroid function, or a liver disorder.
- You may need extra vitamin D and vitamin K while you take a barbiturate.
- Have regular blood, liver, and kidney tests if you take this drug for a long time.
- Use another type of contraception besides birth control pills while you're taking mephobarbital.

MEPROBAMATE

Pregnancy category: NR
No driving

Brand:
Amosene   *Equanil*
Miltown   *Tranmep*

Meprobamate relieves severe anxiety and nervousness.

Possible side effects:
Headache   Drowsiness
Dizziness   Excitement
Vision problems   Lack of coordination
Weakness   Slurred speech
Irregular heartbeat   Fainting
Nausea   Diarrhea
Tingling or prickling feeling

Possible interactions:
* If you take meprobamate along with other tranquilizers, alcohol, antihistamines, or muscle relaxers, the combination may dangerously depress your nervous system.

Other important information:
* If you have liver or kidney problems, epilepsy, alcoholism, or a history of drug abuse, talk with your doctor about your condition before taking this drug.
* You can become dependent on meprobamate. To avoid seizures and other less severe withdrawal symptoms, quit taking the drug gradually under your doctor's supervision.

MERCAPTOPURINE

Pregnancy category: D

Brand:
Purinethol

This drug is used to induce and maintain remission in leukemia.

How to take this drug:
* Drink plenty of fluids while taking this drug.

Possible side effects:
Increased skin pigmentation   Nausea or vomiting
Stomach ulcers

Possible interactions:
* The drug allopurinol increases the effects of this drug. You may need a smaller dose of mercaptopurine if you are taking allopurinol.

- Using the antibacterial combination drug trimethoprim-sulfamethoxazole and mercaptopurine together may increase suppression of bone marrow.

Other important information:

- Don't use if you have previously been resistant to the leukemia drug thioguanine.
- Blood counts should be done weekly throughout treatment.
- Liver functions should be checked weekly when treatment is started.
- Call your doctor if you experience anemia, bleeding, infection, nausea, vomiting, jaundice, fever, or sore throat.
- Mercaptopurine can affect your blood so that your immune system is suppressed, you become anemic, or your blood is thin. Symptoms include fever, sore throat, pneumonia, tiredness, weakness, bruising, or unusual bleeding.

MESALAMINE

Pregnancy category: B

Brand:

Asacol   Pentasa
Rowasa

This anti-inflammatory drug is used to treat certain types of ulcerative colitis, proctosigmoiditis, and proctitis.

How to take this drug:

- Mesalamine is available as tablets, capsules, and rectal suppositories or suspension.
- Tablets should be swallowed whole. If intact or partially intact tablets repeatedly appear in your stool, tell your doctor.

Possible side effects:

Weakness	Stomach pain
Headache	Burping or gas
Nausea	Diarrhea
Fever	Sore throat
Stuffy head and nose	Muscle pain
Dizziness	Indigestion
Constipation	Swollen hands or feet
Itching or rash	Menstrual changes
Sweating	Conjunctivitis
Cough	

Other important information:

- Don't use this drug if you are allergic to aspirin.
- If you are allergic to sulfasalazine, use this drug with extreme caution.

- If you have poor liver or kidney functions or a history of kidney disease, use this drug with caution.
- This drug may worsen colitis in some people. Contact your doctor if you develop rash, fever, stomach pain, cramping, bloody diarrhea, or headache.
- You may not see improvement for up to three weeks.

METAPROTERENOL SULFATE

Pregnancy category: C
MAO warning

Brand:
Alupent   *Prometa*

Metaproterenol is a bronchodilator that works quickly (within five to 30 minutes) to provide temporary relief of the breathing difficulties and wheezing associated with asthma, emphysema, and bronchitis. Some forms of metaproterenol are also used to treat acute asthma attacks in children 6 years and older.

How to take this drug:
- Don't use more often than every three to four hours and don't use more than 12 inhalations a day.

Possible side effects:
Nervousness   Rapid or irregular heartbeat
Nausea or vomiting   Shakiness

Possible interactions:
- Don't use with other bronchodilators.

Other important information:
- Use this drug with extreme caution if you have high blood pressure, an irregular heartbeat, heart disease, overactive thyroid, diabetes, or a history of convulsions.
- Very rarely, this drug can cause bronchospasm or a worsening of your asthma. Contact your doctor immediately if this happens.
- The side effects may be worse for children.
- Don't use this drug more frequently than your doctor recommends. An overdose can cause a heart attack or sudden death. Talk to your doctor if you aren't getting relief from your asthma symptoms.

METFORMIN HYDROCHLORIDE

Pregnancy category: B

Brand:
Glucophage

Metformin hydrochloride is used by type II diabetics to lower the amount of sugar in their bloodstream. In contrast to sulfonylureas, this drug may not cause patients to gain weight.

How to take this drug:
- Take this drug with meals.
- Doses usually start low and gradually increase.
- Never double a missed dose, instead take it as soon as you remember or skip it and go on with your regular schedule.

Possible side effects:

Diarrhea	Nausea or vomiting
Abdominal bloating	Gas
Loss of appetite	Unpleasant taste

Possible interactions:
- Talk to your doctor before taking this drug with furosemide, nifedipine, cimetidine, calcium channel blockers, corticosteroids, estrogens, oral contraceptives, nicotinic acid, thyroid products, diuretics, or isoniazid.
- Talk to your doctor about metformin hydrochloride if you are scheduled for a radiologic study where you will be injected with radioactive iodine (intravenous urogram, intravenous cholangiography, angiography, or CT scans).

Other important information:
- Use this medication along with a controlled diet in order to manage diabetes.
- Don't use this drug if you have kidney problems, liver disease, congestive heart failure, hypoxemia, dehydration, sepsis, or diabetic ketoacidosis.
- Have your doctor monitor your kidneys in order to avoid lactic acidosis (symptoms include abdominal upset, fatigue, sleepiness, and respiratory problems).
- Some oral antidiabetic drugs have been associated with a high risk of death from heart disease.

METHADONE HYDROCHLORIDE

Pregnancy category: NR
No driving   MAO warning

Brand:

Dolophine   *Methadose*

This narcotic painkiller is used to relieve severe pain and to treat drug addiction.

Possible side effects:

Dizziness	Sleepiness
Nausea	Sweating

Possible interactions:

- If you take methadone along with alcohol or tranquilizers, antihistamines, or muscle relaxants, the combination may dangerously depress your nervous system.
- Methadone may increase the effects of the antidepressant desipramine.
- Levels or effects of methadone may be decreased by the tuberculosis drug rifampin.

Other important information:

- Take this drug with caution if you have head injuries, asthma, underactive thyroid, poor kidney or liver function, enlarged prostate, or low blood pressure.
- The major risks of taking this drug are slowed or irregular breathing (some people have stopped breathing) and slowed circulation (some people have had cardiac arrest, which means their circulation has stopped).
- You may become physically and psychologically dependent on this drug. Never take more medicine than you are prescribed.
- This drug can cause very low blood pressure. Be careful when you stand or sit up quickly as you may feel lightheaded and dizzy.

METHOCARBAMOL

Pregnancy category: C
No driving

Brand:

Robaxin   *Robaxin-750*

This muscle relaxant is used to relieve painful muscles. It may also help control neuromuscular symptoms of tetanus.

Possible side effects:

Itching	Rash
Hives	Blurred vision
Stuffy nose	Fever
Headache	Nausea
Dizziness	Drowsiness
Inflamed eyes	

Possible interactions:

- If you take methocarbamol along with alcohol or tranquilizers, antihistamines, or muscle relaxants, the combination may dangerously depress your nervous system.

Other important information:

- The injectable form should not be used by people with kidney problems.

METHOCARBAMOL WITH ASPIRIN

Pregnancy category: C
No driving

Brand:
Robaxisal

This muscle relaxant is combined with aspirin to relieve painful muscles.

Possible side effects:

Dizziness	Nausea
Drowsiness	Blurred vision
Headache	Fever

Possible interactions:
- If you take methocarbamol along with alcohol or tranquilizers, antihistamines, or muscle relaxants, the combination may dangerously depress your nervous system.
- You shouldn't take this drug if you are regularly taking anticoagulants. The combination could dangerously increase your bleeding time.

Other important information:
- If you have any bleeding disorder, a vitamin K deficiency, a stomach ulcer, or severe liver damage, don't take this drug.
- Don't use this drug to treat chicken pox or flu, as it could cause Reye's syndrome.
- People with the following conditions should use this drug with caution: liver or kidney damage, gallbladder disease or gallstones, breathing difficulties, irregular heartbeat, hypothyroidism, enlarged prostate, head injuries, or severe stomach problems. If you have liver or kidney damage, have regular liver and kidney tests while you take this drug.
- Be on the lookout for signs that this drug is depressing your immune system: fever, sore throat, tiredness, weakness, bruising, or unusual bleeding. Have your blood tested regularly.
- Large doses of aspirin can cause heartburn, side effects, or an allergic reaction.

METHOTREXATE SODIUM

Pregnancy category: X

Brand:
Rheumatrex

This drug treats various cancers including certain types of breast and lung cancers, certain skin cancers of the head and neck, non-Hodgkin's lymphomas, and leukemia. It is also used to treat severe psoriasis that does not respond to other treatments. Lower doses are used to treat severe rheumatoid arthritis.

Possible side effects:

Upset stomach	Inflamed mouth
Fever	Chills
Dizziness	Sore throat
Diarrhea	Headache
Loss of appetite	Bleeding ulcers
Blurred vision	Difficulty speaking
Rash, itching, or hives	Hair loss
Sensitivity to light	Acne
Menstrual changes	Pneumonia
Abortion	

Possible interactions:

- Avoid taking this drug with nonsteroidal anti-inflammatory drugs (NSAIDs). The combination may cause severe intestinal problems and bone marrow toxicity, which may be fatal.
- Levels or effects may be increased by the gout drug probenecid, the seizure drug phenytoin, aspirin, the NSAID phenylbutazone, and the sulfonamide antibiotics.

Other important information:

- Methotrexate can be extremely toxic. Symptoms include back pain, fever, headache, confusion, lack of coordination, and, sometimes, convulsions.
- Don't use this drug to treat rheumatoid arthritis in people with blood disorders, alcoholism, or chronic liver disease. Routine blood counts, liver and kidney functions, and a chest X-ray should be performed before treatment begins.
- Take this drug with extreme caution if you have infections, a weak immune system, or poor liver or kidney functions.

METHYCLOTHIAZIDE

Pregnancy category: B

Brand:

Aquatensen *Enduron*

This diuretic reduces blood pressure. It is also used with other drugs to treat swelling and fluid retention associated with congestive heart failure, cirrhosis of the liver, kidney disease, estrogen therapy, and corticosteroid therapy.

Possible side effects:

Loss of appetite	Constipation
Nausea	Stomach pain or cramps
Diarrhea	Blurred vision
Jaundice	Sensitivity to light

Hives	Rash
Dizziness	Headache
Weakness	Restlessness
Muscle cramps or spasms	Tingling

Possible interactions:

- Methyclothiazide may increase the effects of the muscle relaxer tubocurarine.
- Methyclothiazide may decrease the effects of the blood pressure-raising drug norepinephrine.
- Methyclothiazide may decrease the excretion of the antipsychotic drug lithium, which can build up to toxic levels.
- If you take methyclothiazide with the heart drug digitalis, steroids, or the hormone ACTH, the combination may lower your potassium levels.
- Since methyclothiazide may raise blood sugar levels, people with diabetes may need adjustments to their doses of insulin or other glucose-lowering agents if they begin taking methyclothiazide.
- If you have high blood pressure, avoid using over-the-counter cold remedies or diet pills, which can increase blood pressure.

Other important information:

- Don't take methyclothiazide if you are allergic to thiazides or sulfonamide-derived drugs.
- People with poor liver or kidney function should take it with caution.
- Your doctor should check your electrolyte balances frequently if you have heart failure, kidney disease, or liver disease, or if you are taking ACTH or corticosteroids. Your electrolyte balances should also be watched carefully if you get sick and are vomiting or have diarrhea. Weigh daily so you'll know if you're losing too much fluid, which can cause dehydration and possibly blood clots. Warning signs of dehydration include dry mouth, thirst, drowsiness, and weakness. Contact your doctor immediately if you stop urinating.
- This drug may increase cholesterol and triglyceride levels. Use it with caution if you have moderate or high levels.
- Be on the lookout for signs that this drug is depressing your immune system: fever, sore throat, tiredness, weakness, bruising, or unusual bleeding. Have your blood tested regularly.
- Methyclothiazide may increase levels of uric acid in the blood (this puts you at risk for gout), may worsen symptoms of lupus, and may raise blood sugar levels.
- This diuretic may cause dangerously low levels of potassium and other electrolytes. Contact your doctor if you experience any of the symptoms of potassium loss: unusual thirst, tiredness, drowsiness, restlessness, muscle pains or cramps, nausea, or rapid heart rate.

METHYLDOPA

Pregnancy category: B
No driving

Brand:
Aldomet

Methyldopa controls high blood pressure.

Possible side effects:

Sleepiness	Decreased mental sharpness
Stuffy nose	Dry mouth
Weight gain	Bloating

Possible interactions:
* Methyldopa may increase the effects of other high blood pressure drugs and anesthesia.
* It may decrease your body's removal of the antipsychotic drug lithium, allowing the lithium to build up to toxic levels.

Other important information:
* People who have ever developed liver problems from using methyldopa or who currently have liver disease should not take this drug. Have regular liver function tests while you're taking it, and watch for these warning signs: nausea, tiredness, red and itchy skin, yellow eyes and skin (jaundice), and flu-like symptoms.
* Be on the lookout for signs that this drug is depressing your immune system: fever, sore throat, tiredness, weakness, bruising, or unusual bleeding. Have your blood tested regularly.
* This drug can cause very low blood pressure, especially when you first begin to take it. Be careful when you rise quickly — you may feel light-headed and dizzy.

METHYLPHENIDATE HYDROCHLORIDE

Pregnancy category: C
MAO warning

Brand:
Ritalin   *Ritalin-SR*

Methylphenidate is a mild stimulant most often used to treat children with attention deficit disorder (ADD). It increases attention and decreases restlessness in children who are overactive and can't concentrate. Methylphenidate also helps people with narcolepsy (an uncontrollable desire for sleep or sudden attacks of deep sleep).

How to take this drug:
* If you're having trouble sleeping, take your last dose before 6 p.m.

- Take your medicine in two or three divided doses, preferably 30 to 45 minutes before meals.
- If you take the extended-release tablets, don't chew or crush them.

Possible side effects:

Loss of appetite	Nervousness
Trouble sleeping	Stomach pain
Rapid heartbeat	Vision problems
Slow growth rate in children	

Possible interactions:

- Methylphenidate may keep the blood pressure drug guanethidine from working well.
- It may increase levels or effects of anticlotting drugs like warfarin, the anti-inflammatory phenylbutazone, tricyclic antidepressants, and the anticonvulsants phenobarbital, diphenylhydantoin, and primidone.

Other important information:

- People who are very anxious, tense, agitated, or emotionally unstable should not take this drug.
- If you have glaucoma, involuntary muscle movements known as "tics," or Tourette's syndrome (or a family history of it), don't use this drug.
- Methylphenidate may increase the risk of seizures, and you should use it cautiously if you have a history of seizures. If you have a seizure, your doctor should stop your methylphenidate treatment.
- People with high blood pressure should use this drug very cautiously. Have your blood pressure checked regularly while you're taking methylphenidate.
- Have regular blood tests while taking this drug.

METHYLPREDNISOLONE

Pregnancy category: C

Brand:

Medrol

This corticosteroid drug is used to treat or ease the symptoms of various disorders including the following: arthritis and related rheumatic diseases, endocrine disorders, lupus and other collagen diseases, allergic reactions, respiratory diseases, kidney disorders, skin diseases, blood disorders (various anemias), eye diseases, leukemia, colitis, enteritis, meningitis, and trichinosis.

How to take this drug:

- Methylprednisolone is available as tablets, injection, or retention enema.
- Take with food to prevent upset stomach.

Possible side effects:

Sleeplessness
Ulcers
Convulsions
Muscle weakness
Menstrual changes
Cataracts

Bloating
Headache
Slow healing of wounds
Worsening of diabetes
Glaucoma

Possible interactions:

* Methylprednisolone may increase the risk of convulsions if taken with the antibiotic cyclosporin.

Other important information:

* People with fungal infections should not use this drug.
* Corticosteroid drugs may weaken your immune system and decrease your natural resistance to infections. Call your doctor immediately at the first sign of fever or infection.
* Don't get any vaccinations and let your doctor know right away if you are exposed to chicken pox or measles.
* If you have high blood pressure, osteoporosis, diabetes, cirrhosis, underactive thyroid, myasthenia gravis (muscle weakness disease), poor kidney function, or diverticulitis, take this drug with caution.
* Methylprednisolone may cause or aggravate emotional or psychotic problems. Call your doctor if you experience any changes in mood.
* This drug may cause you to lose calcium and potassium and retain salt. You may need to restrict your salt intake and take potassium supplements.
* Most people will experience very few side effects if they take methylprednisolone for 10 days or less. Long-term use can cause many serious side effects.
* If you've been taking high doses of methylprednisolone or you've been taking it for a long time, don't suddenly quit taking it. Withdrawing rapidly could cause nausea, fever, fainting, and even death.

METHYSERGIDE MALEATE

Pregnancy category: X
No driving

Brand:

Sansert

This drug is used to prevent migraine headaches or, at least, reduce their frequency and intensity.

Possible side effects:

Diarrhea
Heartburn

Constipation
Dizziness when standing suddenly

Drowsiness   Nausea or vomiting
Sleeplessness

Possible interactions:
- If you take methysergide along with alcohol or tranquilizers, antihistamines, or muscle relaxants, the combination may dangerously depress
your nervous system.

Other important information:
- Methysergide should only be used to treat frequent, severe migraines
that don't respond to other treatments.
- It should not be used at the beginning of an attack.
- It should not be used by people with severe high blood pressure, coronary artery disease, severe arteriosclerosis, lung disease, poor liver or
kidney function, peripheral vascular disease, disease of the heart valves,
inflammation of the veins or connective tissues in the legs, collagen disease or fibrosis, or serious infections. Long-term treatment may cause
fibrosis, which may affect the heart or lungs.
- Call your doctor immediately if you have any of the following symptoms: leg cramps or swelling, chest pain, back pain, cold or numbness
in hands or feet, or a change in the normal amount of urine.
- A serious risk of using methysergide for long periods of time is scar-
ring inside your chest, stomach, heart valves, lungs, kidneys, and major
blood vessels.

METOCLOPRAMIDE HYDROCHLORIDE

Pregnancy category: B
No driving   MAO warning

Brand:
Reglan

Metoclopramide is used to treat severe heartburn (stomach acid washing
back up into the esophagus), nausea and vomiting after surgery or cancer
chemotherapy, and a condition called diabetic gastroparesis (delayed emptying of the stomach).

Possible side effects:
Restlessness   Drowsiness
Tiredness

Possible interactions:
- If you take metoclopramide along with tranquilizers, alcohol, antihistamines, or muscle relaxers, the combination may dangerously depress
your nervous system.
- Metoclopramide may increase levels or effects of the analgesic acetaminophen, the antibiotic tetracycline, and the antiparkinson drug levodopa.

- Metoclopramide may decrease levels of the heart drug digoxin.
- Effects of metoclopramide may be reduced by narcotic analgesics and anticholinergics.

Other important information:
- People with bleeding in the stomach or some kind of intestinal blockage should not take metoclopramide.
- People with pheochromocytoma (tumor of the adrenal system) should not use metoclopramide because it can cause severe high blood pressure.
- People with epilepsy or people taking drugs that can cause nerve and muscle disorders (such as tardive dyskinesia) shouldn't take this drug. Metoclopramide increases your risk of seizures and nerve disorders.
- Use this drug cautiously if you have a history of depression, Parkinson's disease, or high blood pressure.
- A dangerous but rare side effect is tardive dyskinesia, a disorder where certain muscles or muscle groups move slowly and uncontrollably (like lip smacking, or puffing of cheeks). This side effect may not go away when you quit taking the drug.
- Let your doctor know immediately if you experience any unusual movements, trembling, or spasms since this drug can also cause other nerve or muscle disorders.

METOLAZONE

Pregnancy category: B

Brand:
Zaroxolyn

This diuretic is used to reduce blood pressure and the swelling and fluid retention associated with congestive heart failure and kidney disease.

Possible side effects:
Muscle or joint pain	Muscle spasms
Jaundice	Constipation
Nausea or vomiting	Diarrhea
Loss of appetite	Bloating
Headache	Fainting
Dizziness	Weakness
Tingling	Rapid heartbeat
Chest pain	Skin problems
Sensitivity to light	

Possible interactions:
- Metolazone may increase the effects of other blood-pressure-lowering drugs.
- Metolazone may cause the antipsychotic drug lithium to build up to toxic levels.

- Effects of metolazone may be decreased by the urinary antiseptic methenamine and some nonsteroidal anti-inflammatory drugs (NSAIDs), such as aspirin.
- If you take metolazone along with alcohol or tranquilizers, antihistamines, or muscle relaxers, the combination may dangerously depress your nervous system.
- If you take metolazone with the heart drug digitalis, the combination may cause irregular heartbeat.
- If you take it with corticosteroids, the combination may increase potassium loss and cause salt and water retention.
- If you take it with the muscle relaxer tubocurarine, the combination may cause respiratory depression.
- Since metolazone may raise blood sugar levels, people with diabetes may need adjustments to their doses of insulin or other glucose-lowering agents if they begin taking metolazone.

Other important information:
- Don't use metolazone if you are allergic to thiazides or sulfonamide-derived drugs.
- Don't interchange Zaroxolyn with the related diuretic called Mykrox.
- People with poor kidney function should use metolazone with caution.
- Your doctor should check your electrolyte balances frequently if you get sick and are vomiting or have diarrhea, have heart failure, kidney disease, or liver disease, or if you are taking ACTH or corticosteroids.
- This drug can cause dangerously low levels of potassium. Contact your doctor if you experience unusual thirst, tiredness, drowsiness, restlessness, muscle pains or cramps, nausea, or rapid heart rate. And eat extra potassium-rich foods like bananas.
- Weigh daily so you'll know if you're losing too much fluid, which can cause dehydration and possibly blood clots. Warning signs include dry mouth, thirst, drowsiness, and weakness. Contact your doctor immediately if you stop urinating.
- If you have high blood pressure, avoid using over-the-counter cold remedies or diet pills, which can increase blood pressure.
- Be on the lookout for signs that this drug is depressing your immune system: fever, sore throat, tiredness, weakness, bruising, or unusual bleeding. Have your blood tested regularly.
- Metolazone may increase levels of uric acid in the blood (this puts you at risk for gout) and may worsen symptoms of lupus.

METOPROLOL SUCCINATE

Pregnancy category: C
No driving

Brand:
Toprol-XL

Metoprolol succinate lowers blood pressure, reduces the number of angina attacks, and is used for long-term treatment of angina pectoris.

How to take this drug:
- Do not stop taking this drug abruptly.
- Never double a missed dose, instead take it as soon as you remember or skip it and go on with your regular schedule.
- Do not chew or crush the tablets.

Possible side effects:

Fatigue	Dizziness
Depression	Confusion
Short-term memory loss	Headache
Nightmares	Sleeplessness
Shortness of breath	Slow heartbeat
Diarrhea	Skin rash

Possible interactions:
- Make sure your doctor knows if you are taking digitalis or diuretics to control congestive heart failure before adding metropolol succinate.
- May cause low blood pressure or slowed heart rate if taken with a catecholamine depletor, like reserpine.

Other important information:
- This drug should be used with care by those with bronchitis, asthma, diabetes, hypoglycemia, or liver problems.
- Tell your doctor or dentist you are on this drug before having any kind of surgery.

METOPROLOL TARTRATE

Pregnancy category: C
No driving

Brand:
Lopressor

Metoprolol is a beta blocker that controls high blood pressure and regulates heart rhythm.

How to take this drug:
- Take metoprolol with or after meals.

Possible side effects:

Tiredness	Dizziness
Memory loss	Depression
Mental confusion	Nightmares
Sleeplessness	Irregular heartbeat
Numbness or tingling in hands or feet	Headache
	Fainting

Chest pain	Rash
Itching	Blurred vision
Muscle pain	Ringing in the ears

Possible interactions:
- Taking metoprolol with the blood pressure drug reserpine can cause your blood pressure to drop to a very low level.
- Metoprolol may decrease the effects of the asthma drug epinephrine.

Other important information:
- Don't take this drug if you have emphysema, bronchitis, heart block, cardiac shock, heart failure, or slow heartbeat. It can aggravate asthma symptoms and make congestive heart failure worse.
- If you have diabetes, use this drug cautiously because beta blockers can mask the signs of low blood sugar.
- Metoprolol can also mask signs of an overactive thyroid.
- People with poor liver function should take this drug cautiously.
- Tell your doctor immediately if you have any signs of congestive heart failure such as night cough; swelling of your legs, feet, or hands; or difficulty breathing, especially when lying down or after physical exertion.
- You may have to discontinue this drug before any surgery.
- Never quit taking this drug without talking to your doctor. It could increase your risk of angina and heart attack.

METRONIDAZOLE

Pregnancy category: B

Brand:

Flagyl	*MetroGel*
Noritate	*Protostat*
Metrocream	*MetroGel-Vaginal*
Metrolotion	*Metromidol*

Metronidazole is used to treat many serious bacterial infections, including endocarditis, lower respiratory tract infections, bone and joint infections, skin and skin structure infections, certain stomach infections, cervical and vaginal infections, blood poisoning, and meningitis. The gel form is used to treat rosacea.

How to take this drug:
- Metronidazole is available as a cream, gel, capsule, or injectable drug.
- You can take this drug with or without food. If it upsets your stomach, take it with food.

Possible side effects:

Headache	Nausea
Loss of appetite	Diarrhea
Constipation	Stomach cramps

Seizures	Dizziness
Sleeplessness	Depression
Confusion	Irritability
Urination problems	Painful sexual intercourse
Taste disturbances	Inflamed rectum or anus
Joint pain	

Possible interactions:
- Avoid alcohol while you're taking metronidazole. The combination may cause stomach cramps, vomiting, or headache.
- Metronidazole may increase levels of the anticoagulant warfarin and the seizure drug phenytoin.
- Metronidazole may decrease the excretion of the antipsychotic drug lithium, which can build up to toxic levels.
- Levels or effects of metronidazole may be increased by the ulcer drug cimetidine.

Other important information:
- If you have any disease of the central nervous system, Crohn's disease, or blood disorders, use this drug with caution.
- Metronidazole may lower your red blood cell count and cause anemia, or it may lower your white blood cell count and therefore lower your immunity.
- One possible side effect is the growth of a yeast infection in the mouth or vagina. A furry tongue or inflammation of the mouth or tongue may accompany the yeast infection in the mouth.
- Metronidazole may damage nerve tissues in your extremities. Symptoms include numbness or tingling in the hands or feet, lack of muscle coordination, and weakness.
- Don't be alarmed if the drug turns your urine a deep red-brown color or if you have a metallic taste in your mouth. These harmless side effects will go away when you quit taking the drug.

MEXILETINE HYDROCHLORIDE

Pregnancy category: C

Brand:
Mexitil

Mexiletine is an antiarrhythmic used to correct irregular heartbeats to a normal rhythm.

Possible side effects:

Upset stomach (nausea, vomiting, and heartburn)	Dizziness or lightheadedness
	Shakiness
Lack of coordination	Diarrhea
Constipation	Swelling
Difficulty breathing	Chest pain

Headache	Vision problems
Depression	Numbness or tingling
Sleep disorders	Rash

Possible interactions:
- Mexiletine may increase the effects of the asthma drug theophylline.
- Levels or effects of mexiletine may be decreased by the tuberculosis drug rifampin, the seizure drug phenytoin, and the sedative phenobarbital.

Other important information:
- People with some types of heart rhythm disorders should not use this drug.
- Because mexiletine can make some arrhythmias worse, it should only be used for serious arrhythmias.
- If you have heart disease, heart block or congestive heart failure; low blood pressure; or poor liver function, use this drug very carefully.
- Be on the lookout for signs that this drug is depressing your immune system: fever, sore throat, tiredness, weakness, bruising, or unusual bleeding. Have your blood tested regularly.
- Have regular liver function tests and blood counts while you're taking this drug.

MICONAZOLE NITRATE

Pregnancy category: C

Brand:

Monistat-Derm   *Monistat 3*
Monistat 5

This drug is used to treat fungal infections such as athlete's foot, jock itch, ringworm, tinea versicolor, and yeast infections.

How to take this drug:
- Miconazole is available as a cream, powder, solution, or spray. The vaginal cream and suppositories treat vaginal yeast infections.
- Avoid contact with your eyes, nose, and mouth.
- Clean and dry the infected area before applying the medicine.
- Do not wrap or bandage the area after you apply the medicine (unless your doctor tells you to).
- For the vaginal cream, insert the cream high into the vagina. Continue taking this drug during menstruation, but wear a sanitary napkin instead of a tampon. If you have sexual intercourse during treatment, the male partner should use a condom.

Possible side effects:

Burning and itching	Rash
Hives	Irritation

Other important information:
- Use miconazole cautiously if your skin is blistered, raw, or oozing.
- Use the full course of treatment even if symptoms improve. Contact your doctor if ringworm, jock itch, or yeast infections have not improved within two weeks or if athlete's foot has not improved after four weeks.
- If the vaginal cream causes burning or irritation, contact your doctor.
- Report side effects to your doctor. You may be having an allergic reaction.

MINOCYCLINE HYDROCHLORIDE

Pregnancy category: D
No driving

Brand:
Dynacin   *Minocin*
Vectrin

This antibiotic is used to treat infections caused by various bacteria and microorganisms.

How to take this drug:
- You can take this drug with or without food or milk.
- Never double a missed dose, instead take it as soon as you remember or skip it and go on with your regular schedule.

Possible side effects:

Itching	Swelling
Rash	Joint pain
Sensitivity to sunlight	Loss of appetite
Worsening of lupus	Difficulty swallowing
Nausea	Diarrhea
Darkening of the skin	Colitis

Possible interactions:
- Antacids may decrease absorption of this drug, so take this drug two hours before or after antacids.
- Iron-containing products also reduce absorption, so take these at least three hours before or two hours after taking this drug.
- This drug may increase the levels or effects of anticoagulants and decrease the effects of oral contraceptives.
- Do not take with the antibiotic penicillin.

Other important information:
- Don't use this drug if you are allergic to tetracycline.
- If you have liver or kidney problems, tetracyclines can accumulate to toxic levels in your body.
- Taking an antibiotic for a long time can cause bacteria or fungus to overgrow, leading to another infection (fungal infections of the mouth, anus, or vagina). If you get one of these "superinfections," you may

need to quit taking minocycline and start taking another antibiotic for the second infection.

- Be on the lookout for signs that this drug is depressing your immune system: fever, sore throat, tiredness, weakness, bruising, or unusual bleeding. Have your blood tested regularly.
- Minocycline may cause increased pressure on the brain in adults. Let your doctor know immediately if you develop signs of this high pressure: headache, nausea, and visual disturbances. Minocycline may also cause bulging "soft spots" on babies' heads.
- This drug may make your skin extra-sensitive to sunlight, so protect your skin if you'll be outdoors. Tell your doctor if you develop a severe sunburn or rash.

MINOXIDIL

Pregnancy category: C

Brand:

Loniten

Minoxidil is usually used with a diuretic to control severely high blood pressure. A weaker form is available over-the-counter for male pattern baldness.

Possible side effects:

Thickening, lengthening, and darkening of body hair
Tiredness
Fluid and salt retention

Nausea or vomiting
Headache
Rash

Possible interactions:

- If you take minoxidil with the blood pressure drug guanethidine, the combination may cause dangerously low blood pressure.

Other important information:

- People who have recently had a heart attack should not use minoxidil.
- Minoxidil should not be taken by people with pheochromocytoma, a type of tumor that may be stimulated to grow larger by this drug.
- People with kidney problems may need smaller doses.
- Be on the lookout for signs that this drug is depressing your immune system: fever, sore throat, tiredness, weakness, bruising, or unusual bleeding. Have your blood tested regularly.
- Minoxidil may cause various heart problems, such as a rapid heartbeat and angina. Your doctor may prescribe a beta blocker for this side effect.
- This drug can cause you to retain fluid, which can lead to congestive heart failure. If fluids accumulate in the cavity around the heart, your doctor may take you off the drug for a while. Weigh yourself at least once a week and report to your doctor any gain over 5 pounds.

MIRTAZAPINE

Pregnancy category: C
No driving   MAO warning

Brand:
Remeron

Mirtazapine is used to treat depression.

How to take this drug:
- Take with or without food.
- Continue taking the full course of treatment even if you feel better.

Possible side effects:
Sleepiness	Dizziness
Increased appetite	Weight gain
Dry mouth	Constipation

Possible interactions:
- Avoid taking diazepam while on this drug.
- If you are taking mirtazapine along with other antidepressants and develop nausea, vomiting, flushing, dizziness, tremors, seizures, sweating, or agitation, see your doctor immediately. This could be a serious, even fatal interaction.

Other important information:
- Be careful taking this drug if you have liver or kidney problems.
- Mirtazapine has not been tested for long-term use (longer than six weeks).
- Tell your doctor immediately if you develop signs of an infection (sore throat, fever, flu-like symptoms, etc.). This drug may have affected your white blood count and left you susceptible to infection.
- Mirtazapine may increase your cholesterol or triglyceride levels.
- Use this drug carefully if you have a history of seizures, manic or hypomanic behavior, or suffer from a metabolic disorder.
- Since mirtazapine can cause your blood pressure to drop if you stand up suddenly, be careful if you have a heart condition that could make this side effect worse.

MISOPROSTOL

Pregnancy category: X

Brand:
Cytotec

Misoprostol is used to prevent stomach ulcers in certain people who take nonsteroidal anti-inflammatory drugs (NSAIDs).

How to take this drug:
- To help prevent diarrhea while on this drug, take your doses after meals and at bedtime.

Possible side effects:

Diarrhea	Stomach pain
Nausea	Gas
Constipation	Indigestion
Headache	

Possible interactions:

- Don't take magnesium-containing antacids when you take this medicine.

Other important information:

- Don't take this drug if you are allergic to prostaglandins.
- Your doctor should watch you closely if you have inflammatory bowel disease.
- Women taking misoprostol may experience menstrual problems such as excessive or painful menstruation, spotting or cramps, or postmenopausal vaginal bleeding.
- If you have severe diarrhea or side effects that last longer than eight days, call your doctor.

MODAFINIL

Pregnancy category: C
No driving

Brand:

Provigil

Modafinil helps people suffering from narcolepsy stay awake during the day.

Possible side effects:

Headache	Infection
Nausea	Nervousness
Anxiety	Sleeplessness

Possible interactions:

- Modafinil may interact with diazepam, phenytoin, warfarin, propranolol, methylphenidate, clomipramine, and MAO inhibitors.
- If you are taking steroidal contraceptives, cyclosporine, or theophylline in addition to modafinil, your dosages may have to be adjusted.

Other important information:

- This drug can change your mood, judgment, thinking, feelings, and motor skills.
- If you have severe kidney or liver problems, your dose of modafinil may have to be adjusted.

- Don't use it if you have a history of chest pain, arrhythmia, or mitral valve prolapse.
- Use it cautiously if you've recently suffered from angina or heart attack.
- Methods of birth control besides steroidal contraceptives are recommended while you are on modafinil.
- Modafinil may be slightly addictive. Prescription refills are controlled.

MOLINDONE HYDROCHLORIDE

Pregnancy category: NR
No driving

Brand:
Moban

This drug is a strong tranquilizer used to treat schizophrenia and aggressive or bizarre behavior, without causing muscle relaxation or lack of coordination.

Possible side effects:

Drowsiness	Depression
Blurred vision	Rapid heartbeat
Nausea	Dry mouth
Difficulty urinating	Constipation
Menstrual changes	Swollen breasts
Increased sex drive	Rash

Possible interactions:
- Don't use alcohol or other depressants while taking this drug.
- The molindone tablets contain calcium sulfate, which can decrease the absorption of phenytoin and tetracycline.

Other important information:
- Don't use this drug if you are already heavily sedated.
- This drug contains sulfites. Some people with asthma are sensitive to sulfites.
- There is a small risk of developing nerve problems from this drug. Tell your doctor immediately if you develop muscle weakness or spasms or difficulty speaking or swallowing.

MOMETASONE FUROATE

Pregnancy category: C

Brand:
Elocon

This corticosteroid is used to relieve and heal inflamed or irritated skin conditions including eczema, dermatitis, psoriasis, severe diaper rash, insect bites, minor burns, and sunburn.

How to take this drug:
- It is available as an ointment, cream, or lotion.
- Avoid contact with your eyes.
- Do not wrap or bandage the area after you apply the medicine unless your doctor tells you to. For diaper rash, you should not use tight-fitting diapers or plastic pants after applying this medicine.

Possible side effects:

Irritation	Burning or itching
Dryness	Acne
Skin discoloration	Infection
Weakening and wasting of the skin	Excessive hair growth
	Dermatitis around the mouth
Blocked sweat glands	Streaks on the skin

Other important information:
- Don't use this drug if you are allergic to other steroid creams.
- Don't use this drug for longer than prescribed.
- Very high doses or long-term use in children may cause Cushing's syndrome, a disease of the adrenal gland. Signs of this disease include weight gain and slow growth. Children are also at risk for developing increased pressure in the brain. Signs are headache and bulging "soft spots."
- If your skin is infected, you'll also need an antifungal or antibacterial medicine.
- If you are covering a very large area of your skin and therefore using lots of medicine, you should be tested regularly for hypothalamic-pituitary-adrenal axis suppression. Regular testing could prevent severe side effects and withdrawal symptoms associated with steroids.

MOMETASONE FUROATE MONOHYDRATE

Pregnancy category: C

Brand:
Nasonex

This medication is an anti-inflammatory corticosteroid used to prevent and treat the runny, stuffy nose associated with allergies.

How to take this drug:
- You must use this nasal spray regularly in order for it to be effective.

Possible side effects:

Headache	Viral infection
Sore throat	Cough
Upper respiratory infection	Menstrual pain
Muscle pain	

Possible interactions:
Interactions are rare.

Other important information:
- If you have been treating your allergies with oral steroids, changing to this kind of medication could cause some withdrawal symptoms (joint or muscular pain, depression, fatigue).
- Let your doctor know if you are exposed to chickenpox or measles.
- If you have tuberculosis, ocular herpes simplex, or other systemic infections, talk to your doctor before starting on this medication.
- Don't use this type of nasal spray if you have recently had nasal surgery, an injury to your nose, or some other kind of wound that must heal.
- Nasal corticosteroids have been associated with the development of glaucoma and cataracts. See your eye doctor if you experience any vision problems.

MONTELUKAST SODIUM

Pregnancy category: B

Brand:
Singulair

Montelukast sodium is taken to prevent and treat asthma.

How to take this drug:
- Take with or without food.
- Take it daily even if you have no asthma symptoms.

Possible side effects:

Tiredness	Fever
Stomach pain	Upset stomach
Heartburn	Dizziness
Headache	Cough

Possible interactions:
- If you are aspirin sensitive, don't take aspirin or NSAIDs while you are taking this drug.

Other important information:
- Don't take this drug to relieve an asthma attack.
- Those with PKU (phenylketonuria) who are on a low-phenylalanine diet should know that the chewable tablets contain phenylalanine (a part of aspartame).

MORPHINE SULFATE

Pregnancy category: C
No driving

Brand:
Kadian   *MS Contin*
MSIR

This narcotic analgesic relieves moderate to severe pain.

How to take this drug:
- Don't crush or break the morphine tablets as it may lead to rapid absorption and possible overdose.
- You may want to lie down for a while after you take morphine to help prevent some of the side effects.

Possible side effects:

Breathing problems	Constipation
Dizziness or lightheadedness	Sleepiness
Sweating	Mood changes
Nightmares	Nausea or vomiting
Difficulty urinating	Sweating

Possible interactions:
- If you take morphine along with alcohol or tranquilizers, antihistamines, or muscle relaxants, the combination may dangerously depress your nervous system.

Other important information:
- Don't use morphine if you are allergic to narcotics, have asthma, breathing difficulty, or paralysis of the intestines.
- Morphine should be used with extreme caution by people with head injuries, lesions or increased pressure in the skull, or respiratory depression.
- Use morphine with caution if you have any of the following conditions: inflammation of the pancreas, swelling and fluid retention associated with underactive thyroid, alcoholism or alcohol withdrawal, Addison's disease (progressive weakening of the adrenal gland), enlarged prostate, psychosis resulting from exposure to a toxic substance, coma, curvature of the spine, or liver, kidney, or lung disease.
- The major risks of taking this drug are slowed or irregular breathing (some people have stopped breathing), and slowed circulation (some people have had cardiac arrest, which means their circulation has stopped).
- You may become physically and psychologically dependent on this drug. Never take more medicine than you are prescribed.
- This drug can cause very low blood pressure. Be careful when you stand or sit up quickly — you may feel lightheaded and dizzy.

MUPIROCIN

Pregnancy category: B

Brand:
Bactroban

This antibiotic ointment is used to treat the symptoms of the skin disease impetigo.

How to take this drug:

- Apply a small amount of ointment to the affected area three times a day. You can cover the area with a loose gauze dressing.
- Avoid contact with your eyes.

Possible side effects:

Burning, stinging, or itching	Pain
Contact dermatitis	Swelling
Rash	Dry skin
Nausea	

Other important information:

- People with kidney problems should use this drug with caution.
- If you haven't seen any improvement in three to five days, contact your doctor.

MYCOPHENOLATE MOFETIL

Pregnancy category: C

Brand:

CellCept

Mycophenolate mofetil prevents your body from rejecting transplanted heart and kidneys.

How to take this drug:

- Mycophenolate mofetil is available either as a capsule or as an injectable solution.

Possible side effects:

Body pain	Fever
Headache	Infection
Weakness	Diarrhea
Constipation	Nausea or vomiting
Indigestion	Difficulty breathing
Heart disorders	Weight gain
Cough	Rash
Sleeplessness	Dizziness
Anxiety	Tremors

Possible interactions:

- Don't take this drug with azathioprine or cholestyramine.
- Mycophenolate mofetil may interact with acyclovir, ganciclovir, or oral contraceptives.
- Don't take mycophenolate mofetil and antacids containing magnesium and aluminum hydroxides at the same time.

Other important information:

- This drug is used along with cyclosporine and corticosteroids.

- Taking an immunosuppressant, like mycophenolate mofetil, can make you more likely to develop infections.
- This drug increases your risk of developing skin cancer. Limit your exposure to sunlight and use a sunscreen.
- Tell your doctor of any signs of infection, bruising, or bleeding.
- If you suffer from any serious digestive disorder (ulcers, etc.) use this drug cautiously.
- Be aware that mycophenolate mofetil contains aspartame.
- Your blood must be monitored regularly while on this medication.

NABUMETONE

Pregnancy category: C

Brand:
Relafen

This nonsteroidal anti-inflammatory drug (NSAID) is used to relieve the pain and inflammation associated with arthritis.

How to take this drug:
- Take with food, after meals, or with antacids to help prevent stomach irritation.

Possible side effects:

Nausea	Diarrhea
Constipation	Stomach pain or cramps
Bloody stool	Indigestion
Gas	Loss of appetite
Fluid retention	Ringing in the ears
Itching	Rash
Dizziness	Fatigue
Headache	Dry mouth
Sleeplessness	

Possible interactions:
- Avoid alcohol and any products containing aspirin while taking nabumetone.
- Nabumetone may increase the effects of the anticoagulant warfarin.

Other important information:
- Don't use nabumetone if you are allergic to aspirin or other aspirin substitutes such as NSAIDs.
- People with stomach ulcer should not take this drug. It may cause gastrointestinal bleeding.
- Taking nabumetone is more likely to cause kidney problems if you are elderly, if you take diuretics, or if you have lupus, heart failure, or poor liver or kidney function.

- Take this drug with caution if you have liver abnormalities, high blood pressure, or heart failure.
- Be on the lookout for signs that this drug is depressing your immune system: fever, sore throat, tiredness, weakness, bruising, or unusual bleeding. Have your blood tested regularly.
- Bleeding stomach ulcers and liver or kidney damage are rare but serious reactions to using nabumetone for long periods of time. Warning signs of liver damage include nausea, tiredness, red and itchy skin, yellow eyes and skin (jaundice), and flu-like symptoms.

NADOLOL

Pregnancy category: C
No driving

Brand:
Corgard

Nadolol is a beta blocker used to treat and control high blood pressure and angina.

Possible side effects:

Slow heartbeat	Leg pain
Dizziness	Mental depression
Difficulty breathing	Tiredness
Diarrhea	Nausea
Wheezing	Drowsiness
Cold, tingling fingers and toes	

Possible interactions:
- Taking nadolol and the high blood pressure drug reserpine together may cause very low blood pressure.
- Nadolol may increase the effects of anesthesia.
- Nadolol may decrease the effects of the asthma drug epinephrine.

Other important information:
- People with abnormally slow heartbeat, congestive heart failure, heart block, or cardiogenic shock should not take nadolol.
- If you have circulatory disorders, bronchitis, emphysema, or liver or kidney problems, take nadolol with caution.
- If you have diabetes, use this drug cautiously because beta blockers can mask the signs of low blood sugar.
- Nadolol can also mask signs of an overactive thyroid.
- Nadolol can raise your cholesterol and triglyceride levels.
- Never quit taking this drug without talking to your doctor. It could increase your risk of angina and heart attack.
- Tell your doctor immediately if you have any signs of congestive heart failure such as night cough; swelling of your legs, feet, or hands; or difficulty breathing, especially when lying down or after physical exertion.

Nafarelin acetate

Pregnancy category: X

Brand:
Synarel

This nasal spray is used to treat endometriosis.

Possible side effects:

Hot flashes	Headache
Acne	Muscle pain
Sleeplessness	Vaginal dryness
Nasal irritation	Decreased sex drive
Reduction in breast size	Emotional instability

Possible interactions:
* Do not use a spray decongestant within two hours of this drug.

Other important information:
* Don't use nafarelin acetate if you have any abnormal, undiagnosed vaginal bleeding.
* If you smoke, drink, have a family history of osteoporosis, or use any other drugs, such as corticosteroids or anticonvulsants that may cause bone loss, use this drug with caution.
* This drug may cause cysts to form on the ovaries.
* Nafarelin acetate should cause menstruation to stop. Notify your doctor if regular menstrual periods persist.
* Avoid sneezing while using this spray or immediately afterwards as the drug may not be absorbed correctly.

Naltrexone hydrochloride

Pregnancy category: C

Brand:
ReVia

Naltrexone hydrochloride is part of a treatment program for alcoholism or drug dependence.

How to take this drug:
* Don't start taking this product unless you have gone 7 to 10 days without opioids.
* This drug is available in tablet form or as an injectable solution.

Possible side effects:

Nausea or vomiting	Headache
Dizziness	Nervousness
Tiredness	Sleeplessness
Anxiety	Abdominal pain
Joint or muscle pain	

Possible interactions:
- Naltrexone hydrochloride and thioridazine may cause dullness and sleepiness.
- Taking this drug with cough and cold medicines, antidiarrheals, and narcotic painkillers could cause breathing difficulties.

Other important information:
- Don't take naltrexone hydrochloride if you are taking narcotic painkillers, are dependent on opioids, are in acute opioid withdrawal, have acute hepatitis or liver failure.
- After going through this drug treatment program, you may be more sensitive to lower doses of opioids.
- Use this drug cautiously if you have kidney problems.
- While on this medication, carry an identification card to alert medical personnel that you are taking naltrexone hydrochloride.
- See your doctor immediately if you develop abdominal pain, white bowel movements, dark urine, or yellow eyes.
- Monitor your liver regularly while you are on this drug.

NAPROXEN

Pregnancy category: B
No driving

Brand:
Naprosyn	EC-Naprosyn
Anaprox	Anaprox DS
Naprelan	

This nonsteroidal anti-inflammatory drug (NSAID) relieves the pain and symptoms of rheumatoid arthritis, juvenile arthritis, osteoarthritis, tendinitis, bursitis, gout, and ankylosing spondylitis. It is also used to relieve painful menstruation and mild to moderate pain from other conditions.

Possible side effects:
Nausea	Diarrhea
Constipation	Stomach pain or cramps
Indigestion	Inflamed mouth or tongue
Headache	Dizziness
Rapid heartbeat	Drowsiness
Itching	Sweating
Skin problems	Ringing in the ears
Vision abnormalities	Thirst
Water retention	

Possible interactions:
- Naproxen and naproxen sodium drugs should not be taken at the same time.
- Avoid alcohol and any products containing aspirin while taking naproxen.

- Naproxen may increase the risk of bleeding if taken with the anticoagulant warfarin.
- Naproxen may increase the levels or effects of the antipsychotic drug lithium and the cancer drug methotrexate, possibly increasing them to toxic levels.
- Naproxen may decrease the effects of the diuretic furosemide and the beta blocker propranolol.
- The gout drug probenecid may increase the effects of naproxen, which may increase the risk of intestinal problems.

Other important information:
- Anaprox, Anaprox DS, and Naprelan contain naproxen and sodium. If you are on a low-sodium diet, talk to your doctor before taking these drugs.
- Don't use naproxen if you are allergic to aspirin or other aspirin substitutes such as NSAIDs.
- People with stomach ulcers should not take this drug. It may cause gastrointestinal bleeding.
- Taking naproxen is more likely to cause kidney problems if you are elderly, if you take diuretics, or if you have lupus, heart failure, or poor liver or kidney function.
- Take this drug with caution if you have liver abnormalities, high blood pressure, or heart failure.
- Be on the lookout for signs that this drug is depressing your immune system: fever, sore throat, tiredness, weakness, bruising, or unusual bleeding. Have your blood tested regularly.
- Bleeding stomach ulcers and liver or kidney damage are rare but serious reactions to using naproxen for long periods of time. Warning signs of liver damage include nausea, tiredness, red and itchy skin, yellow eyes and skin (jaundice), and flu-like symptoms.

NARATRIPTAN HYDROCHLORIDE

Pregnancy category: C

Brand:
Amerge

This drug is used for the short-term treatment of migraines. It is not meant to prevent migraines or to decrease the number of migraine attacks. It has not been proven to treat cluster headaches.

How to take this drug:
- Take naratriptan hydrochloride with fluids any time after headache begins.
- Don't take a second tablet without checking with your doctor to make sure that your symptoms are not being caused by a more serious condition.
- Don't take more than 5 mg within any 24-hour period.

Possible side effects:

Pain or tightness in the chest or throat (if severe call your doctor)
Drowsiness
Nausea or vomiting

Numbness, prickling, or tingling
Dizziness
Fatigue
Ear, nose, and throat infections

Possible interactions:

- If you have taken other migraine medications containing naratriptan, or medications containing ergotamine, dihydroergotamine, or methysergide within the past 24 hours, do not take this drug.
- Selective serotonin reuptake inhibitors (SSRIs) like fluoxetine, fluvoxamine, paroxetine, or sertraline, may cause side effects if taken with this drug.

Other important information:

- Don't take naratriptan hydrochloride if you have a history of heart or circulatory disease, including heart attack, angina (chest pain), or stroke, uncontrolled high blood pressure, severe kidney or liver disease, hemiplegic or basilar migraine.
- Talk to your doctor about this drug if you are obese, postmenopausal, have diabetes, smoke, or are a male over 40.

NEFAZODONE HYDROCHLORIDE

Pregnancy category: C
No driving   MAO warning

Brand:

Serzone

Nefazodone hydrochloride is used to treat depression.

How to take this drug:

- Never double a missed dose, instead take it as soon as you remember or skip it and go on with your regular schedule.

Possible side effects:

Headache
Dry mouth
Dizziness or lightheadedness
Constipation
Diarrhea
Weakness
Sore throat
Memory problems

Sleepiness
Nausea
Sleeplessness
Indigestion
Confusion
Nervousness
Vision problems

Possible interactions:

- Don't take nefazodone hydrochloride with triazolam (Halcion), alprazolam (Xanax), cisapride (Propulsid), or pimozide (Orap).

- If you take buspirone, your dose may need to be lowered.
- Nefazodone hydrochloride may interact with other central nervous system drugs. Talk to your doctor.
- Have your doctor monitor you carefully if you take nefazodone hydrochloride with digoxin, simvastatin, or cyclosporine.
- If you combine this drug with lovastatin, simvastatin, or atorvastatin, you may develop a rare but often fatal muscle disease call rhabdomyolysis.

Other important information:
- Use this drug carefully if you have heart or blood vessel disorders.
- Since nefazodone hydrochloride can cause postural hypotension (dizziness upon standing up suddenly), be careful taking it if you are dehydrated, have low blood volume, or are taking medication for high blood pressure.
- If you have a history of mania, talk to your doctor before taking this drug.
- If you have cirrhosis of the liver, you may need your dose of nefazodone hydrochloride adjusted.
- It may be several weeks before you see any improvement. Be sure and continue taking your medication even after you feel better.
- Stop taking nefazodone hydrochloride before surgery requiring general anesthesia.

NEOSTIGMINE BROMIDE

Pregnancy category: C

Brand:
Prostigmin

This muscle stimulant is used to treat myasthenia gravis (nerve/muscle weakness disease). It is also used after surgery to prevent urinary retention and to reverse the effects of muscle relaxants used during surgery.

Possible side effects:

Increased saliva	Muscle spasms
Stomach cramps	Diarrhea
Frequent urination	Small pupils
Extra mucus in your lungs	Increased sweating
Gas	Watery eyes

Possible interactions:
- Effects of neostigmine may be increased by the antibiotics neomycin, streptomycin, and kanamycin.
- Effects of neostigmine may be decreased by anesthetics, drugs that regulate heart rhythm, and drugs that relax muscles or relax the nervous system.

Other important information:
- Neostigmine should not be used by people with allergies to bromides, with intestinal or urinary obstructions, or with peritonitis.

- Neostigmine should be used with caution by people with ulcers, asthma, slow or irregular heartbeat, epilepsy, overactive thyroid, hypersensitivity of the parasympathetic nervous system, or by people who have recently had a blood clot in the heart.
- Check with your doctor immediately if you develop any other side effects.
- If you are taking the drug for myasthenia gravis, you may want to keep a daily record of your condition (when you are the most tired, when you have the most energy, etc.) to help your doctor determine the best dosing schedule for you.

NIACIN

Pregnancy category: C

Brand:
Nicolar   *Niaspan*
Niacor   *Slo-Niacin*

Niacin, or vitamin B3, controls cholesterol or triglyceride levels in some people when diet and exercise are not effective. It is a potent medicine, not just a vitamin.

How to take this drug:
- Take niacin with meals to reduce upset stomach, itching, and flushing.

Possible side effects:
Rapid or irregular heartbeat
Headache
Dry skin
Inflammatory disease of the
  skin (acanthosis nigricans)
Vomiting

Weakened vision
Abnormal pigmentation of the skin
Flushing
Itching
Diarrhea
Indigestion

Possible interactions:
- If you take niacin with the cholesterol-lowering drug lovastatin, your risk of rhabdomyolysis, a muscle disease, is increased.
- Niacin combined with blood-pressure-lowering drugs may cause very low blood pressure.
- Aspirin may increase levels or effects of niacin.
- Avoid alcohol and hot drinks as these may increase some side effects including itching and flushing.

Other important information:
- Niacin should not be used by alcoholics or people with poor liver function, bleeding from an artery, or stomach ulcer.
- This drug may cause the dangerous and sometimes fatal disease called rhabdomyolysis that destroys muscle tissue. Notify your doctor immediately if you develop any pain, tenderness, or weakness in your muscles.

- Niacin may cause stomach ulcers or aggravate diabetes or gout. If you already have diabetes, gout, gallbladder disease, heart disease, angina, jaundice, or have had a recent heart attack, take niacin with extreme caution.
- Liver function and blood sugar levels should be checked frequently.
- Time-release forms of niacin may cause severe liver damage. Warning signs include nausea, tiredness, red and itchy skin, yellow eyes and skin (jaundice), and flu-like symptoms.

NICARDIPINE HYDROCHLORIDE

Pregnancy category: C

Brand:

Cardene   *Cardene SR*

Nicardipine is a calcium channel blocker that lowers blood pressure and treats some forms of angina.

Possible side effects:

Headache	Dizziness
Weakness	Swelling
Flushing	Worsening of angina
Indigestion	Nausea
Dry mouth	Rash
Muscle pain	Rapid heartbeat
Prickling or tingling sensation	

Possible interactions:

- If you take nicardipine with beta blockers or the anesthetic fentanyl, the combination may cause very low blood pressure or heart irregularities.
- This drug may increase levels or effects of the immunosuppressant cyclosporine and the heart drug digoxin.
- The ulcer drug cimetidine may increase the levels or effects of nicardipine.

Other important information:

- People with narrowing of the aorta should not take this drug.
- Your doctor should prescribe this drug cautiously and monitor you carefully if you have heart failure, poor liver or kidney function, decreased blood supply to the brain (cerebral infarction), or hemorrhage in the brain.
- If you stop taking calcium channel blockers suddenly, your angina could get worse. Stop taking the drug gradually under your doctor's supervision.
- Your angina may get worse when you first start taking this drug or any time your doses are increased.

NICOTINE TRANSDERMAL SYSTEM

Pregnancy category: D

Brand:
Habitrol   *Nicoderm CG*
ProStep

This drug is used to help reduce nicotine withdrawal symptoms in people trying to quit smoking cigarettes.

How to take this drug:
- When you apply a new patch, choose a different area on your skin. Don't apply the patch to a previously used area for at least a week.
- Dispose of used patches carefully. There is still enough nicotine in a used patch to poison a child or a pet.

Possible side effects:
Rash, itching, or burning	Local swelling
Diarrhea	Indigestion
Muscle or joint pain	Abnormal dreams
Sleepiness	Headache

Possible interactions:
- This drug may increase levels of the pain reliever acetaminophen, the asthma drug theophylline, the blood pressure drug propranolol, the antianxiety and alcohol withdrawal drug oxazepam, the stimulant caffeine, the antidepressant imipramine, and the pain reliever pentazocine.
- For diabetics who use insulin, this drug may increase insulin levels, requiring a decrease in dose.
- Levels of the beta blocker labetalol and the blood pressure drug prazosin may also be increased while taking this drug.
- This drug may decrease levels or effects of the nervous system stimulant phenylephrine and the beta blocker/asthma drug isoproterenol.

Other important information:
- Don't use this drug if you have an allergy to nicotine or to any component of the transdermal patch, such as adhesive material. If skin irritation develops at the patch site, call your doctor.
- The use of this drug may seriously aggravate the following medical conditions: angina, heart attack, high blood pressure, diabetes, kidney or liver disease, overactive thyroid, stomach ulcer, and irregular heartbeat.
- Don't use any form of tobacco while you are being treated with this drug.

NIFEDIPINE

Pregnancy category: C

Brand:
Adalat   *Procardia*

Nifedipine is a calcium channel blocker used to treat angina.

Possible side effects:

Headache	Dizziness
Weakness	Nervousness
Rapid heartbeat	Wheezing and shortness of breath
Heartburn	Muscle cramps
Flushing	Swollen hands and feet
Nausea	

Possible interactions:

- If you take nifedipine with the anesthetic fentanyl, the combination may cause very low blood pressure.
- The ulcer drug cimetidine may increase the levels or effects of nifedipine.
- Nifedipine may increase the levels or effects of anticoagulants and the heart drug digoxin.
- Don't suddenly stop taking beta blockers before or during treatment with calcium channel blockers. It can make your angina worse.

Other important information:

- Your doctor should prescribe this drug cautiously and monitor you carefully if you have liver disease or kidney disease.
- Your angina may get worse when you first start taking this drug or any time your doses are increased.
- Tell your doctor immediately if you have any signs of congestive heart failure such as night cough; swelling and fluid retention in your legs, feet, or hands; or difficulty breathing, especially when lying down or after physical exertion.
- Have your blood pressure tested regularly, especially when you first start taking nifedipine.
- Be on the lookout for signs that this drug is depressing your immune system: fever, sore throat, tiredness, weakness, bruising, or unusual bleeding. Have your blood tested regularly.

NITROFURANTOIN

Pregnancy category: B

Brand:

Furadantin   *Macrobid*
Macrodantin

This antibacterial drug is used to treat urinary tract infections.

How to take this drug:

- Take with food or milk to help prevent upset stomach and to help your body absorb the drug.

Possible side effects:

Headache	Nausea
Gas	

Possible interactions:
* Antacids that contain magnesium trisilicate may increase the effects of this drug.
* Probenecid and sulfinpyrazone, drugs used to treat gout, may increase the effects of nitrofurantoin.

Other important information:
* People with poor kidney function, hemolytic anemia, or decreased urine output should not use this drug.
* This drug may cause hemolysis, a destruction of red blood cells, particularly in people with G6PD deficiency. Your doctor will stop your drug treatment if you have this side effect.
* People with poor liver function should use this drug with caution. It can cause liver damage, so watch out for warning signs like nausea, tiredness, red and itchy skin, yellow eyes and skin (jaundice), and flu-like symptoms.
* Don't be alarmed if the color of your urine becomes brownish.
* Taking an antibiotic for a long time can cause bacteria or fungus to overgrow, leading to another infection (such as a yeast infection of the mouth or skin). If you get one of these "superinfections," you may need to stop taking nitrofurantoin and start taking another antibiotic for the second infection.
* Nitrofurantoin may cause increased pressure on the brain. Signs of this high pressure include headache, nausea, and blurred vision. Let your doctor know immediately if you develop these symptoms.
* If you take nitrofurantoin for many months, you may be at risk for lung complications. Report any unusual tiredness, chest pain, difficulty breathing, fever, chills, or cough to your doctor.
* Be on the lookout for signs that this drug is depressing your immune system: fever, sore throat, tiredness, weakness, bruising, or unusual bleeding. Have your blood tested regularly.

NITROGLYCERIN

Pregnancy category: C

Brand:
Nitrostat

Nitroglycerin tablets prevent or relieve angina (chest pain) caused by coronary artery disease. It is also available as a patch (see next entry).

How to take this drug:
* Always store nitroglycerin tablets in the original glass container with the cap on.
* Sit quietly while taking this drug.
* Dissolve one tablet under your tongue or in the side of your cheek as soon as you feel the symptoms of an angina attack. Repeat as instructed by your doctor.

- You can take this drug five to 10 minutes before an activity that could bring on an attack.

Possible side effects:

Fainting	Nausea
Increased heart rate	Frequent headaches
Lightheadedness	

Possible interactions:

- Taking nitroglycerin with blood pressure-lowering drugs, beta blockers, tranquilizers, or anti-nausea drugs may cause dangerously low blood pressure.
- Aspirin may increase the effects of nitroglycerin in your system.

Other important information:

- People with allergies to nitrates should not take this drug.
- People with low blood pressure, a recent heart attack, or heart failure should take nitroglycerin with extreme caution.
- Stop taking nitroglycerin and call your doctor if you develop blurred vision or dry mouth.
- Since this drug can cause very low blood pressure and dizziness, sit or stand up slowly, and be careful on stairs.

NITROGLYCERIN TRANSDERMAL SYSTEM

Pregnancy category: C

Brand:

Minitran   *Nitro-Dur*
Transderm-Nitro

Nitroglycerin prevents angina (chest pain) caused by coronary artery disease.

How to take this drug:

- Don't place the patch on your arms below the elbow or on your legs below the knee.
- The patch area should be without hair, but do not shave.
- The patch area must be clean and very dry. Do not apply it just after showering or bathing.

Possible side effects:

Skin irritation	Frequent headaches
Lightheadedness	

Possible interactions:

- Nitroglycerin may interact with calcium channel blockers, causing dangerously low blood pressure.

Other important information:

- People with allergies to nitrates or adhesives should not use this drug.

- Talk to your doctor before using transdermal nitroglycerin if you have congestive heart failure or low blood pressure, or have suffered a recent heart attack.
- Nitroglycerin can cause a slow heartbeat and a worsening of your angina.
- You can become physically dependent on nitroglycerin, so don't stop taking it suddenly. You may experience withdrawal symptoms.
- Since this drug can cause very low blood pressure and dizziness, sit or stand up slowly, and be careful on stairs.

NIZATIDINE

Pregnancy category: C

Brand:
Axid

Nizatidine decreases the amount of acid your stomach produces. It helps stomach ulcers heal, treats gastroesophageal reflux disease (severe heartburn), controls bleeding in the stomach or intestines, and treats Zollinger-Ellison disease, a condition in which your stomach produces too much acid.

Possible side effects:

Hives	Irregular heartbeat
Sweating	Rash
Confusion	Headache
Diarrhea	Dizziness

Possible interactions:
- No significant interactions have been reported.

Other important information:
- Don't take nizatidine if you are allergic to any anti-ulcer drugs.
- Your doctor may have to adjust your dosage if you have liver or kidney problems.

NORFLOXACIN

Pregnancy category: C
No driving

Brand:
Chibroxin   *Noroxin*

Noroxin, the tablet form of this antibacterial drug, is used to treat urinary tract infections, sexually transmitted diseases, and inflammation of the prostate. The ointment, Chibroxin, is used to treat eye infections.

How to take this drug:
- Take norfloxacin on an empty stomach — one hour before or two hours after meals.

- Drink plenty of fluids while you are taking this drug.
- Never double a missed dose, instead take it as soon as you remember or skip it and go on with your regular schedule.
- When applying the eye ointment, don't let the container touch your eye.

Possible side effects:

Dizziness	Nausea
Stomach pain or cramping	Loss of appetite
Tiredness	Rash
Sweating	Eye irritation
Dilated pupils	Irritated eyelids

Possible interactions:

- This drug may increase the effects of caffeine, the anticoagulant warfarin, the immunosuppressant cyclosporine, and the asthma drug theophylline.
- Levels of this drug may be increased by probenecid, a drug used to treat gout.
- Levels or effects of this drug may be decreased by the antibacterial drug nitrofurantoin.
- Take antacids, vitamins, or any products containing iron or zinc four hours before or two hours after taking norfloxacin.

Other important information:

- Don't use this drug if you are allergic to fluoroquinolones or quinolone antibacterials, are under 18 years of age, a pregnant woman, or a nursing mother.
- If you have any disorders of the central nervous system, such as epilepsy, which may increase your risk of seizures, use this drug with caution.
- Check your kidney and liver functions, and have blood tests done periodically while you are taking this drug.
- Serious, sometimes fatal, allergic reactions can occur, causing swelling of the face or throat, difficulty breathing, itching, hives, tingling, or loss of consciousness.
- Taking an antibiotic for a long time can cause bacteria or fungus to overgrow, leading to another infection. If you get one of these "superinfections," you may need to quit taking norfloxacin and start taking another antibiotic for the second infection.
- Quit using the eye ointment and call your doctor if your eyes become very irritated or if you develop a skin rash or another sign of allergic reaction.
- This drug will increase your skin's sensitivity to the sun. Always use a sunscreen and wear protective clothes when you will be exposed to the sun for a while.

NORTRIPTYLINE HYDROCHLORIDE

Pregnancy category: D
No driving   MAO warning

Brand:
Pamelor

Nortriptyline is a tricyclic antidepressant with mild sedative effects that treats the symptoms of depression.

How to take this drug:
- This drug is available as capsules or liquid.

Possible side effects:
Dizziness	Drowsiness
Dry mouth	Rapid heartbeat
Vision problems	Constipation
Headache	Increased appetite
Nausea	Urination problems
Increased sweating	Unpleasant taste
Black tongue	

Possible interactions:
- Any of the type of antidepressants called selective serotonin reuptake inhibitors (fluoxetine, sertraline, and paroxetine) can cause nortriptyline to reach dangerously high levels in your body. You may need lower than normal doses of both drugs. You also should not quickly switch from fluoxetine to a tricyclic antidepressant like nortriptyline. You may need to wait five weeks for the fluoxetine to clear out of your body.
- Some blood pressure-lowering drugs may not work as well if you also take nortriptyline.
- If you take nortriptyline along with tranquilizers, alcohol, antihistamines, or muscle relaxants, the combination may dangerously depress your nervous system.
- Your doctor should supervise you closely for side effects if you take nortriptyline along with any anticholinergic drugs such as some antihistamines and muscle relaxants, or along with any sympathomimetic drugs such as some decongestants.
- Cimetidine, an ulcer drug, can increase the levels of nortriptyline in your body.
- Taking reserpine and nortriptyline at the same time can cause a "stimulating" effect for some depressed people.
- For diabetics taking chlorpropamide, taking nortriptyline can cause hypoglycemia.

Other important information:
- Don't use this drug if you are recovering from a heart attack.

- If you have a history of seizures, liver problems, urinary retention, thyroid problems, increased pressure in the eye, or heart problems, talk with your doctor about your condition before you take nortriptyline.
- When possible, quit taking nortriptyline several days before surgery.
- If you suddenly quit taking this drug, you could experience nausea, headache, and a general feeling of fatigue. If you gradually quit taking the drug, you may still experience irritability, restlessness, and dream and sleep disturbances.

NYSTATIN

Pregnancy category: C

Brand:
Mycostatin   *Nilstat*
Nystex   *Nystop*

This drug is used to treat yeast infections of the skin and mucous membranes.

How to take this drug:
- It is available as a tablet, oral suspension, powder, cream, ointment, or lozenge (also called a troche).
- Hold the oral suspension or lozenge in your mouth as long as possible. Do not chew or swallow the lozenge.
- Apply the cream and ointment twice a day or as directed.
- Do not wrap or bandage the area after you apply the medicine (unless your doctor tells you to).
- Clean and dry the infected area before applying the medicine.
- For fungal infections of the feet, the powder should be dusted on the feet and in shoes and socks.

Possible side effects:
Skin irritation or rash   Stomach pain
Nausea

Other important information:
- Use nystatin cautiously if your skin is blistered, raw, or oozing.
- Avoid contact with your eyes, nose, and mouth.
- Continue using the medicine for at least two days after your symptoms have disappeared (or as long as your doctor prescribes).
- Nystatin usually relieves your symptoms within 24 to 72 hours.

OFLOXACIN

Pregnancy category: C
No driving

Brand:
Floxin

This antibiotic is used to treat infections of the lower respiratory tract, urinary tract, skin, and skin structures. It is also used to treat sexually transmitted diseases and an inflamed prostate gland.

How to take this drug:
- Take one hour before or two hours after meals.
- Never double a missed dose, instead take it as soon as you remember or skip it and go on with your regular schedule.

Possible side effects:

Headache	Nausea
Diarrhea	Dizziness
Sleeplessness	Rash or itching
Altered sense of taste	Chest pain
Dry mouth	Nervousness
Fever	Sore throat
Loss of appetite	Gas
Fatigue	Constipation

Possible interactions:
- This drug may increase the effects of the anticoagulant warfarin and the immunosuppressant cyclosporine.
- Levels or effects of ofloxacin may be decreased by the antibacterial drug nitrofurantoin.
- Take antacids, vitamins, or any products containing iron or zinc four hours before or two hours after taking ofloxacin.
- If taken with nonsteroidal anti-inflammatory drugs (NSAIDs), ofloxacin may increase the risk of seizure.

Other important information:
- Don't take ofloxacin if you're allergic to fluoroquinolones or quinolone medications.
- Use this drug cautiously if you have diabetes, poor kidney or liver function, or any disorders of the central nervous system, such as epilepsy, that may increase your risk of seizures.
- Blood glucose levels and liver and kidney functions should be checked periodically. If low blood sugar occurs in diabetics, stop taking the drug and call your doctor.
- You may become more sensitive to sunlight on this drug even when using sunscreen. This side effect may persist after treatment is stopped.
- Taking an antibiotic for a long time can cause bacteria or fungus to overgrow, leading to another infection. If you get one of these "superinfections," you may need to quit taking ofloxacin and start another antibiotic for the second infection.

OLANZAPINE

Pregnancy category: C
No driving

Brand:
Zyprexa

Olanzapine is used to manage the symptoms of psychotic disorders, such as schizophrenia.

How to take this drug:
* Take with or without food.
* Never double a missed dose, instead take it as soon as you remember or skip it and go on with your regular schedule.

Possible side effects:
Dizziness when standing suddenly	Rapid heartbeat
Headache	Sleepiness
Nervousness	Sleeplessness
Dizziness	Dry mouth
Constipation	Weight gain

Possible interactions:
* Because olanzapine can lower your blood pressure, be careful about taking it with other antihypertensives.
* Your doctor needs to monitor you closely if you combine olanzapine with omeprazole, rifampin, fluvoxamine, levodopa, drugs that boost the effect of dopamine (Mirapex, Parlodel, Permax, or Requip), or carbamazepine.

Other important information:
* Be careful taking this drug if you have a history of seizures, Alzheimer's disease, heart disease, or liver problems.
* If you plan on exercising strenuously or are exposed to extreme heat while on this medication, you are at greater risk of over-heating your body. Drink plenty of fluids.

OLSALAZINE SODIUM

Pregnancy category: C

Brand:
Dipentum

This drug is used to reduce the risk that ulcerative colitis will recur in people who cannot take sulfasalazine.

How to take this drug:
* Take this drug with food in evenly divided doses.

Possible side effects:
Nausea	Diarrhea

Stomach pain or cramps
Indigestion
Inflamed mouth
Rash
Headache
Depression
Dizziness

Loss of appetite
Bloating
Itching
Muscle or joint pain
Fatigue
Sleeplessness

Possible interactions:
- Olsalazine may increase the effects of the anticoagulant warfarin.

Other important information:
- Don't use this drug if you are allergic to salicylates.
- If you have kidney disease, use this drug with caution.
- This drug may worsen the symptoms of colitis: bloody diarrhea, stomach cramps, and fever.

OMEPRAZOLE

Pregnancy category: C

Brand:
Prilosec

Omeprazole decreases the amount of acid your stomach produces. It helps stomach ulcers heal, treats gastroesophageal reflux disease (severe heartburn), controls bleeding in the stomach or intestines, and treats Zollinger-Ellison disease, a condition in which your stomach produces too much acid.

How to take this drug:
- Take your medicine before you eat.
- Swallow the capsules whole. Don't crush, chew, or open.

Possible side effects:
Headache
Stomach pain
Dizziness
Constipation
Weakness
Irregular heartbeat

Diarrhea
Nausea
Rash
Cough
Chest pain
Back pain

Possible interactions:
- This drug may increase levels or effects of the anticoagulant warfarin, the tranquilizer diazepam, and the seizure drug phenytoin.

Other important information:
- There is a chance that long-term (two-year) therapy with omeprazole could cause the growth of cancerous tumors.

- Be on the lookout for signs that this drug is depressing your immune system: fever, sore throat, tiredness, weakness, bruising, or unusual bleeding. Have your blood tested regularly.

ORLISTAT

Pregnancy category: B

Brand:
Xenical

Orlistat is prescribed to treat and manage obesity.

How to take this drug:
- Take orlistat within one hour of meals.

Possible side effects:
Changes in bowel movements   Abdominal pain
Respiratory infection   Headache
Back pain   Menstrual changes
Anxiety

Possible interactions:
- Orlistat may interact with cyclosporine or pravastatin.

Other important information:
- You must stick to a low-calorie diet in addition to taking this drug. About 30 percent of your calories should come from fat.
- If you eat a meal that is very high in fat, you may experience worse side effects.
- Before beginning this medication, your doctor must rule out other causes for your weight problem, such as hypothyroidism.
- Don't take orlistat if you have conditions that interfere with how your body absorbs nutrients, like lactose intolerance, irritable bowel syndrome, cholestasia, etc.
- Certain vitamins won't be absorbed as well while you are on this medication, therefore, take a multivitamin containing fat-soluble vitamins. Take it once a day, at least two hours before or after taking orlistat.
- Vitamin K levels may drop while you are on orlistat. Talk to your doctor about bleeding problems this could cause.
- You may have a higher risk of developing kidney stones while on this drug.
- If you're diabetic, you may have to adjust your medication while taking orlistat.

ORPHENADRINE CITRATE

Pregnancy category: C
No driving

Brand:
Norflex

This muscle relaxant is used to relieve mild to moderate pain and discomfort associated with muscle disorders such as sprains, strains, and other injuries.

Possible side effects:

Rapid heartbeat	Dry mouth
Blurred vision	Dilated pupils
Increased pressure in the eyes	Difficulty urinating
Nausea or vomiting	Dizziness
Hallucinations	Tremors
Constipation	

Possible interactions:
• Taking orphenadrine with the pain reliever propoxyphene may cause confusion, anxiety, and tremors.

Other important information:
• Don't take this drug if you have the nerve/muscle weakness disease called myasthenia gravis, glaucoma, enlarged prostate, stomach ulcers, difficulty swallowing because of dilation of the esophagus, or obstruction of the stomach, intestines, or bladder.
• Take this drug with caution if you have asthma, an irregular or rapid heartbeat, or heart failure.
• This medicine should not take the place of rest, physical therapy, exercise, or any other treatment your doctor recommends.
• If you use this medicine for a long time, you should have your blood, urine, and liver functions monitored periodically.

OXAPROZIN

Pregnancy category: C

Brand:
Daypro

This nonsteroidal anti-inflammatory drug (NSAID) relieves the pain and symptoms of arthritis.

Possible side effects:

Nausea	Indigestion
Stomach pain	Weight loss
Sleeplessness	Constipation
Diarrhea	Gas

Depression   Sleepiness
Rash   Ringing in the ears
Frequent urination

Possible interactions:
- Avoid aspirin while taking this drug.
- Oxaprozin may increase the risk of bleeding if taken with the anticoagulant warfarin.
- Oxaprozin may decrease the effects of the beta blocker metoprolol.
- Levels or effects of oxaprozin may be increased by the ulcer drugs cimetidine and ranitidine.

Other important information:
- Don't use this drug if you have nasal polyps, water retention or swelling, or allergies to aspirin or other aspirin substitutes such as NSAIDs.
- Don't take it if you have a stomach ulcer. Alcoholics and smokers also have an increased risk of stomach and intestinal problems.
- Taking oxaprozin is more likely to cause kidney problems if you are elderly, if you take diuretics, or if you have lupus, heart failure, or poor liver or kidney function.
- Take this drug with caution if you have liver abnormalities, high blood pressure, blood clotting disorders, or poor heart function.
- Be on the lookout for signs that this drug is depressing your immune system: fever, sore throat, tiredness, weakness, bruising, or unusual bleeding. Have your blood tested regularly.
- Bleeding stomach ulcers and liver or kidney damage are rare but serious reactions to using oxaprozin for long periods of time. Warning signs of liver damage include nausea, tiredness, red and itchy skin, yellow eyes and skin (jaundice), and flu-like symptoms.
- This drug may make your skin extra-sensitive to sunlight, so protect your skin if you'll be outdoors.

OXAZEPAM

Pregnancy category: NR
No driving

Brand:
Serax

This benzodiazepine treats anxiety, tension, agitation, irritability, and anxiety associated with depression. It also helps treat the symptoms of alcohol withdrawal.

Possible side effects:
Drowsiness   Lightheadedness
Dizziness   Headache
Fainting   Excitement

Possible interactions:
- If you take oxazepam along with tranquilizers, alcohol, antihistamines, or muscle relaxers, the combination may dangerously depress your nervous system.

Other important information:
- People with some kinds of glaucoma shouldn't use this drug.
- You can become dependent on oxazepam, especially if you take more than 4 mg per day for longer than eight to 12 weeks. To avoid seizures and other less severe withdrawal symptoms, quit taking the drug gradually under your doctor's supervision.
- Very rarely, oxazepam has caused low blood pressure. Take this drug cautiously if a drop in blood pressure could cause heart trouble for you.
- Have regular blood counts and liver function tests while you're taking this drug.

OXYBUTYNIN CHLORIDE

Pregnancy category: B
No driving

Brand:
Ditropan

Oxybutynin chloride treats the symptoms of an overactive bladder: incontinence, the urgent need to urinate, and having to urinate frequently.

How to take this drug:
- It is available as a regular tablet, an extended release tablet, or as syrup.
- Take the extended release tablets once a day.
- You can take this drug with or without food.
- Don't break, split, or chew the extended release tablets.

Possible side effects:

Dry mouth	Constipation
Headache	Diarrhea
Nausea	Sleepiness
Vision problems	Dizziness
Indigestion	Weakness
Body pain	Rapid heartbeat
Rash	Impotence

Possible interactions:
- Oxybutynin chloride may interact with drugs, like bisphosphonates, which can irritate your esophagus.
- Taking it with other nerve-blocking drugs may make the side effects more severe.

Other important information:
- Don't use it if you retain urine or suffer from glaucoma or obstruction disorders in your intestines.
- Be careful using this drug if you have GERD, kidney or liver problems, ulcerative colitis, muscle weakness, or any condition that slows down the digestive process.
- It can make these conditions worse: hyperthyroidism, heart disease, congestive heart failure, arrhythmia, hiatal hernia, high blood pressure, and sudden drops in blood pressure.
- Take this drug carefully if you have trouble swallowing pills.
- If you are in a hot environment, you will be more susceptible to fever and heat stroke while taking this medication.
- This drug may affect how your body absorbs other medication.
- Taking alcohol or other sedatives with oxybutynin chloride will make you even more drowsy.

PAROXETINE

Pregnancy category: B
No driving   MAO warning

Brand:
Paxil

Paroxetine, a selective serotonin reuptake inhibitor (SSRI), treats the symptoms of depression.

Possible side effects:
Weakness	Sweating
Nausea	Decreased appetite
Sleepiness	Dizziness
Sleeplessness	Shakiness
Nervousness	Sexual problems

Possible interactions:
- This drug interacts dangerously with MAO inhibitors like Eldepryl, Marplan, Nardil, and Parnate.
- Tryptophan and paroxetine together can cause agitation, restlessness, and upset stomach. You may want to avoid foods high in tryptophan, such as meats, poultry, fish, liver, kidney, eggs, nuts, peanut butter, broad beans, and wheat germ.
- Paroxetine may cause increased bleeding if you take it while you are taking warfarin.
- The ulcer drug cimetidine may increase levels or effects of paroxetine.
- The sedative phenobarbital may lower levels of paroxetine in your body.
- Phenytoin and paroxetine may interact.
- If you are taking phenothiazines; certain antiarrhythmics such as propafenone, flecainide, and encainide; or any antidepressant, you may need to adjust your dose.

Other important information:
- You may need a lower than normal dosage of paroxetine if you have liver or kidney disease. Your doctor should monitor you closely for side effects.
- Take this drug with caution if you have a history of seizures.
- Most people notice an improvement in their depression after one to four weeks on paroxetine.

PENBUTOLOL SULFATE

Pregnancy category: C
No driving

Brand:
Levatol

Penbutolol is a beta blocker used to treat and control high blood pressure.

Possible side effects:

Nausea	Diarrhea
Indigestion	Headache
Weakness	Dizziness
Hallucinations	Abnormal dreams
Prickling or tingling sensation	Slow heartbeat
Sleeplessness	Chest pain
Cough or wheezing	Difficulty breathing
Sweating	

Possible interactions:
- Penbutolol may decrease the effects of the asthma drug epinephrine and the heart rhythm drug lidocaine.
- Nonsteroidal anti-inflammatories (NSAIDs), such as indomethacin, may decrease effects of penbutolol.

Other important information:
- Don't take this drug if you have a very slow heartbeat, heart failure, heart block, shock, bronchitis, emphysema, or asthma. The drug may worsen heart failure, heart disease, or angina.
- Penbutolol can make asthma symptoms worse.
- If you have diabetes, use this drug cautiously because beta blockers can mask the signs of low blood sugar.
- Penbutolol can also mask signs of an overactive thyroid.
- Never quit taking this drug without talking to your doctor. It could increase your risk of angina and heart attack.
- Tell your doctor immediately if you have any signs of congestive heart failure such as night cough; swelling of your legs, feet, or hands; or difficulty breathing, especially when lying down or after physical exertion.

PENICILLIN V POTASSIUM

Pregnancy category: B

Brand:
Ledercillin VK

Pen Vee K

Betapen-VK

V-Cillin K

Beepen-VK

Veetids

This penicillin antibiotic is used to treat a wide variety of mild to moderate systemic infections by killing the bacteria that cause the infections.

How to take this drug:
- Take one hour before or two hours after meals.
- Take all of the prescription, even after the infection goes away.
- You can take penicillin V with food to help prevent upset stomach.

Possible side effects:
Stomach pain or cramps

Diarrhea

Black tongue

Nausea

Gas

Skin eruptions

Possible interactions:
- This drug may decrease the effectiveness of birth control pills.
- Levels or effects of this drug may be decreased by the antibiotics neomycin, erythromycin, chloramphenicol, and tetracycline.

Other important information:
- Don't use this drug if you are allergic to penicillin or other antibiotics. Call your doctor if you develop a rash, fever, or chills.
- If you are vomiting or have diarrhea, do not use this drug.
- Be on the lookout for signs that this drug is depressing your immune system: fever, sore throat, tiredness, weakness, bruising, or unusual bleeding. Have your blood tested regularly.

PENTOXIFYLLINE

Pregnancy category: C

Brand:
Trental

Pentoxifylline makes the blood less sticky and improves the flow of blood through blood vessels. It eases calf pain caused by poor blood circulation.

How to take this drug:
- Swallow the tablet whole. Don't crush, break, or chew before swallowing.
- Take this medicine with meals to help avoid stomach upset.

Possible side effects:
Indigestion

Nausea

Dizziness	Headache
Chest pain	Belching
Gas	Bloating
Tremors	Blurred vision
Nervousness	Irregular heartbeat
Flushing	

Possible interactions:
- Pentoxifylline may increase the effects of the anticoagulant warfarin.

Other important information:
- Pentoxifylline should not be used by people allergic to methylxanthines (such as caffeine, theophylline, theobromine).
- Use pentoxifylline with caution if you have any condition in which there is a risk of bleeding: stomach ulcers, rectal bleeding, recent stroke, or recent surgery.

PERGOLIDE MESYLATE

Pregnancy category: B

Brand:
Permax

Pergolide, prescribed with levodopa/carbidopa, treats Parkinson's disease.

Possible side effects:

Sleepiness	Nausea
Constipation	Diarrhea
Upset stomach	Runny or stuffy nose
Hallucinations	Sleeplessness

Possible interactions:
- Effects of this drug may be decreased by phenothiazines, a type of tranquilizer.

Other important information:
- Don't use this drug if you are allergic to ergot derivatives.
- If you have irregular heart rhythms, talk with your doctor before you take this drug. It can cause irregular heartbeats.
- This drug causes more than half of the people who take it to have abnormal, involuntary muscle movements. Report tremors or movements you can't control to your doctor.
- Ten percent of the people taking the drug experience low blood pressure (which causes dizziness) when they stand up. Make sure you change positions slowly, especially when you first start taking the drug.

PERPHENAZINE

Pregnancy category: NR
No driving

Brand:
Trilafon

Perphenazine, a phenothiazine-type tranquilizer, treats mental illnesses and controls severe nausea and vomiting.

How to take this drug:
- The concentrate form of perphenazine is best taken in liquids such as orange, grapefruit, tomato, pineapple, apricot, or prune juice; carbonated orange drink; homogenized milk; or water. Don't use caffeinated drinks, including tea, or apple juice.

Possible side effects:
Sleepiness	Dry mouth
Urine retention	Confusion

Possible interactions:
- The combination of perphenazine along with large amounts of any drug that depresses your nervous system, such as other tranquilizers, alcohol, antihistamines, pain relievers, or muscle relaxers, may dangerously depress your nervous system. Talk to your doctor about adjusting your dose.
- Perphenazine may increase the effects of atropine.

Other important information:
- Use this drug cautiously if you have a history of seizures, poor kidney function, lung infections, asthma, or emphysema.
- Be careful with this drug if you work in extreme heat or around phosphorus insecticides.
- Have your blood counts and liver and kidney functions checked regularly while you're taking this drug.
- Don't quit taking this drug suddenly. If you do, you may experience stomach pain, nausea, dizziness, and shakiness.
- There is a small risk of developing nerve problems from this drug. Tell your doctor immediately if you develop muscle weakness or spasms or difficulty speaking or swallowing.
- If your body temperature goes up, that may be a signal that you can't tolerate this drug.

PHENAZOPYRIDINE HYDROCHLORIDE

Pregnancy category: B

Brand:
Prodium   *Pyridium*

This drug is used to relieve the pain, burning, and frequent urination caused by urinary tract infection, illness, or medical procedures affecting the urinary tract.

How to take this drug:
- Take this drug after meals since it may upset your stomach.

Possible side effects:
Itching	Rash
Upset stomach	Headache

Other important information:
- People with decreased kidney function should not take this drug.
- If your skin or the whites of your eyes become yellow, call your doctor. Your kidneys may be allowing the drug to accumulate in your body.
- Phenazopyridine may cause your urine to become a red-orange color. It could also stain soft contact lenses.
- If you have a urinary tract infection, you should only use this drug for two days.

PHENELZINE SULFATE

Pregnancy category: C

Brand:
Nardil

Phenelzine is a monoamine oxidase (MAO) inhibitor. It treats depression, usually mixed with anxiety, phobias, or hypochondria.

Possible side effects:
Drowsiness	Headache
Tremors	Twitching
Dizziness	Dry mouth
Constipation	Stomach problems
Weight gain	Rash
Sweating	Blurred vision
Nervousness	Difficulty urinating
Prickling or tingling in hands or feet	Sexual problems

Possible interactions:
- Taking any of the following drugs while taking MAO inhibitors can cause extremely high blood pressure: buspirone, epinephrine, norepinephrine, amphetamines, methylphenidate, phenylalanine, dopamine, methyldopa, tryptophan, and tyrosine.
- Over-the-counter medicines you should avoid while taking phenelzine include: cough and cold preparations (including any containing dextromethorphan), nasal decongestants, hay fever medications, sinus

medications, asthma inhalers, weight-reducing medicines, or appetite-controlling medicines.

- You can experience extremely high blood pressure when you eat any foods high in tyramine or dopamine while taking MAO inhibitors: yogurt, aged cheese, liver, avocados, bananas, broad beans, sauerkraut, wine, beer, and pickled, dried, or smoked meats, fish or vegetables (including salami and pepperoni). Avoid large amounts of caffeine and chocolate.
- Foods high in tryptophan can cause confusion, delirium, and agitation: meats, poultry, fish, liver, kidney, eggs, nuts, peanut butter, broad beans, and wheat germ.
- Phenelzine may dangerously increase the effects of depressants and sedatives, including alcohol.
- Taking phenelzine with meperidine (Demerol) may cause high fever, seizures, and coma.
- Taking phenelzine with other antidepressants could cause a negative drug interaction. Wait at least 10 days after you quit taking phenelzine before you begin taking another antidepressant or the anti-anxiety buspirone. You should wait 14 days before you begin taking bupropion.
- After taking the antidepressant fluoxetine, you should wait five weeks before you begin taking phenelzine.
- You should not take phenelzine while taking guanethidine. If you take other high blood pressure drugs, such as thiazide diuretics and beta blockers, you should take phenelzine cautiously.

Other important information:
- Don't take this drug if you have poor liver function, heart failure, or a tumor that produces adrenaline (pheochromocytoma).
- Quit taking phenelzine 10 days before having surgery that requires anesthesia.
- For diabetics, phenelzine may cause hypoglycemia.
- Tell your doctor if you have dizziness or lightheadedness when you get up from a lying or sitting position.
- The most serious reaction to phenelzine is severe, even deadly, high blood pressure. Have your blood pressure checked often, and tell your doctor immediately about any heart palpitations or frequent headaches you have. Other symptoms of unusually high blood pressure are severe chest pain, enlarged pupils, increased sensitivity of eyes to light, increased sweating, nausea, and stiff or sore neck.
- You may not notice any improvement in your depression until you've been taking phenelzine for four weeks.

PHENTERMINE HYDROCHLORIDE

Pregnancy category: NR
No driving   MAO warning

Brand:
Adipex-P   *Fastin*

Oby-Trim   *Ona-Mast*

Phentermine hydrochloride is used to reduce appetite and aid in weight loss over short periods of time.

How to take this drug:
- Take phentermine hydrochloride on an empty stomach.
- Don't take it late in the day.
- Never double a missed dose, instead take it as soon as you remember or skip it and go on with your regular schedule.
- Don't take this medication longer than prescribed.

Possible side effects:

Rapid heartbeat	Dizziness
Headache	Tremors
Restlessness or anxiety	Sleeplessness
Depression	Hives
Impotence	Dry mouth
Bad taste	Constipation
Diarrhea	

Possible interactions:
- This drug may increase the effects of insulin; your dosage may need to be adjusted.
- It may decrease the effects of the blood pressure drug guanethidine.
- Check with your doctor before combining phentermine hydrochloride with antidepressants.

Other important information:
- Don't take phentermine hydrochloride if you have a history of drug abuse, high blood pressure, arteriosclerosis or heart disease, overactive thyroid, glaucoma, alcoholism, or psychotic disorders such as schizophrenia.
- This drug is not a substitute for a healthy diet and exercise.

PHENYLEPHRINE, PHENYLPROPANOLAMINE, AND GUAIFENESIN
Pregnancy category: C
MAO warning

Brand:
Entex

This drug combines two decongestants and an expectorant and is used when you have a cold, bronchitis, or sinusitis. It relieves a congested nose and thick mucus in the chest.

Possible side effects:

Nervousness	Sleeplessness
Restlessness	Headache
Nausea	Stomach pain

Possible interactions:
- You shouldn't take this drug if you are taking other drugs that stimulate the sympathetic nervous system, such as epinephrine or other decongestants.

Other important information:
- Don't use this drug if you have very high blood pressure.
- If you have mildly high blood pressure, diabetes, heart or blood vessel disease, increased pressure in the eye, an overactive thyroid, or an enlarged prostate, talk to your doctor about your condition before taking this drug.
- This drug may make urinating more difficult if you have an enlarged prostate.

PHENYTOIN SODIUM

Pregnancy category: D
No driving

Brand:
Dilantin Kapseals

Phenytoin is used by people with epilepsy to treat and prevent certain types of seizures.

How to take this drug:
- Stay on the exact dose schedule your doctor advises.

Possible side effects:

Lack of coordination	Slurred speech
Confusion	Vision problems
Nausea or vomiting	

Possible interactions:
- This drug interacts dangerously with cyclosporine (Sandimmune).
- A large amount of alcohol can increase levels of phenytoin in your body. However, chronic alcohol abuse can decrease phenytoin levels.
- The following drugs may increase the effects of phenytoin: the heart rhythm drug amiodarone, the antibiotic chloramphenicol, the anti-anxiety drugs chlordiazepoxide and diazepam, the anticoagulant dicumarol, the anti-alcoholic drug disulfiram, estrogens, the tuberculosis drug isoniazid, phenothiazine tranquilizers, the nonsteroidal anti-inflammatory drug phenylbutazone, salicylates such as aspirin, sulfonamide antibacterials, the antidiabetic drug tolbutamide, and the antidepressant trazodone.
- The following drugs may decrease effects of phenytoin: antacids, the seizure drug carbamazepine, the blood pressure drug reserpine, the ulcer drug sucralfate, and the antipsychotic drug molindone.
- If you take phenytoin along with phenobarbital, valproic acid, or sodium valproate, your doctor may need to adjust your dosages of both drugs. They can affect the levels of each other.

- Certain drugs may not work as well when you are also taking phenytoin: birth control pills, corticosteroids, anticoagulants, the heart drug digitoxin, the antibiotic doxycycline, the diuretic furosemide, the tuberculosis drug rifampin, and the asthma drug theophylline.
- Don't take antacids containing calcium within two to three hours of taking phenytoin. They could keep you from absorbing the phenytoin properly.

Other important information:

- Phenytoin can reach toxic levels more quickly if you have poor liver function and if you are an older adult.
- Unless you're having an allergic reaction to the drug and under your doctor's supervision, never quit taking phenytoin suddenly. You could bring on a seizure.
- You may need vitamin D and vitamin K supplements. Some people taking phenytoin may need folic acid supplements to help prevent anemia.
- This drug can cause gum problems, so it is important to keep your teeth and gums clean and flossed, and visit your dentist regularly.
- Phenytoin may cause some lymph node diseases. Signs to look for are enlarged glands in your neck or underarms, fever, or a rash.
- Tell your doctor right away if you develop a skin rash. If it is a mild, measles-like rash, you'll be able to take phenytoin again once the rash has cleared up.
- For people with diabetes, phenytoin may raise your blood sugar levels.
- Be on the lookout for signs that this drug is depressing your immune system: fever, sore throat, tiredness, weakness, bruising, or unusual bleeding. Have your blood tested regularly.

PILOCARPINE HYDROCHLORIDE, ORAL

Pregnancy category: C
No driving

Brand:

Salagen

Pilocarpine hydrochloride tablets treat dry mouth from Sjogren's syndrome or from radiotherapy for cancer of the head and neck. (Also available as an ointment to treat glaucoma; see next entry.)

Possible side effects:

Sweating	Nausea or vomiting
Runny or stuffy nose	Diarrhea
Chills	Frequent urination
Dizziness	Weakness
Headache	Indigestion
Watery eyes	Swelling
Vision problems	

Possible interactions:
- Pilocarpine hydrochloride can interact with beta adrenergic antagonists.

Other important information:
- Don't take Salagen tablets if you have asthma, narrow-angle glaucoma, or an inflamed iris.
- Have your doctor monitor you closely if you have heart disease, liver or gallbladder problems, chronic bronchitis, or chronic obstructive pulmonary disease.
- It may cause problems with your night vision.
- If any of the side effects become severe, you may be experiencing pilocarpine toxicity. See your doctor immediately.
- Drink lots of fluids while on this medication.

PILOCARPINE HYDROCHLORIDE, TOPICAL

Pregnancy category: C
No driving

Brand:
Pilopine HS Ophthalmic Gel

This ophthalmic gel is used to control eye pressure from glaucoma.

How to take this drug:
- Don't allow the tube to touch your eye or any other surface. If the tip or the contents become contaminated, you could develop an eye infection.
- Never double a missed dose, instead take it as soon as you remember or skip it and go on with your regular schedule.

Possible side effects:
Watery eyes	Burning eyes
Headache	Reduced night vision
Vision problems	Detached retina

Other important information:
- You can use this medication with other drugs.
- Don't use if you have inflammation of the iris (acute iritis).
- This will affect your night vision.

PINDOLOL

Pregnancy category: B
No driving

Brand:
Visken

Pindolol is a beta blocker that treats and controls high blood pressure.

Possible side effects:

Sleeplessness	Muscle or joint pain
Nausea	Stomach pain
Chest pain	Strange dreams
Prickling or tingling sensation	Itching

Possible interactions:

- Pindolol may increase effects of the antipsychotic drug thioridazine.
- Pindolol may decrease the effectiveness of the asthma drug theophylline.
- Effects of pindolol may be increased by the blood pressure drug reserpine and birth control pills.
- Nonsteroidal anti-inflammatory drugs (NSAIDs), such as aspirin, may decrease the effects of pindolol.

Other important information:

- People with asthma, very slow heartbeat, heart block, shock, or heart failure should not take this drug.
- Take pindolol cautiously if you have bronchitis, emphysema, or poor liver or kidney function.
- If you have diabetes, use this drug cautiously because beta blockers can mask the signs of low blood sugar.
- Pindolol can also mask signs of an overactive thyroid.
- Tell your doctor immediately if you have any signs of congestive heart failure such as night cough; swelling of your legs, feet, or hands; or difficulty breathing, especially when lying down or after physical exertion.
- Never quit taking this drug without talking to your doctor. It could increase your risk of angina and heart attack.
- Discuss your medication with your doctor before having surgery. He may want to discontinue the drug before your surgery.

PIRBUTEROL

Pregnancy category: C
MAO warning

Brand:

Maxair Autohaler   *Maxair Inhaler*

Pirbuterol is a bronchodilator. It prevents and reverses bronchospasm caused by asthma.

How to take this drug:

- Don't take more medicine than you are prescribed or stop taking your medicine without consulting your doctor.

Possible side effects:

Nervousness	Tremors
Headache	Dizziness

Rapid heartbeat   Coughing
Nausea

Possible interactions:
*   Don't use with other beta adrenergic aerosol bronchodilators.

Other important information:
*   People with a history of seizures, diabetes, overactive thyroid, high blood pressure, irregular heartbeat, or heart disease should use this drug with caution.
*   Pirbuterol can affect your blood pressure. Have it tested regularly while taking the drug.
*   Pirbuterol can be used along with theophylline and/or steroid therapy.
*   Call your doctor if your asthma symptoms get worse.

PIROXICAM

Pregnancy category: C/D
No driving

Brand:
Feldene

This nonsteroidal anti-inflammatory drug (NSAID) is used to relieve the symptoms of arthritis.

Possible side effects:
Nausea   Stomach pain
Loss of appetite   Constipation
Indigestion   Diarrhea
Inflamed mouth   Headache
Ringing in the ears   Dizziness
Sleepiness   Water retention

Possible interactions:
*   Avoid alcohol while taking all NSAIDs including piroxicam.
*   It may interact with anticoagulants.
*   Piroxicam may increase the antipsychotic drug lithium to toxic levels.
*   Effects of this drug may be decreased by aspirin.

Other important information:
*   Don't take this drug if you are allergic to aspirin or other NSAIDs.
*   Take piroxicam with caution if you have low platelet counts, poor kidney or liver function, heart failure, high blood pressure, or any disorder that causes fluid retention.
*   Be on the lookout for signs that this drug is depressing your immune system: fever, sore throat, tiredness, weakness, bruising, or unusual bleeding. Have your blood tested regularly.

- This drug can cause liver damage. Warning signs include nausea, tiredness, red and itchy skin, yellow eyes and skin (jaundice), and flu-like symptoms.
- Bleeding stomach ulcers and kidney damage are rare but serious reactions to using piroxicam for long periods of time.

POTASSIUM CHLORIDE

Pregnancy category: C

Brand:

Micro-K	*Micro-K 10*
K+10	*K-Dur 20*
Klor-Con	*Klor-Con M 20*
Slow-K	

This drug is used to maintain the body's supply of potassium when you don't get enough through your diet or any time potassium is depleted due to illness or drugs.

How to take this drug:
- Swallow tablets whole. Don't crush or chew.
- Take this drug with a full glass of water or liquid.
- To avoid upset stomach, take potassium chloride with food.

Possible side effects:

Nausea or vomiting	Gas
Diarrhea	Upset stomach
Rash	

Possible interactions:
- This drug may lead to dangerously high levels of potassium if taken with ACE inhibitors or potassium-sparing diuretics.

Other important information:
- If you have poor kidney function or heart disease, use this drug with caution.
- Blood levels of potassium should be checked frequently.
- The capsules and tablets can cause ulcers and bleeding in the stomach and intestines. If you have very dark stools, stomach pain, or vomiting, contact your doctor.

PRAVASTATIN

Pregnancy category: X

Brand:
Pravachol

Pravastatin is used to reduce total cholesterol and LDL cholesterol levels.

Possible side effects:

Nausea	Chest pain
Rash	Diarrhea
Stomach pain	Heartburn
Gas	Constipation
Headache	Inflamed nasal passages
Dizziness	Flu-like symptoms

Possible interactions:

- The following drugs may increase the risk of rhabdomyolysis when you take them with pravastatin: the blood fat reducer gemfibrozil, the antibiotic erythromycin, or the ulcer drug cimetidine.

Other important information:

- Pravastatin should not be used by people with liver disease or suspected liver problems.
- Use pravastatin with caution if you have a history of high alcohol consumption or poor kidney function.
- Pravastatin may alter some hormone levels.
- This drug may cause rhabdomyolysis, a dangerous and sometimes fatal disease that destroys muscle tissue. Notify your doctor immediately if you develop any pain, tenderness, or weakness in your muscles.
- This drug can also lead to kidney failure (caused by rhabdomyolysis) in people with severe infections, uncontrolled seizures, low blood pressure, any kind of trauma such as major surgery, or severe metabolic, electrolyte, or endocrine disorders.
- This drug can cause liver damage. Warning signs include nausea, tiredness, red and itchy skin, yellow eyes and skin (jaundice), and flu-like symptoms. You should have regular liver function tests while you're taking this drug.

PRAZOSIN HYDROCHLORIDE

Pregnancy category: C
No driving

Brand:

Minipress   *Minipress XL*

Prazosin controls high blood pressure.

How to take this drug:

- Take your first dose at bedtime to help reduce the "first-dose" effect.

Possible side effects:

Rapid heartbeat	Weakness
Headache	Drowsiness
Nausea	Constipation
Diarrhea	Fluid retention

Difficulty breathing	Frequent urination
Blurred vision	Rash
Dry mouth	Stuffy nose

Possible interactions:
* Don't drink alcohol while taking this drug.
* If you take prazosin with other blood pressure drugs, you're more likely to experience very low blood pressure and fainting.

Other important information:
* Take this drug cautiously if you have poor liver function.
* Prazosin may cause you to have very low blood pressure when you first start taking it. Your blood pressure can drop so low that you faint or lose consciousness. This is known as the "first-dose" effect. This can also occur if your dose is increased quickly, if your treatment is restarted after you've missed several doses, or if you begin taking another antihypertensive drug.
* Because of the drop in blood pressure, you can feel dizzy or lightheaded after standing up. Move slowly and carefully.
* A very rapid heartbeat can be a dangerous side effect.

PREDNISOLONE

Pregnancy category: C

Brand:
Prelone

This drug is a corticosteroid used to treat or ease the symptoms of various disorders including the following: allergic reactions, blood disorders, lupus, endocrine system disorders, eye allergies and inflammatory conditions, fluid retention in diseases of the kidneys, intestinal diseases, leukemia, respiratory diseases, arthritis, bursitis, and skin diseases and eruptions.

How to take this drug:
* Take with food to prevent upset stomach.

Possible side effects:

Sleeplessness	Headache
Bloating	Muscle weakness

Possible interactions:
* Prednisolone may interact with aspirin or other NSAIDs, barbiturates, phenytoin (Dilantin), rifampin, blood thinners, diuretics, and salicylates.

Other important information:
* People with fungal infections should not use this drug.
* Corticosteroid drugs may weaken your immune system and decrease your natural resistance to infections. Call your doctor immediately at the first sign of fever or infection.

- Don't get any vaccinations, and take extra care to avoid exposure to people with chicken pox or measles. If you are exposed, let your doctor know right away.
- If you have high blood pressure, osteoporosis, diabetes, cirrhosis, underactive thyroid, herpes simplex of the eye, myasthenia gravis (muscle weakness disease), poor kidney function, colitis, diverticulitis, or ulcer, take prednisolone with caution.
- Most people will experience very few side effects if they take prednisolone for 10 days or less. Long-term use can cause many serious side effects.
- Prednisolone may cause or aggravate emotional or psychotic problems. Call your doctor if you experience any changes in mood.
- This drug may cause you to lose calcium and potassium and retain salt. You may need to restrict your salt intake and take potassium supplements.
- If you've been taking high doses of prednisolone or you've been taking it for a long time, don't suddenly quit taking it. Withdrawing rapidly could cause nausea, fever, fainting, and even death.

PREDNISONE

Pregnancy category: C

Brand:
Deltasone

This drug is a corticosteroid used to treat or ease the symptoms of various disorders including the following: endocrine system disorders, arthritis, bursitis, lupus, skin diseases, allergic reactions, eye allergies and inflammatory conditions, respiratory diseases, blood disorders, leukemia, intestinal diseases, and multiple sclerosis.

How to take this drug:
- Take with food to avoid upset stomach.

Possible side effects:
Sleeplessness	Euphoria
Mood changes or depression	Bloating

Possible interactions:
- Prednisone can interact with the following drugs: aspirin, blood thinners, barbiturates like phenobarbital, phenytoin (Dilantin), rifampin, carbamazepine (Tegretol), estrogen and oral contraceptives, ketoconazole (Nizoral), and diuretics.

Other important information:
- People with fungal infections should not use this drug.
- Corticosteroids may weaken your immune system and decrease your natural resistance to infections. Call your doctor immediately at the first sign of fever or infection.

- Using corticosteroids for a long period of time can cause eye disease or infection.
- This drug may cause you to lose calcium and potassium and retain salt. You may need to restrict your salt intake and take potassium supplements. It can also raise your blood pressure.
- Don't get any vaccinations, and take extra care to avoid exposure to people with chicken pox or measles. If you are exposed, let your doctor know right away.
- If you've been taking high doses of prednisone or you've been taking it for a long time, don't suddenly quit taking it. Withdrawing rapidly could cause nausea, fever, fainting, and even death.
- If you have high blood pressure, osteoporosis, diabetes, cirrhosis, underactive thyroid, herpes simplex of the eye, myasthenia gravis (muscle weakness disease), poor kidney function, colitis, diverticulitis, or ulcer, take prednisone with caution.
- Prednisone may cause or aggravate emotional or psychotic problems. Call your doctor if you experience any changes in mood.
- Most people will experience very few side effects if they take prednisone for 10 days or less. Long-term use can cause many serious side effects.

PRIMIDONE

Pregnancy category: NR
No driving

Brand:
Mysoline

People with epilepsy use primidone to control many types of seizures.

Possible side effects:
Lack of coordination	Dizziness
Nausea or vomiting	Loss of appetite
Vision changes	Drowsiness

Possible interactions:
- Primidone is partly converted to phenobarbital in the body. See the entry for phenobarbital for possible interactions with other drugs.

Other important information:
- Don't stop taking anticonvulsants suddenly or change the dose without consulting your doctor.
- You may need folic acid to treat anemia, a rare side effect of primidone.

PROBENECID

Pregnancy category: B

Brand:
Benemid   *Probalan*

Probenecid treats gout and is also used along with some antibiotics to make them more effective.

How to take this drug:
- While you're taking this drug, drink 10 to 12 glasses of fluid per day to help prevent kidney stones.
- If the medicine upsets your stomach, you should let your doctor know. You may need a lower dose.

Possible side effects:
Nausea
Headache
Flushing
Frequent urination

Loss of appetite
Dizziness
Sore gums

Possible interactions:
- Probenecid may increase the effects of anesthetics.
- It may cause low blood sugar if used with anti-diabetic drugs.
- Probenecid may increase the risk of toxicity of nonsteroidal anti-inflammatory drugs (NSAIDs), acetaminophen, the anti-anxiety drug lorazepam, the cancer drug methotrexate, and the tuberculosis drug rifampin.
- Effects of probenecid may be decreased by aspirin and the tuberculosis drug pyrazinamide.
- Don't use probenecid with penicillin if you have poor kidney function.

Other important information:
- Don't start taking probenecid during a gout attack. However, you may experience a gout attack after you begin taking it.
- People with blood diseases or kidney stones should not take probenecid.
- Take probenecid with caution if you have a history of ulcers or poor kidney function.
- Be on the lookout for signs that this drug is depressing your immune system: fever, sore throat, tiredness, weakness, bruising, or unusual bleeding. Have your blood tested regularly.
- Call your doctor if you have blood in your urine, pain in your ribs or back, or yellow eyes and skin (jaundice).
- This drug may cause kidney stones.

PROCAINAMIDE HYDROCHLORIDE

Pregnancy category: C

Brand:
Procan SR
Procanbid

Pronestyl

Procainamide is an antiarrhythmic used to bring irregular heartbeats to a normal rhythm.

How to take this drug:
- Take this medicine on time and exactly as your doctor prescribes.

Possible side effects:

Nausea	Diarrhea
Loss of appetite	Stomach pain
Bitter taste	Swelling
Flushing	Itching
Hives or rash	Weakness
Dizziness	Depression
Hallucinations	

Possible interactions:
- Procainamide may increase the effects of neuromuscular blocking agents.
- If you take procainamide with the heartbeat regulator disopyramide, the combination may cause very low blood pressure or worsen irregular heartbeat.

Other important information:
- Procainamide should not be used by people with complete heart block, the irregular heart rhythm called "torsade de pointes," asthma, allergic reaction, or lupus.
- Use procainamide with caution if you have heart disease, heart block, heart failure, poor kidney or liver function, or myasthenia gravis (muscle weakness disease).
- Be on the lookout for signs that this drug is depressing your immune system: fever, sore throat, tiredness, weakness, bruising, or unusual bleeding. Have your blood tested regularly.
- At least 20 percent of the people who take procainamide eventually get lupus erythematosus-like syndrome. Some symptoms are fever, skin eruptions, and joint and muscle pain. Call your doctor immediately if you have any of these symptoms.

PROCHLORPERAZINE

Pregnancy category: NR
No driving

Brand:
Compazine

This phenothiazine is usually used to relieve severe nausea and vomiting, but it is occasionally prescribed as a tranquilizer to treat anxiety and mental disorders.

Possible side effects:

Sleepiness	Dry mouth
Urine retention	Confusion

Possible interactions:
- If you take prochlorperazine along with tranquilizers, alcohol, antihistamines, or muscle relaxers, the combination may dangerously depress your nervous system.
- This drug may decrease the effectiveness of anticoagulants and blood-pressure-lowering medicines.
- If you take prochlorperazine with a diuretic, you may experience dizziness and very low blood pressure when you stand up or exercise.

Other important information:
- This drug can cause very low blood pressure, so take it with caution if you have a history of heart disease. Be careful when you stand up suddenly since you can become dizzy.
- Use prochlorperazine with caution if you have a history of epilepsy or glaucoma. This drug may increase the risk of seizures.
- This drug can make you become overheated if you are exposed to hot weather.
- Prochlorperazine can cause liver damage. Warning signs include nausea, tiredness, red and itchy skin, yellow eyes and skin (jaundice), and flu-like symptoms.
- Be on the lookout for signs that this drug is depressing your immune system: fever, sore throat, tiredness, weakness, bruising, or unusual bleeding. Have your blood tested regularly.
- There is a small risk of developing nerve problems from this drug. Tell your doctor immediately if you develop muscle weakness or spasms or difficulty speaking or swallowing.

PROGESTERONE, ORAL

Pregnancy category: B
No driving

Brand:
Prometrium

Prometrium capsules are used to prevent endometrial hyperplasia (abnormal cell growth in the lining of the uterus) in postmenopausal women on conjugated estrogen and to correct menstrual irregularities.

How to take this drug:
- Taking Prometrium with food makes it absorb more quickly.

Possible side effects:

Dizziness	Breast pain
Headache	Cramps or abdominal pain
Tiredness	Bloating
Joint or muscle pain	Depression
Irritability	Upper respiratory infection

Possible interactions:

- Progesterone is not metabolized by your body well if you are also taking ketoconazole.

Other important information:

- Be careful using this drug if you have a history of depression.
- If you're diabetic, progesterone can affect your blood sugar levels.
- Don't use progesterone if you have unusual vaginal bleeding; kidney or liver problems; breast, cervical, or uterine cancer; or blood clotting disorders.
- Prometrium capsules contain peanut oil. Don't take them if you're allergic to peanuts.
- Stop taking Prometrium immediately and see your doctor if you develop vision problems or migraines.
- Have a thorough gynecological exam before beginning progesterone.
- Be careful taking this drug if you have epilepsy, migraines, asthma, or heart problems. These conditions could become worse.

PROGESTERONE, TOPICAL

Pregnancy category: NR
No driving

Brand:

Crinone

Crinone is a vaginal gel prescribed in fertility treatments and to correct menstrual irregularities.

How to take this drug:

- If you must use Crinone with another vaginal medication, wait at least six hours between applications.

Possible side effects:

Breast enlargement	Sleepiness
Constipation	Nausea
Cramps or abdominal pain	Headache
Nervousness	Breast pain
Depression	Urination problems
Decreased sex drive	Vaginal discharge
Joint pain	

Possible interactions:

- Don't use Crinone if you are using another vaginal medication.

Other important information:

- Be careful using Crinone if you have a history of depression.
- If you're diabetic, progesterone can affect your blood sugar levels.

- Don't use progesterone if you have unusual vaginal bleeding; kidney or liver problems; breast, cervical, or uterine cancer; or blood clotting disorders.
- Have a thorough gynecological exam before beginning progesterone.
- Be careful taking this drug if you have epilepsy, migraines, asthma, or heart problems. These conditions could become worse.

PROMETHAZINE HYDROCHLORIDE

Pregnancy category: C
No driving

Brand:

Phenergan Plain   *Prometh Plain*

Promethazine is a sedating antihistamine that relieves symptoms of food allergies, hay fever, and other allergies. It helps relieve sneezing, runny nose, itching, rashes, hives, swelling, and difficulty breathing. Promethazine can be used in addition to epinephrine to treat severe allergic reactions. It treats motion sickness and prevents or controls nausea and vomiting. Promethazine is also used as a sedative before or after some surgeries and given along with some pain relievers after surgery.

How to take this drug:

- For motion sickness, take the first dose a half-hour to an hour before you travel.

Possible side effects:

Sleepiness   Rash
Nausea

Possible interactions:

- While taking promethazine, avoid alcohol and other depressants such as sleeping pills, tranquilizers, and tricyclic antidepressants. Doctors will usually reduce your dose of barbiturates or analgesic depressants such as morphine by one-half if you are taking promethazine.

Other important information:

- Don't use promethazine if you have a lower respiratory disease, such as asthma, bronchitis, or pneumonia. It can dry out and thicken the mucus in your airways, making it more difficult to remove.
- Don't use promethazine if you are allergic to any phenothiazine or have sleep apnea.
- Don't take this drug if you have certain kinds of glaucoma, bladder neck obstruction, obstruction of the pylorus (opening from the stomach to the intestine), stomach ulcer, or an enlarged prostate.
- People with seizure disorders, poor liver function, or heart disease should use it cautiously.

- This drug may affect pregnancy test results and may increase blood sugar levels.
- Call your doctor if you experience any involuntary muscle movements or abnormal sensitivity to sunlight.

PROPAFENONE HYDROCHLORIDE

Pregnancy category: C

Brand:
Rythmol

Propafenone hydrochloride is given in a hospital setting to treat life-threatening arrhythmias.

Possible side effects:

Unusual taste	Nausea or vomiting
Dizziness	Constipation
Headache	Tiredness
Vision problems	Weakness
Difficulty breathing	Dry mouth
Diarrhea	

Possible interactions:
- Propafenone hydrochloride may interact with these drugs: local anesthetics, digoxin, beta-blockers, warfarin, desipramine, cyclosporin, theophylline, and rifampin.

Other important information:
- Don't use this drug if you suffer from several specific heart disorders, some lung disorders, or mineral imbalances. Talk to your doctor about your condition.
- Don't take this drug if you have a respiratory condition like chronic bronchitis or emphysema.
- If you have a pacemaker, get regular checkups while on propafenone hydrochloride.
- Tell your doctor if you develop any signs of infection, like chills, fever, sore throat, etc.
- Be careful taking this drug if you have liver or kidney problems.

PROPOXYPHENE HYDROCHLORIDE

Pregnancy category: C/D
No driving

Brand:

Darvon	*Dolene*
Kesso-Gesic	

This narcotic analgesic is used to relieve mild to moderate pain.

Possible side effects:

Dizziness	Sleepiness
Nausea	Headache
Constipation	Hallucinations
Depression	Anxiety
Rash	Stomach pain

Possible interactions:

- If you take propoxyphene along with alcohol or tranquilizers, antihistamines, or muscle relaxants, the combination may dangerously depress your nervous system.
- Propoxyphene may increase the effects of anticoagulants and anticonvulsants.
- If you take propoxyphene with high doses of aspirin, the combination may cause kidney damage.

Other important information:

- High doses or long-term use of propoxyphene can lead to drug dependence. Take this drug with caution if you are prone to addiction or if you are taking other depressants. Never take more than you are prescribed.
- People with liver or kidney problems may need a reduced dose.
- You may avoid some of the side effects if you lie down after taking this drug.

PROPRANOLOL HYDROCHLORIDE

Pregnancy category: C

Brand:

Inderal   *Inderal LA*

Propranolol is a beta blocker that controls high blood pressure, treats angina, various heart rhythm problems, and some kinds of muscle tremors, and is used after heart attacks to prevent further heart attacks. This drug is also used to treat and to prevent migraine headaches.

Possible side effects:

Prickling or tingling of the hands	Lightheadedness
Slow heartbeat	Depression
Vision changes	Hallucinations
Disorientation	Short-term memory loss
Vivid dreams	Hair loss
Dry eyes	Impotence
Nausea	Diarrhea
Constipation	

Possible interactions:

- Propranolol may increase the effects of antipyrine (drug that tests liver function) and the heart drug lidocaine.

- Propranolol may decrease the effects of the hormone thyroxine and the asthma drug theophylline.
- Effects of propranolol may be increased by the ulcer drug cimetidine and the antipsychotic drug chlorpromazine.
- Effects of propranolol may be decreased by alcohol, aluminum hydroxide gel (antacid), the seizure drug phenytoin, and the tuberculosis drug rifampin.
- If you take propranolol with the blood pressure drug reserpine, the combination may cause very low blood pressure, very slow heartbeat, or fainting.
- If you take propranolol with the antipsychotic drug haloperidol, the combination may cause very low blood pressure and heart attack.
- If you take propranolol with the angina drug verapamil, the combination may cause further weakening of the heart.

Other important information:
- People with heart failure, heart block, or asthma should not take propranolol. It can aggravate asthma symptoms.
- If you have diabetes, use this drug cautiously because beta blockers can mask the signs of low blood sugar.
- Propranolol can also mask signs of an overactive thyroid.
- Propranolol may decrease pressure in the eyes, which can alter glaucoma tests.
- People with poor liver or kidney function, bronchitis, or emphysema should take this drug with caution.
- Be on the lookout for signs that this drug is depressing your immune system: fever, sore throat, tiredness, weakness, bruising, or unusual bleeding. Have your blood tested regularly.
- Lupus is a rare side effect. Some signs of lupus are sore throat, fever, muscle and joint aches, and skin rash. Call your doctor immediately if you develop any of these signs.
- Tell your doctor immediately if you have any signs of congestive heart failure such as night cough; swelling of your legs, feet, or hands; or difficulty breathing, especially when lying down or after physical exertion.
- Never quit taking this drug without talking to your doctor. It could increase your risk of angina and heart attack.

PROTRIPTYLINE HYDROCHLORIDE

Pregnancy category: NR
No driving   MAO warning

Brand:
Vivactil

Protriptyline hydrochloride treats the symptoms of depression. It is a nonsedating tricyclic antidepressant, and it works particularly well for depressed people who are withdrawn and lack energy.

How to take this drug:

- Protriptyline may cause insomnia, so try not to take the medicine late in the day.

Possible side effects:

Agitation   Anxiety
Rapid heartbeat   Confusion
Dizziness   Seizures
Changes in sexual abilities   Drowsiness
Difficulty urinating   Headache
Nausea or vomiting   Loss of appetite
Unpleasant taste   Sun sensitivity
Breast enlargement

Possible interactions:

- Some blood-pressure-lowering drugs such as guanethidine may not work as well if you also take protriptyline.
- If you take protriptyline along with tranquilizers, alcohol, antihistamines, or muscle relaxants, the combination may dangerously depress your nervous system.
- Your doctor should supervise you closely for side effects if you take protriptyline along with any anticholinergic drugs such as some antihistamines and muscle relaxants or along with any sympathomimetic drugs such as some decongestants.
- The ulcer drug cimetidine can increase the levels of protriptyline in your body.

Other important information:

- Don't take this drug if you are recovering from a heart attack.
- Take this drug very cautiously if you have heart disease, urinary retention, glaucoma, thyroid disease, or a history of seizures.
- When possible, quit taking protriptyline several days before surgery.
- Be careful in hot weather. This drug could make you sweat less in high temperatures, so you're more likely to get a high fever or heatstroke.
- This drug is very likely to cause dry mouth and constipation, so drink plenty of fluids and eat a high-fiber diet.
- If you suddenly quit taking this drug, you could have nausea, headache, and a general feeling of fatigue. If you gradually quit taking the drug, you may still experience irritability, restlessness, and dream and sleep disturbances.

PYRAZINAMIDE

Pregnancy category: C

Brand:

Pyrazinamide

This drug is used to treat active tuberculosis.

How to take this drug:
- Never double a missed dose, instead take it as soon as you remember or skip it and go on with your regular schedule.

Possible side effects:

Nausea	Loss of appetite
Joint or muscle pain	Gout
Painful or difficult urination	

Possible interactions:
- This drug may interfere with certain urine tests.

Other important information:
- Don't use pyrazinamide if you have gout or severe liver damage.
- If you have mild liver disease or diabetes, use this drug with caution. Liver functions should be closely monitored. Contact your doctor if you develop nausea, tiredness, red and itchy skin, yellow eyes and skin (jaundice), and flu-like symptoms.
- Your uric acid levels should be checked regularly while you are taking this drug. High uric acid levels can cause gout.
- This drug may make your skin extra-sensitive to sunlight, so protect your skin if you'll be outdoors.

PYRIDOSTIGMINE BROMIDE

Pregnancy category: C

Brand:

Mestinon   *Regonol*

This muscle stimulant is used to treat myasthenia gravis (nerve/muscle weakness disease).

Possible side effects:

Increased saliva	Muscle spasms
Stomach cramps	Diarrhea
Frequent urination	Small pupils
Mucus in your lungs	Increased sweating
Gas	Watery eyes

Possible interactions:
- The heartbeat regulator atropine may decrease the effects of pyridostigmine.

Other important information:
- People with intestinal or urinary obstructions should not take this drug.
- Take this drug with caution if you have asthma.
- If you develop other side effects, contact your doctor immediately.

QUAZEPAM

Pregnancy category: X
No driving

Brand:
Doral

Quazepam is a sleep-inducing drug used to treat insomnia. It is a benzodiazepine.

Possible side effects:

Daytime drowsiness	Headache
Tiredness	Dizziness
Dry mouth	Upset stomach
Aggressiveness	Agitation

Possible interactions:
- If you take quazepam along with tranquilizers, alcohol, antihistamines, or muscle relaxants, the combination may dangerously depress your nervous system.

Other important information:
- You can become dependent on quazepam. To avoid seizures and other less severe withdrawal symptoms, quit taking the drug gradually under your doctor's supervision.
- People with poor liver, kidney, or lung function should use quazepam cautiously. The drug may stay in your body longer and increase your risk of side effects.
- You may have trouble sleeping for the first couple of nights after you stop taking this drug.
- With chronic use, quazepam is likely to accumulate in your body and cause daytime sleepiness and other side effects.
- Some people have memory loss for several hours after taking a benzodiazepine. Make sure you'll be able to get a full night's sleep after taking your medicine.

QUINAPRIL HYDROCHLORIDE

Pregnancy category: C/D

Brand:
Accupril

This angiotensin converting enzyme (ACE) inhibitor treats high blood pressure.

Possible side effects:

Dizziness	Coughing
Tiredness	Nausea
Chest pain	Diarrhea
Headache	Back pain

Possible interactions:

- Quinapril may increase levels of the antipsychotic drug lithium, possibly to toxic levels.
- Quinapril may decrease levels of the antibiotic tetracycline.

Other important information:

- People with poor kidney and liver functions should take this drug very cautiously.
- Quinapril may cause a severe drop in blood pressure after the first dose, particularly in people taking diuretics, on dialysis, or with congestive heart failure. Be careful when you rise quickly — you may feel lightheaded and dizzy. If you faint, stop taking the drug and immediately contact your doctor.
- Quinapril may cause dangerously high, even fatal levels of potassium in the blood. Don't use potassium-sparing diuretics or take potassium supplements without talking to your doctor.
- Be on the lookout for signs that this drug is depressing your immune system: fever, sore throat, tiredness, weakness, bruising, unusual bleeding. Have your blood tested regularly.
- Mild swelling can occur in the throat, face, lips, tongue, mucous membranes, hands, or feet, but swelling of the throat can be extremely dangerous. Contact your doctor immediately.
- If you develop jaundice (yellow eyes or skin), contact your doctor immediately.

RALOXIFENE HYDROCHLORIDE

Pregnancy category: X

Brand:

Evista

Raloxifene hydrochloride helps prevent osteoporosis in postmenopausal women.

How to take this drug:

- Take this drug with or without meals.

Possible side effects:

Hot flashes	Sinusitis
Sore throat	Cough
Weight gain	Joint or muscle pain
Nausea	Indigestion
Depression	Sleeplessness

Possible interactions:

- Cholestyramine affects how well raloxifene hydrochloride is absorbed.
- If you take this drug along with warfarin, have your doctor check your blood for clotting time.

Other important information:

- You may still need to take calcium supplements and vitamin D in addition to this medication.
- Don't take it if you are at risk of developing life-threatening blood clots.
- This drug is not recommended if you are premenopausal and are taking estrogen.
- Raloxifene hydrochloride may lower your cholesterol levels. Take this into account if you are taking other medications for high cholesterol.
- Talk to your doctor immediately if you experience breast pain or uterine bleeding.
- This medication won't treat hot flashes.
- There is no proven increased risk of endometrial or breast cancer with this drug.

RAMIPRIL

Pregnancy category: C/D

Brand:

Altace

This angiotensin converting enzyme (ACE) inhibitor treats high blood pressure.

Possible side effects:

Coughing	Headache
Dizziness	Fatigue
Nausea	

Possible interactions:

- This drug may increase levels of the antipsychotic drug lithium, possibly to toxic levels.

Other important information:

- People with poor kidney and liver functions should take this drug very cautiously.
- Ramipril may cause a severe drop in blood pressure after the first dose, particularly in people taking diuretics, on dialysis, or with congestive heart failure. Be careful when you rise quickly — you may feel lightheaded and dizzy. If you faint, stop taking the drug and immediately contact your doctor.
- Ramipril may cause dangerously high, often fatal levels of potassium in the blood. Don't use potassium-sparing diuretics or take potassium supplements without talking to your doctor.
- Be on the lookout for signs that this drug is depressing your immune system: fever, sore throat, tiredness, weakness, bruising, unusual bleeding. Have your blood tested regularly.

- Mild swelling can occur in the throat, face, lips, tongue, mucous membranes, hands, or feet, but swelling of the throat can be extremely dangerous. Contact your doctor immediately.

Ranitidine hydrochloride

Pregnancy category: B

Brand:
Zantac

Ranitidine hydrochloride helps stomach ulcers heal, treats gastro-esophageal reflux disease (severe heartburn), controls bleeding in the stomach or intestines, and treats Zollinger-Ellison disease, a condition in which your stomach produces too much acid.

Possible side effects:
Headache	Diarrhea
Sleepiness	Dizziness
Breast enlargement in men	Impotence

Possible interactions:
- No significant interactions have been reported.

Other important information:
- Don't take ranitidine if you are allergic to any anti-ulcer drugs.
- Your doctor may need to adjust your dose if you have liver or kidney problems.
- Be on the lookout for signs that this drug is depressing your immune system: fever, sore throat, tiredness, weakness, bruising, unusual bleeding. Have your blood tested regularly.
- Ranitidine may cause itching or peeling skin. Rare reactions are serious skin disorders in which dark red rings or raised spots erupt on your skin (Stevens-Johnson syndrome) or parts of your skin deteriorate.
- You can take antacids while you take ranitidine.

Recombinant OspA

Pregnancy category: C
Refrigerate

Brand:
LYMErix

This drug is a 3-dose vaccine against Lyme disease, which is caused by the Borrelia burgdorferi bacterium and carried by Ixodes ticks.

How to take this drug:
- The vaccine is given in three doses over a 12-month period.
- You must receive all three injections.

Possible side effects:

Pain at injection site
Headache
Tiredness

Muscle or joint pain
Upper respiratory infection
Rash

Possible interactions:

- If you are receiving medication to suppress your immune system, the vaccine may not be effective.
- Don't take this vaccine if you are also taking an anticoagulant.

Other important information:

- Even if you've had Lyme disease before, you can get it again.
- This vaccine is not a treatment for Lyme disease.
- There is no guarantee that the vaccine will protect everyone from the disease.
- This is recommended for people between the ages of 15 and 70.
- It will not protect you against other tick-borne diseases (babesiosis or ehrlichiosis).
- Consider taking steps to protect yourself from tick bites, such as wearing pants and long-sleeved shirts, using a commercial tick repellent, etc.
- Don't take this medication if you have a clotting disorder.

REPAGLINIDE

Pregnancy category: C

Brand:

Prandin

Repaglinide is a drug used to lower blood glucose levels in type II diabetics.

How to take this drug:

- Take repaglinide before meals. If you skip a meal, skip that dose. If you add a meal, add a dose.

Possible side effects:

High blood sugar levels
(hyperglycemia)
Upper respiratory infection
Joint pain

Low blood sugar levels
(hypoglycemia)
Sinusitis

Possible interactions:

- These drugs may affect how repaglinide is absorbed in your body: ketoconazole, miconazole, erythromycin, troglitazone, rifampicin, barbiturates, and carbamazepine.
- Watch for signs of hypoglycemia if you take repaglinide with NSAIDs, salicylates, sulfonamides, chloramphenicol, coumarins, probenecid, MAO inhibitors, or beta-blockers.

- These drugs may raise your blood sugar levels: thiazides, other diuretics, corticosteroids, phenothiazines, thyroid products, estrogens, oral contraceptives, phenytoin, nicotinic acid, sympathomimetics, calcium channel blockers, and isoniazid.

Other important information:
- If you have kidney or liver problems, your doctor will need to monitor this drug carefully.
- Use repaglinide in addition to a diet and exercise program.
- Don't use this medication if you suffer from diabetic ketoacidosis or have type I diabetes.
- Using drugs to lower blood sugar levels can increase your risk of heart disease.
- Know the warning signs of low blood sugar levels (hypoglycemia): fatigue, weakness, irritability.
- If you develop fever or infection, undergo surgery, or experience a traumatic accident, you may need to discontinue repaglinide for a period of time.
- Your blood glucose must be checked regularly on this medication.

RIFAMPIN

Pregnancy category: C

Brand:
Rifadin   *Rimactane*

This drug is used to treat all forms of tuberculosis and certain other bacterial infections.

How to take this drug:
- Preferably, take this drug on an empty stomach — at least one hour before or two hours after meals. If the drug irritates your stomach, you can take it with food.
- Never double a missed dose, instead take it as soon as you remember or skip it and go on with your regular schedule.

Possible side effects:

Dizziness	Headache
Drowsiness	Lack of coordination
Vision problems	Weakness
Confusion	Menstrual changes
Nausea	Heartburn
Gas	Stomach cramps
Flushing	Itching
Rash	Sore mouth or tongue
Flu-like symptoms	

Possible interactions:
- This drug may decrease levels or effects of the following drugs: anticoagulants, anticonvulsants, barbiturates, beta blockers, corticosteroids, birth control pills, the immunosuppressant cyclosporine, diabetic drugs, the anti-anxiety drug diazepam, the antifungal drug ketoconazole, and the asthma drug theophylline.
- Effects of this drug may be increased by the gout drug probenecid.
- Avoid alcoholic beverages while taking this drug. The combination could cause liver damage.

Other important information:
- People with liver disease should use this drug with caution. Even so, liver functions should be closely monitored. Watch yourself for signs of liver damage such as fatigue, loss of appetite, yellow skin and eyes, and dark urine.
- Blood counts should be done before and throughout treatment.
- This drug may color urine, stools, sweat, saliva, and tears red-orange. Soft contact lenses may be permanently stained.
- Be on the lookout for signs that this drug is depressing your immune system: fever, sore throat, tiredness, weakness, bruising, unusual bleeding. Have your blood tested regularly.

RIFAPENTINE

Pregnancy category: C

Brand:
Priftin

Rifapentine is an antibiotic used to treat pulmonary tuberculosis (TB).

How to take this drug:
- You must follow a very strict schedule with this drug.
- Take your medication exactly as prescribed for the entire time that you are being treated, and don't skip doses. Otherwise, TB can return.
- If you have a problem with nausea, vomiting, or upset stomach, taking this drug with food may help.

Possible side effects:

Fever	Loss of appetite
General discomfort	Nausea or vomiting
Darkened urine	Yellow skin or eyes
Pain or swelling in your joints	Bloody urine
Rash	Itching
Skin breakouts	Permanently stained contact lenses

Possible interactions:
- Many medications can interact with rifapentine.

- This drug may affect the reliability of birth control pills, so other methods of birth control should be used.

Other important information:
- Rifapentine should never be taken alone; it will be prescribed in combination with other anti-TB drugs based on your condition.
- Don't take rifapentine if you have a history of allergic reaction to any of the rifamycins (e.g., rifampin and rifabutin).
- Anti-TB drugs can cause serious liver problems; have your doctor monitor your liver function.
- If you begin having severe and/or constant diarrhea, stop taking rifapentine immediately, and contact your health care provider for treatment.
- If you have a history of poor nutrition, alcoholism, diabetes, or you are a teenager; your doctor may want you to add vitamin B6 as a supplement to your diet.
- Notify your doctor if you develop any of the listed side effects.
- You must have regular checkups while taking this drug.

RISEDRONATE SODIUM

Pregnancy category: C

Brand:
Actonel

Risedronate sodium is used to treat Paget's disease of the bone.

How to take this drug:
- This drug works best without food. For maximum absorption, fast 10 hours prior or four hours after taking it. If you are unable to follow this type of schedule, take it at least 30 minutes before the first food or drink of the day.
- Do not lie down for 30 minutes after taking risedronate sodium.
- If you take aspirin or NSAIDs with this drug, you are more likely to suffer from stomach or intestinal problems.

Possible side effects:

Flu-like symptoms	Chest pain
Weakness	Diarrhea
Abdominal pain	Nausea
Constipation	Joint pain
Headache	Dizziness
Rash	

Possible interactions:
- Do not take calcium supplements or antacids at the same time as this drug.

Other important information:
- Don't take risedronate sodium if you have low blood calcium levels (hypocalcemia) or severe kidney problems.

- Tell your doctor if you have a history of stomach problems because this drug can cause difficulty swallowing, inflammation of the esophagus, esophageal ulcer, and stomach ulcer.
- This drug can interfere with bone-imaging tests.

RISPERIDONE

Pregnancy category: C
No driving

Brand:
Risperdal

Risperidone is prescribed to treat psychotic disorders, especially schizophrenia.

Possible side effects:

Sleeplessness	Tremors
Headache	Anxiety
Sleepiness	Dizziness
Constipation	Nausea
Indigestion	Runny or stuffy nose
Rash	Irregular heartbeat

Possible interactions:
- If you take risperidone with medications to lower your blood pressure, you are more likely to suffer from dizziness when you stand up suddenly.
- If you take this drug along with tranquilizers, alcohol, antihistamines, or muscle relaxants, the combination may dangerously depress your nervous system.
- Risperidone may affect how your body uses levodopa, dopamine agonists, carbamazepine, clozapine, and fluoxetine.

Other important information:
- Your dose of risperidone must be adjusted if you have kidney or liver disease.
- Some antipsychotic drugs can bring on Neuroleptic Malignant Syndrome (NMS), a sometimes fatal combination of symptoms (muscle rigidity, unstable pulse and blood pressure, kidney failure, unconsciousness, and fever).
- Because of the risk of developing tardive dyskinesia, a muscle movement disorder that is often irreversible, risperidone should only be prescribed in the smallest doses, for the shortest amount of time, and only if other medications are ruled out.
- This drug can make you dizzy or faint when you stand up suddenly.
- Use this drug cautiously if you are recovering from a heart attack, have heart disease, high blood pressure, seizures, or are exposed to extreme temperatures.

RIZATRIPTAN BENZOATE

Pregnancy category: C
No driving   MAO warning

Brand:
Maxalt

Rizatriptan benzoate is used for the short-term treatment of most types of migraine attacks in adults. It will not prevent migraines and has not been shown to treat hemiplegic or basilar migraines, or cluster headaches.

How to take this drug:
- If taken with food, it may take an additional hour for this drug to reach its peak effectiveness.
- Wait at least two hours before taking a second dose.
- Do not take more than 30 mg within any 24-hour period.

Possible side effects:
Sleepiness or fatigue	Dizziness
Pain, pressure or tightness in your chest or throat	Nausea

Possible interactions:
- Don't take rizatriptan benzoate if you have taken other migraine medications similar to it, or medications containing ergotamine, dihydroergotamine, or methysergide within the past 24 hours.
- Phenylketonuric patients should not take this drug because it contains phenylalanine.
- Talk to your doctor before combining this drug with selective serotonin reuptake inhibitors (SSRIs) like fluoxetine, fluvoxamine, paroxetine, or sertraline.
- If you are also taking propranolol, use the 5-mg dose of rizatriptan benzoate, and don't take more than three doses within a 24-hour period.

Other important information:
- Don't take this drug if you have a history of heart or circulatory disease, including heart attack, angina (chest pain), or stroke.
- Since this drug may increase blood pressure, don't take it if you have uncontrolled high blood pressure.
- Talk to your doctor before taking this drug if you have any of these heart disease risk factors: high cholesterol, high blood pressure, obesity, diabetes, smoking, strong family history of heart disease, or if you are postmenopausal or a male over 40.
- Use extra caution with this drug if you are on dialysis or have liver disease.
- If you develop pain or pressure in your chest as a side effect, talk to your doctor immediately.

SACROSIDASE

Pregnancy category: NR
Refrigerate

Brand:
Sucraid

Sacrosidase is used as a replacement for those who do not have the enzymes needed to properly break down and absorb sucrose (table sugar) and iso-maltose (a type of starch) in the intestines.

How to take this drug:
- Because this drug contains no preservatives, bacteria will grow in it. Reseal and store it properly, write down the date you open a bottle, and throw away any open bottle after four weeks.
- Mix sacrosidase with water, milk, or infant formula. Don't mix it with fruit juice because the acids may reduce its effectiveness.
- This drug does not work if it is heated before or after mixing.
- Take half the dose at the beginning of each meal or snack and the other half at the end of the meal or snack.
- Use the measuring scoop or dropper that comes with your prescription in order to get the most accurate dose each time. Don't use a household measuring spoon.

Possible side effects:
Stomach pain	Nausea or vomiting
Diarrhea	Constipation
Difficulty sleeping	Headache
Nervousness	Dehydration

Other important information:
- Don't take sacrosidase if you are allergic to yeast, yeast products, or glycerin (glycerol).
- This drug may cause an allergic reaction. If you develop swelling of the face, wheezing, or difficulty breathing, get help right away. You may have to take your first and second doses in your doctor's office to observe how your body reacts, or you may be tested in advance to check your sensitivity to the drug.
- Talk to your doctor about your diet if you are diabetic and plan on taking this drug.

SALMETEROL XINAFOATE

Pregnancy category: C
MAO warning

Brand:
Serevent

Salmeterol xinafoate is a maintenance drug used to treat asthma over a long period of time. It can also prevent asthma attacks brought on by exercise. The inhaler may be used to treat breathing problems from emphysema and chronic bronchitis.

How to take this drug:
- Salmeterol xinafoate is available as an inhaled powder (Serevent Diskus) or as an inhaler (Serevent Inhalation Aerosol).
- Don't take this drug more than twice a day.
- You must take salmeterol xinafoate regularly in order for it to work.
- Never double a missed dose, instead take it as soon as you remember or skip it and go on with your regular schedule.
- The Serevent Diskus is disposable.
- Read and follow the instructions for using this medication carefully.
- If you are using salmeterol xinafoate to prevent exercise-induced asthma, take it 30 minutes before starting to exercise.

Possible side effects:
Headache
Bronchitis
Rapid heartbeat

Runny or stuffy nose
Flu
Sore throat

Possible interactions:
- Be very careful using these drugs with salmeterol xinafoate: MAO inhibitors, tricyclic antidepressants, beta-blockers, loop or thiazide diuretics.

Other important information:
- This medication will not stop an asthma attack.
- Tell your doctor if your medications are no longer helping your asthma. This can be a serious warning sign.
- Take this drug along with any other asthma medications (steroids) your doctor has prescribed.
- Allergic reactions can be serious. Call your doctor immediately if you develop difficulty breathing, hives, swelling, or a rash.
- Some people develop heart-related side effects after taking salmeterol xinafoate. Have your doctor monitor your heart rate and blood pressure, especially if you already have heart problems.

SCOPOLAMINE

Pregnancy category: C
No driving

Brand:
Transderm-Scop

This circular, flat patch is placed behind the ear several hours before you travel to prevent nausea and vomiting due to motion sickness. It works for up to three days.

Possible side effects:

Dry mouth	Drowsiness
Blurred vision	Dilated pupils

Possible interactions:

- If you take scopolamine along with alcohol or tranquilizers, antihistamines, or muscle relaxers, the combination may dangerously depress your nervous system.

Other important information:

- People with glaucoma should not use scopolamine.
- People with stomach, intestinal, or bladder obstruction, poor liver or kidney functions, or problems with metabolism should use this drug cautiously.
- If it comes in contact with your eyes, this drug can cause blurred vision and dilation of your pupils. Wash your hands with soap and water after you handle the patch. If the drug does get in your eyes and they feel itchy, dry or painful, remove the patch and call your doctor.
- When you remove the patch, you may have withdrawal symptoms including nausea, vomiting, headache, and dizziness.
- If you have any unusual side effects, remove the patch and call your doctor.
- When you throw the patch away, fold it in half with the sticky side together to avoid accidental contact with children or pets.

SECOBARBITAL SODIUM

Pregnancy category: D
No driving

Brand:

Seconal Sodium

This barbiturate is used to promote sleep and to relieve anxiety and tension.

Possible side effects:

Daytime sleepiness

Possible interactions:

- If you take secobarbital along with tranquilizers, alcohol, antihistamines, or muscle relaxants, the combination may dangerously depress your nervous system.
- Secobarbital may increase the effects of corticosteroids.
- This drug may decrease the effectiveness of anti-clotting drugs like warfarin, the anti-fungal drug griseofulvin, birth control pills, and doxycycline.
- Secobarbital may increase the effects of phenytoin.
- Sodium valproate, valproic acid, and monoamine oxidase (MAO) inhibitors may increase the depressant effects of secobarbital.

Other important information:

- You can become addicted to this drug so don't increase your dose without talking to your doctor.

- Withdraw from secobarbital slowly. If you quit taking the drug quickly, you may have nightmares, insomnia, anxiety, dizziness, and nausea. If you're addicted to the drug and you quit taking it suddenly, delirium, convulsions, and death may result.
- Secobarbital is a short-acting barbiturate — it begins working in 10 to 15 minutes and lasts about three to four hours.
- Secobarbital loses its ability to promote sleep after two weeks of taking it regularly.
- You should have regular blood, liver, and kidney tests if you take this drug for a long time.
- Don't rely on birth control pills as a means of contraception while you're taking secobarbital.

SELEGILINE HYDROCHLORIDE

Pregnancy category: C

Brand:

Eldepryl

Selegiline hydrochloride is used along with levodopa and carbidopa to treat Parkinson's disease. It works with levodopa to improve walking ability, speech, and shaking muscles.

Possible side effects:

Nausea	Hallucinations
Confusion	Depression
Sleeplessness	Uncontrolled muscle movements
Irregular heartbeat	Agitation
Chest pain	Swelling
Burning lips or mouth	Constipation
Drowsiness	Increased sweating
Hair loss	Shakiness
Weakness	Weight loss

Possible interactions:

- This drug interacts dangerously with serotonin-based antidepressants like Paxil, Prozac, and Zoloft.
- Taking selegiline with the pain medicine meperidine (Demerol) may cause high fever, seizures, and coma.
- After taking the antidepressant fluoxetine, you should wait five weeks before you begin taking selegiline. You should wait 14 days after you quit taking selegiline before you begin taking fluoxetine.
- Your doctor may reduce your dose of levodopa after you begin taking selegiline.

Other important information:

- Never take more than 10 mg of selegiline a day. Taking more than this amount could cause dangerously high blood pressure. Call your doctor if you develop a severe headache — it could be a sign of high blood pressure.

SERTRALINE

Pregnancy category: B
No driving   MAO warning

Brand:
Zoloft

Sertraline, a selective serotonin reuptake inhibitor, treats the symptoms of depression.

How to take this drug:
* You can take your dose in the morning or the evening.

Possible side effects:

Nausea	Diarrhea
Stomach pain	Shakiness
Dizziness	Sleeplessness
Sleepiness	Increased sweating
Dry mouth	Decreased appetite
Ejaculation problems	

Possible interactions:
* This drug interacts dangerously with MAO inhibitors like Eldepryl, Marplan, Nardil, and Parnate.
* Sertraline may cause increased bleeding if you take it while you are taking warfarin. It may affect levels of warfarin and digitoxin in your body, and vice versa.
* The ulcer drug cimetidine may increase levels or effects of sertraline.
* If you take lithium, your lithium levels should be closely monitored after you begin taking sertraline.

Other important information:
* You may need a lower than normal dose of sertraline if you have liver or kidney disease. Your doctor should monitor you closely for side effects.
* Take this drug with caution if you have a history of seizures.

SEVELAMER HYDROCHLORIDE

Pregnancy category: C

Brand:
Renagel

Sevelamer hydrochloride is used to lower the level of phosphorus in patients on hemodialysis with end-stage kidney disease.

How to take this drug:
* Take this drug with meals.

- Don't chew or take apart the capsules because the contents expand in water.

Possible side effects:

Diarrhea	Infection
Pain	Vomiting
Indigestion	Headache
Blood clots	

Possible interactions:

- Talk to your doctor about all prescription and nonprescription drugs you are taking. You may need to take them one hour before or three hours after your dose of sevelamer hydrochloride.

Other important information:

- Don't take sevelamer hydrochloride if you have hypophosphatemia (low levels of phosphorus) or bowel obstruction.
- Stick to your prescribed diet.

SIBUTRAMINE HYDROCHLORIDE

Pregnancy category: C
No driving   MAO warning

Brand:

Meridia

Sibutramine hydrochloride monohydrate is used along with a low-calorie diet to manage obesity.

How to take this drug:

- Take this drug with or without food.

Possible side effects:

Dry mouth	Loss of appetite
Sleeplessness	Constipation
Dizziness	Anxiety
Headache	Depression
Runny or stuffy nose	Sore throat
Rash	Back pain
Flu-like symptoms	Nausea
Joint pain	Menstrual pain
Weakness	Abdominal pain
Chest pain	

Possible interactions:

- Tell your doctor if you are taking any weight loss products, decongestants, antidepressants, cough medicines, lithium, dihydroergotamine, sumatriptan (Imitrex), or tryptophan.

Other important information:
- Don't use this drug if you have severe kidney or liver conditions, suffer from anorexia nervosa, or are taking other drugs to suppress your appetite.
- Because sibutramine hydrochloride monohydrate can increase your blood pressure and heart rate, you must have your doctor monitor you regularly while on this drug. If you have a history of high blood pressure, heart disease, congestive heart failure, arrhythmias, or stroke, don't take this medication.
- Be careful if you have glaucoma since this drug can cause an eye condition called mydriasis (abnormal pupil dilation).
- Use this drug cautiously if you have a history of seizures.
- Sibutramine hydrochloride monohydrate is a controlled substance that can lead to some physical or psychological dependence.

SILDENAFIL CITRATE

Pregnancy category: B

Brand:
Viagra

Sildenafil citrate is used to treat impotence in men.

How to take this drug:
- Sildenafil citrate may be taken anywhere from 30 minutes to four hours before sexual activity.
- Don't take it more than once a day.
- If you take this drug with a high-fat meal, it won't be absorbed as easily.

Possible side effects:

Heart-related problems including heart attack, sudden death, irregular heartbeat, stroke, chest pain and increased blood pressure	Headache Flushing Upset stomach Stuffy nose
Urinary tract infection	Vision changes such as
Diarrhea	color or light sensitivity

Possible interactions:
- Several medications interact with this drug, so be sure to tell your doctor about all prescription and nonprescription medications you are on.
- Sildenafil citrate has not been studied with other treatments for impotence, so combining it with another treatment is not recommended.

Other important information:
- This drug does not protect you from getting sexually transmitted diseases.
- It should not be used by women or children.
- Don't take it if you are currently using medicines that contain nitrates, such as nitroglycerin.

- Because of possible serious side effects, talk to your doctor if you have recent heart problems, extremes in blood pressure, chest pain, or eye disorders.
- Before taking sildenafil citrate, have your doctor determine the cause of your impotence and if sexual activity is advisable.
- If your erection lasts longer than four hours, you may have developed priapism. Contact your doctor immediately.
- Conditions like sickle cell anemia, leukemia, multiple myeloma, or an abnormally shaped penis may prevent you from taking this drug.
- If you have kidney or liver disease, your doctor may need to adjust your dose.

SIMVASTATIN

Pregnancy category: X

Brand:
Zocor

Simvastatin is used to reduce total cholesterol and LDL cholesterol levels.

Possible side effects:

Headache	Stomach pain
Upper respiratory infection	Nausea
Gas	Indigestion
Constipation	Diarrhea
Weakness	

Possible interactions:
- The following drugs may increase the risk of rhabdomyolysis (a muscle-destroying disease) when you take them with simvastatin: the blood fat-reducer gemfibrozil, the antibiotic erythromycin, immunosuppressant drugs, and niacin.
- Simvastatin may increase the effects of the anticoagulant warfarin.

Other important information:
- Simvastatin should not be used by people with liver disease or suspected liver problems.
- Use simvastatin with caution if you have a history of high alcohol consumption or poor kidney function.
- Simvastatin may alter some hormone levels.
- This drug can also lead to kidney failure (caused by the rhabdomyolysis) in people with severe infections, uncontrolled seizures, low blood pressure, any kind of trauma such as major surgery, or severe metabolic, electrolyte, or endocrine disorders.
- A serious possible side effect is the dangerous disease that destroys muscle tissue called rhabdomyolysis. Contact your doctor if you develop any muscle pain, tenderness, or weakness, especially if accompanied by fever.

- Since simvastatin can cause severe liver damage, you should have regular liver function tests while you're taking this drug.

SPIRONOLACTONE

Pregnancy category: NR
No driving

Brand:

Aldactone

This diuretic helps control high blood pressure. It is also used to help stabilize potassium levels in people taking digitalis and to reduce fluid retention and swelling in conditions such as cirrhosis of the liver, congestive heart failure, and kidney disease. Doctors may use spironolactone to diagnose an overactive adrenal gland.

Possible side effects:

Vomiting	Stomach cramps
Diarrhea	Menstrual problems
Postmenopausal bleeding	Erection problems
Breast tumors	Unusual hair growth
Deepening of the voice	Breast enlargement in men
Confusion	Headache
Lack of coordination	Tiredness
Drowsiness	Drug fever
Rash or hives	

Other important information:

- People with kidney problems should not take this drug.
- Weigh daily so you'll know if you're losing too much fluid. Losing too much fluid can cause dehydration and possibly blood clots. Warning signs of dehydration include dry mouth, thirst, drowsiness, and weakness. Contact your doctor immediately if you stop urinating.
- If you have high blood pressure, avoid using over-the-counter cold remedies or diet pills that can increase blood pressure.
- This drug can cause dangerously high levels of potassium in your body. So don't take supplements that contain potassium unless your doctor tells you otherwise, and watch for these warning signs: prickling or tingling sensation, muscle weakness, tiredness, and slow heartbeat. Very high potassium levels can cause serious heart rhythm problems and death.
- Your doctor should regularly check your electrolyte levels (levels of salt, potassium, etc.).
- It can also cause bleeding or ulceration in the stomach.

SUCRALFATE

Pregnancy category: B

Brand:
Carafate

Sucralfate is used to treat stomach and duodenal ulcers.

How to take this drug:
* Take your medicine on an empty stomach at least one hour before meals.

Possible side effects:

Constipation	Nausea or vomiting
Diarrhea	Stomach pain
Gas	Indigestion
Dry mouth	Headache
Sleepiness	Sleeplessness
Dizziness	Back pain

Possible interactions:
* Sucralfate may decrease your body's absorption of ciprofloxacin, keto-conazole, the seizure drug phenytoin, the ulcer drugs cimetidine and ranitidine, the heart drug digoxin, the antibiotic tetracycline, and the asthma drug theophylline.

Other important information:
* People with kidney failure and those on dialysis should use this drug cautiously.
* If you have kidney problems, make sure you avoid aluminum-containing antacids. Your body could absorb too much aluminum. Otherwise, you can take antacids while you take sucralfate, but don't take them within 30 minutes of taking sucralfate.

SULFAMETHOXAZOLE

Pregnancy category: C
Refrigerate

Brand:
Gantanol

This sulfa drug is used to treat various infections of the urinary tract, ears, and eyes. It is also used to treat meningitis, malaria, nocardiosis, and toxoplasmosis.

How to take this drug:
* Take your medicine on an empty stomach with a full glass of water.
* Throw away any medicine you haven't used after 14 days.

Possible side effects:

Nausea	Diarrhea
Loss of appetite	Stomach pain

Headache   Depression
Sleeplessness   Drowsiness
Convulsions   Hallucinations
Ringing in the ears   Hearing loss
Dizziness   Lack of coordination
Joint pain   Fever
Chills   Hair loss
Inflamed mouth or tongue

Possible interactions:
- This drug may increase levels or effects of the seizure drug phenytoin and the anticoagulant warfarin.
- It may also cause the cancer drug methotrexate to build up to toxic levels.
- You should not use sulfamethoxazole with methenamine, a drug used to relieve discomfort of the lower urinary tract. Methenamine may increase your chances of dangerous, and possibly fatal, reactions to sulfa drugs. Sulfamethoxazole can also increase levels of methenamine in your body.

Other important information:
- People with poor liver or kidney function, asthma, or G6PD deficiency should use this drug with caution. It may cause the destruction of red blood cells in people with G6PD.
- Blood and urine should be tested regularly during treatment.
- This drug may cause blood disorders in elderly people who are taking diuretics.
- To help prevent kidney stones, drink plenty of fluids while taking this drug.
- This drug may make your skin extra-sensitive to sunlight, so protect your skin if you'll be outdoors.
- Take all of the prescription, even after you begin to feel better.
- Be on the lookout for signs that this drug is depressing your immune system: fever, sore throat, tiredness, weakness, bruising, unusual bleeding. Have your blood tested regularly.
- Liver and kidney damage and allergic reactions such as rashes and other skin problems are some of the possible risks of taking this drug. Allergic reactions can be serious and even fatal. Discontinue drug and call your doctor if fever, rash, or other allergic reaction occurs.

SULFAMETHOXAZOLE AND TRIMETHOPRIM

Pregnancy category: C

Brand:
Bactrim   *Bactrim DS*
Cotrim   *Cotrim DS*
Septra   *Septra DS*
Sulfamethoprim   *Sulfamethoprim DS*

This combination drug is used to treat infections of the intestines (such as traveler's diarrhea), urinary tract, ears, and lungs (such as frequently recurring bronchitis).

How to take this drug:
* Take with food or milk if this drug upsets your stomach. If it doesn't upset your stomach, take it one hour before or two hours after a meal.

Possible side effects:

Nausea	Diarrhea
Loss of appetite	Stomach pain
Inflamed mouth or tongue	Headache
Depression	Sleeplessness
Drowsiness	Convulsions
Hallucinations	Ringing in the ears
Hearing loss	Dizziness
Lack of coordination	Joint pain
Fever	Chills
Hair loss	

Possible interactions:
* This drug may increase levels or effects of the seizure drug phenytoin and the anticoagulant warfarin.
* It may increase levels of the cancer drug methotrexate to toxic levels.
* This drug may cause blood disorders in elderly people who are taking diuretics.

Other important information:
* People with poor liver or kidney function, asthma, folate deficiency, malnutrition, or G6PD deficiency should use it with caution. This drug may cause destruction of red blood cells in people with G6PD.
* Blood and urine should be tested regularly during treatment.
* To help prevent kidney stones, drink at least four to six glasses of water every day while taking this drug.
* This drug may make your skin extra-sensitive to sunlight, so protect your skin if you'll be outdoors.
* Be on the lookout for signs that this drug is depressing your immune system: fever, sore throat, tiredness, weakness, bruising, unusual bleeding. Have your blood tested regularly.
* Taking an antibiotic for a long time can cause bacteria or fungus to overgrow, leading to another infection. If you get one of these "super-infections," you may need to quit taking this drug and start taking another antibiotic for the second infection.
* Liver and kidney damage and allergic reactions such as rashes and other skin problems are some of the possible risks of taking this drug. Allergic reactions can be serious and even fatal. Discontinue drug and call your doctor if you experience difficulty breathing, fever, chills,

hallucinations, a skin rash or hives, tiredness, nervousness, muscle weakness, or low back pain.

SULFASALAZINE

Pregnancy category: B

Brand:
Azulfidine

This anti-inflammatory drug is used to treat ulcerative colitis.

How to take this drug:
* Take this drug with food or milk to avoid upset stomach.

Possible side effects:
Nausea	Vomiting
Headache	Loss of appetite
Upset stomach	Infertility in men
Itching	Rash
Hives	Fever

Possible interactions:
* Sulfasalazine may decrease levels of folic acid and the heart drug digoxin.

Other important information:
* Don't use this drug if you have obstructions of the intestines or urinary tract.
* People with poor liver or kidney functions, asthma, blood diseases, or G6PD deficiency should use it with caution. This drug may cause destruction of red blood cells in people with G6PD deficiency.
* Blood and urine should be tested regularly throughout treatment.
* Don't stop taking this drug because you feel better. Take the full course of treatment.
* Avoid prolonged exposure to the sun, and wear a sunscreen and protective clothing.
* Drink extra fluids while you're taking sulfasalazine to help prevent kidney stones.
* Be on the lookout for signs that this drug is depressing your immune system: fever, sore throat, tiredness, weakness, bruising, unusual bleeding. Have your blood tested regularly.

SULFISOXAZOLE

Pregnancy category: C
Refrigerate

Brand:
Sosol

Sulfisoxazole is used to treat various infections of the urinary tract, ears, and eyes. It is also used to treat meningitis, malaria, nocardiosis, and toxoplasmosis.

How to take this drug:
* Take your medicine on an empty stomach with a full glass of water.
* Throw away any medicine you haven't used after 14 days.

Possible side effects:

Nausea	Diarrhea
Loss of appetite	Stomach pain
Inflamed mouth or tongue	Headache
Depression	Sleeplessness
Drowsiness	Convulsions
Hallucinations	Ringing in the ears
Hearing loss	Dizziness
Lack of coordination	Joint pain
Fever	Chills
Hair loss	

Possible interactions:
* This drug may increase levels or effects of the anesthetic thiopental and the anticoagulant warfarin.
* It may also increase levels of the cancer drug methotrexate to toxic levels.

Other important information:
* People who have poor liver or kidney functions, asthma, or G6PD deficiency should use this drug with caution. It may cause destruction of red blood cells in people with G6PD.
* Blood and urine should be tested regularly during treatment.
* To help prevent kidney stones, drink plenty of fluids while taking this drug.
* This drug may make your skin extra-sensitive to sunlight, so protect your skin if you'll be outdoors.
* Take all of the prescription, even after you begin to feel better.
* Be on the lookout for signs that this drug is depressing your immune system: fever, sore throat, tiredness, weakness, bruising, unusual bleeding. Have your blood tested regularly.
* Liver and kidney damage and allergic reactions including rashes and other skin problems are some of the possible risks of taking this drug. Allergic reactions can be serious and even fatal. Discontinue drug and call your doctor if fever, rash, or other allergic reaction occurs.

SULINDAC

Pregnancy category: NR

Brand:
Clinoril

This nonsteroidal anti-inflammatory drug (NSAID) relieves the symptoms of arthritis, bursitis, gout, and ankylosing spondylitis.

How to take this drug:
- Take with food, after meals, or with antacids to help prevent stomach irritation.

Possible side effects:

Nausea	Diarrhea
Constipation	Gas
Stomach cramps	Loss of appetite
Ringing in the ears	Itching
Rash	Water retention or swelling
Headache	Nervousness
Dizziness	

Possible interactions:
- Avoid alcohol and aspirin while taking NSAIDs such as sulindac.
- Sulindac may prolong bleeding time if used at the same time as anticoagulants.
- It may increase levels of the cancer drug methotrexate and the immunosuppressant cyclosporine to toxic levels.
- Effects of this drug may be decreased by the arthritis drug diflunisal.
- If you need to stop taking corticosteroids while you're taking sulindac, be sure to withdraw slowly from the steroids instead of stopping suddenly.

Other important information:
- Don't take this drug if you are allergic to aspirin or other NSAIDs.
- Take this drug with caution if you have intestinal disease, poor liver or kidney function, poor heart function, high blood pressure, fluid retention, diabetes, or kidney stones.
- Be on the lookout for signs that this drug is depressing your immune system: fever, sore throat, tiredness, weakness, bruising, unusual bleeding. Have your blood tested regularly.
- Bleeding stomach ulcers and liver or kidney damage are rare but serious reactions to using sulindac for long periods of time. Warning signs of liver damage include nausea, tiredness, red and itchy skin, yellow eyes and skin (jaundice), and flu-like symptoms.

SUMATRIPTAN SUCCINATE

Pregnancy category: C
MAO warning

Brand:
Imitrex

This drug is used to relieve a migraine attack but is not meant to prevent or reduce the number of attacks you experience.

How to take this drug:
- You should take the medicine as soon as your migraine symptoms appear, but you can take it at any time during an attack.
- For the injection form, you can give yourself a second injection if you still have pain, but wait an hour after the first injection, and talk to your doctor first.

Possible side effects:

Tingling	Warm or hot sensation
Flushing	Heaviness
Chest, jaw, and neck tightness	Head tightness

Possible interactions:
- Don't use sumatriptan and any headache drugs containing ergotamine within 24 hours of each other.

Other important information:
- People with angina, ischemia, uncontrolled high blood pressure, or past heart attacks should not take sumatriptan.
- Find out what kind of migraine you have before you take sumatriptan. It is not meant for people with basilar or hemiplegic migraines.
- People with poor liver or kidney function should take it with caution.
- Sumatriptan may increase the risk of seizure for people with epilepsy.
- If you have had an allergic reaction to drugs before, you are more likely to be allergic to sumatriptan.
- Tell your doctor immediately if you have any of these rare reactions: shortness of breath, wheezing, skin rash or lumps, heart throbbing, hives, or swelling of the eyelids, face, or lips.
- Rarely, sumatriptan causes heart problems such as angina or transient ischemia (temporary deficiency of blood supply to a body part).
- If you have severe or prolonged chest pain, get emergency help immediately.

TAMOXIFEN CITRATE

Pregnancy category: D

Brand:
Nolvadex

This drug is used to treat and decrease the risk of some forms of breast cancer.

How to take this drug:
- You can take this drug with or without food.
- Take the tablets whole.
- Never double a missed dose, instead take it as soon as you remember or skip it and go on with your regular schedule.

Possible side effects:

Nausea or vomiting	Hot flashes

Vaginal discharge	Menstrual changes
Swelling	Loss of appetite
Mood changes	Tiredness
Bone or muscle pain	Rash
Hair loss	Cough

Possible interactions:
- This drug may increase the effects of anticoagulants.
- The effects of this drug may be increased by the antiparkinson drug bromocriptine.

Other important information:
- This drug may cause eye problems, uterine abnormalities, and liver disorders.
- People with blood disorders or a history of blood clots should take this drug only with extreme caution. It can increase your risk of developing blood clots and suffering a stroke. Have your blood checked regularly during treatment. Notify your doctor if menstrual disorders, swelling in your legs, chest pain, shortness of breath, difficulty walking, numbness, or abnormal bleeding occurs.
- Have a breast exam, a mammogram, and a gynecologic exam regularly throughout treatment.

TAMSULOSIN HYDROCHLORIDE

Pregnancy category: B
No driving

Brand:
Flomax

Tamsulosin hydrochloride treats the symptoms of an enlarged prostate, benign prostatic hyperplasia (BPH).

How to take this drug:
- Don't cut, crush, or chew the capsules.
- Take this drug at the same time every day, about 30 minutes before a meal.
- Never double a missed dose, instead take it as soon as you remember or skip it and go on with your regular schedule.

Possible side effects:

Headache	Weakness
Dizziness	Runny or stuffy nose
Diarrhea	Abnormal ejaculation
Back or chest pain	

Possible interactions:
- Tamsulosin hydrochloride may interact with warfarin (Coumadin), cimetidine (Tagamet), or blood pressure drugs such as alpha-blockers.

Other important information:
- Don't take this medication to treat high blood pressure.
- While on this drug, you are more likely to experience a sudden drop in blood pressure when standing up. You may feel dizzy or faint. Be careful to avoid injury from falling.
- Before starting on this drug, make sure your doctor determines that you have BPH and not another condition with similar symptoms, like prostate cancer.
- Women or children should not use this drug.

TELMISARTAN

Pregnancy category: C/D

Brand:
Micardis

This drug is an angiotensin II receptor blocker (ARB), one in the newest class of drugs to treat high blood pressure.

How to take this drug:
- You can take this drug with or without food.

Possible side effects:

Upper respiratory infection	Back pain
Sinusitis	Diarrhea

Possible interactions:
- Digoxin may interact with telmisartan.

Other important information:
- You can use telmisartan alone or with other blood pressure drugs.
- If you are taking high doses of diuretics, you are more likely to suffer from sudden drops in blood pressure. Talk to your doctor about the risk.
- Be careful using this drug if you have severe kidney or liver problems.

TEMAZEPAM

Pregnancy category: X
No driving

Brand:
Restoril

Temazepam is a sleep-inducing drug used to treat insomnia. It is a benzodiazepine.

How to take this drug:
- Take temazepam at least 30 minutes before bedtime.

Possible side effects:

Daytime drowsiness	Tiredness
Headache	Nervousness
Dizziness	Nightmares
Weakness	Blurred vision
Dry mouth	Diarrhea
Upset stomach	Aggressiveness
Agitation	

Possible interactions:

- If you take temazepam with other tranquilizers, alcohol, antihistamines, or muscle relaxants, the combination may dangerously depress your nervous system.
- Never drink alcohol while taking any benzodiazepine.

Other important information:

- You can become dependent on temazepam. To avoid seizures and other less severe withdrawal symptoms, such as heightened senses, muscle cramps, diarrhea, and blurred vision, quit taking the drug gradually under your doctor's supervision.
- People with poor liver, kidney, or lung function should use temazepam cautiously. The drug may stay in your body longer and increase your risk of side effects.
- Daytime sleepiness may last for several days after you quit taking the drug.
- Some people have memory loss for several hours after taking a benzodiazepine. Make sure you'll be able to get a full night's sleep after taking your medicine.
- You may have trouble sleeping for the first couple of nights after you stop taking this drug.
- It's best not to take sleep-inducing drugs for more than seven to 10 days.

TERAZOSIN

Pregnancy category: C
No driving

Brand:

Hytrin

Terazosin is prescribed to control high blood pressure.

Possible side effects:

Rapid heartbeat	Weakness
Headache	Drowsiness
Nausea	Constipation
Diarrhea	Fluid retention

Difficulty breathing	Frequent urination
Blurred vision	Rash
Dry mouth	Stuffy nose

Possible interactions:
- Don't drink alcohol while taking this drug.
- If you take terazosin with other blood pressure drugs, you're more likely to experience very low blood pressure and fainting.

Other important information:
- Take this drug cautiously if you are taking other blood-pressure-lowering drugs or if you have poor liver function.
- Terazosin may cause you to have very low blood pressure when you first start taking it. Your blood pressure can drop so low that you faint or lose consciousness. This is known as the "first-dose" effect. It can also occur if your dose is increased quickly, if your treatment is restarted after you've missed several doses, or if you begin taking another antihypertensive drug. Taking the first dose at bedtime may help reduce the "first-dose" effect.
- Very low blood pressure is a common side effect. This can cause dizziness after standing up, lightheadedness, and fainting.
- A very rapid heartbeat can be a dangerous side effect.

TERBINAFINE HYDROCHLORIDE

Pregnancy category: B

Brand:
Lamisil

Terbinafine hydrochloride fights several kinds of bacteria that cause skin infections. The tablet is prescribed for the nail fungus, onychomycosis. The spray solution and the cream both treat athlete's foot, jock itch, and ringworm.

How to take this drug:
- It is available as a tablet, a spray solution, and a cream.

Possible side effects:

Headache	Diarrhea
Indigestion	Rash or itching
Abdominal pain	Nausea
Changes in taste	Skin irritation

Possible interactions:
- Terbinafine may interact with cyclosporine, rifampin, cimetidine, or terfenadine.

Other important information:
- Stop using this medication immediately if you develop a skin reaction.

- Don't take Lamisil tablets if you have liver problems.
- If you begin to have nausea, loss of appetite, or fatigue while taking Lamisil tablets, have your doctor test your liver function.
- If your immune system is deficient, have your blood tested regularly.
- It may take up to six weeks to see results.

TERBUTALINE SULFATE

Pregnancy category: B
MAO warning

Brand:
Brethaire

Terbutaline is a bronchodilator that works quickly to relieve wheezing and the bronchial spasms that accompany asthma, bronchitis, and emphysema.

How to take this drug:
- Don't take more medicine than you are prescribed or stop taking your medicine without consulting your doctor.

Possible side effects:

Rapid or irregular heartbeat	Headache
Tremors	Nervousness
Drowsiness	Dizziness
Nausea	Stomach pain
Chest pain	Sweating
Flushing	Sleeplessness
Dry mouth	

Possible interactions:
- Taking other bronchodilators or epinephrine while taking terbutaline increases your risk of heart problems such as cardiac arrest. You can use an aerosol inhaler and a tablet or syrup bronchodilator at the same time if you are under the close supervision of your doctor.
- Taking beta-blockers (a type of blood pressure drug) while taking terbutaline can reduce the effectiveness of both drugs.

Other important information:
- If you have heart disease, an irregular heartbeat, low potassium levels, high blood pressure, diabetes, or an overactive thyroid, talk to your doctor about your condition before using this drug.
- Your doctor should monitor your blood pressure and your heart condition while you are taking terbutaline.
- Call your doctor if your asthma symptoms get worse.
- After you've taken terbutaline for a while, each dose may not relieve your symptoms for as long as it once did.

TERCONAZOLE

Pregnancy category: C

Brand:
Terazol 3   *Terazol 7*

Terconazole is used to treat vaginal yeast infections.

How to take this drug:
* This drug is available as a suppository or cream.

Possible side effects:
Headache	Menstrual changes
Stomach pain	Vaginal burning or itching

Other important information:
* Don't get this drug in your eyes or mouth.
* Continue taking this drug during menstruation, but wear a sanitary napkin instead of a tampon.
* Insert the cream or suppository high into the vagina.
* If you have sexual intercourse during treatment, the male partner should use a condom.

TETRACYCLINE HYDROCHLORIDE

Pregnancy category: D

Brand:
Achromycin V	*Bristacycline*
Panmycin	*Robitet*
Sumycin	*Tetracyn*

This antibiotic is used to treat many infections by various microorganisms.

How to take this drug:
* Take on an empty stomach with a full glass of water one hour before or two hours after meals.
* Never double a missed dose, instead take it as soon as you remember or skip it and go on with your regular schedule.

Possible side effects:
Sensitivity to light	Difficulty swallowing
Loss of appetite	Nausea
Diarrhea	Inflamed tongue
Rash	Itching
Swollen hands or feet	Dizziness
Ringing in the ears	

Possible interactions:
* Tetracycline may increase the effects of anticoagulants.
* This drug may decrease the effects of the antibiotic penicillin.

- Levels of this drug may be decreased by antacids.

Other important information:
- Tetracycline may accumulate to toxic levels in people with kidney problems.
- Be on the lookout for signs that this drug is depressing your immune system: fever, sore throat, tiredness, weakness, bruising, unusual bleeding. Have your blood tested regularly.
- Taking an antibiotic for a long time can cause bacteria or fungus to overgrow, leading to another infection (fungal infections of the mouth, anus, or vagina). If you get one of these "superinfections," you may need to quit taking tetracycline and start taking another antibiotic for the second infection.
- Tetracycline may cause increased pressure on the brain in adults. Signs of this include headache, nausea, and blurred vision. Let your doctor know immediately if you develop these symptoms. Tetracycline may cause bulging "soft spots" on babies' heads too.
- Liver tests should be performed regularly during treatment.

THEOPHYLLINE

Pregnancy category: C

Brand:
Slo-Bid	Elixophyllin
Theolair	Aquaphyllin
Slo-Phyllin	Theoclear-80
Quibron-T	Theo-Dur
Theochron	

Theophylline is a bronchodilator that comes in capsules, elixir, oral solution, and syrup, and tablets. It relieves acute asthma and the wheezing and bronchial spasms that accompany bronchitis and emphysema.

How to take this drug:
- Don't split, crush, dissolve, or chew tablets.
- Don't take the tablets more often than your doctor prescribes.
- Taking theophylline after a high-fat meal may slightly slow down the rate your body absorbs the drug. However, unless your doctor tells you otherwise, you can take the drug without regard to when you eat.
- Take your medicine at the same time every day.

Possible side effects:
Nausea	Diarrhea
Stomach pain	Vomiting blood
Rapid heartbeat	Respiratory problems
Flushing	Hair loss
Rash	Headache

Sleeplessness	Irritability
Restlessness	Convulsions
Muscle spasms	

Possible interactions:
- Theophylline may decrease blood levels of the seizure drug phenytoin and the antipsychotic drug lithium.
- The ulcer drug cimetidine, birth control pills, the beta-blocker propranolol, the gout drug allopurinol, the antibiotics erythromycin and troleandomycin, and the antibacterial drug ciprofloxacin may increase blood levels of theophylline.
- The tuberculosis drug rifampin and the seizure drug phenytoin may decrease blood levels of theophylline.
- If you take another bronchodilator or ephedrine along with theophylline, the effects of both drugs may be increased.

Other important information:
- Don't take this drug if you have stomach ulcers or a seizure disorder, unless it is being controlled by a seizure drug.
- Don't use if you are allergic or hypersensitive to caffeine or any of the other bronchodilators that are "xanthine derivatives."
- Use this drug cautiously if you have high blood pressure.
- Theophylline can accumulate to toxic levels if you have poor liver function or heart failure, or if you are over 55 with lung disease, or if you are taking other bronchodilators or ephedrine. Toxicity can cause serious side effects, even death, without warning. Contact your doctor immediately if you experience nausea, restlessness, irregular heartbeat, or convulsions.

THIORIDAZINE HYDROCHLORIDE

Pregnancy category: NR
No driving

Brand:
Mellaril

This tranquilizer is used to treat depression, anxiety, sleep disturbances, and fears. It also treats severe hyperactivity and other behavior problems in children.

How to take this drug:
- Add the concentrated form to water or juice (not apple juice) just before you drink it.

Possible side effects:

Sleepiness	Dry mouth
Urine retention	Confusion
Dizziness when standing suddenly	

Possible interactions:
- If you take this drug with other tranquilizers, alcohol, antihistamines, or muscle relaxers, the combination may dangerously depress your nervous system.
- This drug may increase the effects of atropine.
- Levels of thioridazine may be increased by the beta-blockers propranolol and pindolol.

Other important information:
- Take this drug very cautiously if you have heart disease with blood pressure problems.
- Be careful with this drug if you work in extreme heat or around phosphorus insecticides.
- Nerve disorders are a rare side effect with any antipsychotic. Tell your doctor if you develop difficulty speaking or swallowing, loss of balance, muscle spasms, stiff arms or legs, trembling, shaking, restless leg syndrome, weak or tired muscles, or uncontrolled movements.
- Don't quit taking this drug suddenly, or you may experience stomach pain, nausea, headache, insomnia, dizziness, and shakiness.

THIOTHIXENE

Pregnancy category: NR
No driving

Brand:
Navane

Thiothixene is a tranquilizer used to treat mental illness, such as loss of contact with reality and personality disorders.

Possible side effects:

Sleepiness	Dry mouth
Urine retention	Confusion

Possible interactions:
- If you take thiothixene along with other tranquilizers, alcohol, antihistamines, or muscle relaxers, the combination may dangerously depress your nervous system and cause very low blood pressure.
- This drug may increase the effects of atropine.

Other important information:
- Don't take this drug if you have circulatory collapse, if your central nervous system is depressed for any reason, or if you have certain kinds of blood disorders.
- Take this drug very cautiously if you have heart disease, a history of seizures, or if you work in extreme heat.
- Nerve disorders are a rare side effect with any antipsychotic. Tell your doctor if you develop difficulty speaking or swallowing, loss of balance,

muscle spasms, stiff arms or legs, trembling, shaking, restless leg syndrome, weak or tired muscles, or uncontrolled movements.
- Thiothixene commonly causes low blood pressure.
- This drug can cause pregnancy test results to be unreliable.
- It may make you extra-sensitive to sunlight, so protect your skin if you'll be outdoors.

THYROID, DESICCATED

Pregnancy category: A

Brand:

Armour Thyroid

This drug is used to replace thyroid hormones when the thyroid gland does not produce enough. It is also used to treat some forms of goiter and thyroid cancer.

How to take this drug:
- Never double a missed dose, instead take it as soon as you remember or skip it and go on with your regular schedule.

Possible interactions:
- This drug may increase the effects of the anticoagulant warfarin and decrease the levels or effects of insulin in diabetics.
- Levels of this drug may be reduced by the cholesterol reducers cholestyramine (Questran) and colestipol (Colestid).
- Taking this drug along with the asthma drug epinephrine may cause heart problems.

Other important information:
- Don't use this drug if you have abnormal adrenal or thyroid gland function.
- If you have heart or blood vessel abnormalities such as angina, or diabetes or adrenal gland abnormalities, use with extreme caution.
- Diabetics may need their dosage of antidiabetic medication adjusted.
- Periodic lab tests should be done to reassess thyroid function and speed of blood clotting.
- Call your doctor if any signs of overdose occur: diarrhea, nervousness, stomach cramps, rapid heartbeat, headache, weight loss, palpitations, fever, sweating, chest pain, insomnia, or irregular heartbeat.

TICLOPIDINE HYDROCHLORIDE

Pregnancy category: B

Brand:

Ticlid

Ticlopidine helps prevent strokes caused by blood clots. It is meant for people who have already had a stroke or are at high risk of stroke and cannot take aspirin.

How to take this drug:
- Take your medicine after meals or with food to help avoid stomach upset.

Possible side effects:

Diarrhea	Indigestion
Nausea	Gas
Rash	Itching
Hives	Dizziness
Loss of appetite	Nosebleed
Bleeding of the eye	Bloody urine
Headache	Ringing in the ears
Weakness	

Possible interactions:
- Don't take aspirin while taking this drug.
- Ticlopidine may increase levels of the asthma drug theophylline and the liver-function-testing drug antipyrine.
- Ticlopidine may decrease levels of the heart drug digoxin.
- The ulcer drug cimetidine may increase levels of ticlopidine.
- Antacids may decrease levels of ticlopidine. Don't take antacids within two hours of taking your dose of ticlopidine.

Other important information:
- People with blood or bleeding disorders or severe liver problems should not take this drug.
- Take this drug cautiously if you have poor kidney function or any condition that may increase the risk of internal bleeding.
- This drug can also cause hepatitis with jaundice. Watch for yellow eyes and skin, rashes, light-colored stools, or dark urine.
- Ticlopidine can raise your cholesterol and triglyceride levels.
- Be on the lookout for signs that this drug is depressing your immune system: fever, sore throat, tiredness, weakness, bruising, unusual bleeding. Have your blood tested regularly.

TIMOLOL MALEATE

Pregnancy category: C
No driving

Brand:
Timoptic-XE   *Timoptic*

Timolol maleate is an eye medication that reduces pressure within the eyeball caused by glaucoma or high blood pressure.

How to take this drug:
- Don't allow the tip of the container to touch your eye or any other surface. If the bottle or its contents become contaminated, you could develop a severe eye infection.

- If you are taking other eye medications, use them at least 10 minutes apart.

Possible side effects:

Blurred vision	Burning, stinging, or itching eyes
Watery eyes	Headache
Dizziness	Upper respiratory infection

Possible interactions:

- Timolol maleate may interact with beta-blockers, digitalis, calcium antagonists, and catecholamine-depleting drugs like reserpine.

Other important information:

- Don't use this if you have bronchial asthma, severe breathing disorders like chronic bronchitis or emphysema, or heart-flow problems. Life-threatening breathing or heart reactions are possible.
- Talk to your doctor about withdrawing from this drug before having surgery.
- Use this drug cautiously if you have diabetes. It can hide the symptoms of low blood sugar.
- If you are at risk of thyroid problems, don't stop taking this drug suddenly.
- It may take several weeks to see improvements.

TOLAZAMIDE

Pregnancy category: C

Brand:
Tolinase

People with noninsulin dependent (type II) diabetes use this drug to lower their blood sugar levels when they can't control it by diet alone.

Possible side effects:

Heartburn	Feelings of fullness
Itching	Hives
Skin eruptions	Sensitivity to sunlight
Weakness	Tiredness
Dizziness	Numbness or tingling
Headache	Ringing in the ears

Possible interactions:

- Tolazamide is more likely to cause low blood sugar if you are also taking aspirin, beta blockers, the antibiotic chloramphenicol, anticoagulants, monoamine oxidase (MAO) inhibitors, the antifungal drug miconazole, non-steroidal anti-inflammatory drugs (NSAIDs), or the gout drug probenecid.
- You increase your risk of high blood sugar if you take this drug along with birth control pills, corticosteroids, diuretics, estrogen, the tuberculosis drug isoniazid, phenothiazine tranquilizers, thyroid drugs, or the seizure drug phenytoin.

Other important information:

- While on this drug, you are at a higher risk of developing fatal heart problems.
- Don't use this drug if you have diabetes complicated by ketoacidosis.
- If you have liver or kidney problems or congestive heart failure, use this drug with caution.
- This drug shouldn't be used as the only therapy for type I diabetes.
- Check your blood and urine periodically for abnormal sugar levels while taking this drug.
- Combine tolazamide with a healthy weight loss and exercise program.
- Be on the lookout for signs that this drug is depressing your immune system: fever, sore throat, tiredness, weakness, bruising, unusual bleeding. Have your blood tested regularly.
- Since this drug can cause low blood sugar, especially when you haven't eaten enough, when you've exercised, or when you've consumed alcohol, learn to recognize the signs of hypoglycemia and know how to treat it.
- This drug can lose its effectiveness when you've taken it for a long period of time.
- Tell your doctor about any stressful events you experience, such as surgery, trauma, infection, or fever. You may need insulin or some other special treatment.

TOLBUTAMIDE

Pregnancy category: C

Brand:

Tolbutamide

People with noninsulin dependent (type II) diabetes use this drug to lower their blood sugar levels when they can't control it by diet alone.

How to take this drug:

- Never double a missed dose, instead take it as soon as you remember or skip it and go on with your regular schedule.

Possible side effects:

Nausea   Heartburn
Bloating

Possible interactions:

- Tolbutamide is more likely to cause low blood sugar if you are also taking aspirin, beta blockers, the antibiotic chloramphenicol, anticoagulants, monoamine oxidase (MAO) inhibitors, the antifungal drug miconazole, nonsteroidal anti-inflammatory drugs (NSAIDs), or the gout drug probenecid.
- You increase your risk of high blood sugar if you take this drug along with birth control pills, corticosteroids, diuretics, estrogen, the tuberculosis

drug isoniazid, phenothiazine tranquilizers, thyroid drugs, or the seizure drug phenytoin.

Other important information:
- Don't use this drug if you have diabetes complicated by ketoacidosis.
- If you have liver or kidney problems or congestive heart failure, use this drug with caution.
- This drug shouldn't be used as the only therapy for type I diabetes.
- Check your blood and urine regularly for abnormal sugar levels.
- Combine tolbutamide with a healthy weight loss and exercise program.
- Be on the lookout for signs that this drug is depressing your immune system: fever, sore throat, tiredness, weakness, bruising, unusual bleeding. Have your blood tested regularly.
- Since tolbutamide can cause low blood sugar, especially when you haven't eaten enough, when you've exercised, or when you've consumed alcohol, learn to recognize the signs of hypoglycemia and know how to treat it.
- This drug can lose its effectiveness when you've taken it for a long period of time.
- Tell your doctor about any stressful events you experience, such as surgery, trauma, infection, or fever. You may need insulin or some other special treatment.

TOLCAPONE

Pregnancy category: C
No driving   MAO warning

Brand:
Tasmar

Tolcapone is used together with carbidopa/levodopa to treat Parkinson's disease.

How to take this drug:
- Take tolcapone in addition to your current levodopa/carbidopa medications. However, your doctor may need to lower the dose of these medications to get the best response for your symptoms.
- Tolcapone can be taken with or without food.

Possible side effects:

Muscle tenderness or pain	High fever
Confusion	Diarrhea
Hallucinations	Dizziness when standing suddenly
Abnormal jerky movements	Nausea or vomiting
Sleep disorders	Loss of appetite
Headache	Abdominal pain
Tiredness	Jaundice
Itching	

Possible interactions:

- Be especially careful when taking other sleep inducing drugs.
- Check with your doctor before combining tolcapone and warfarin.

Other important information:

- This drug is not prescribed without a signed patient consent form to make sure you understand the potential risks and benefits.
- Because there is the risk of serious liver injury with this drug, your doctor must monitor your liver function on a very strict schedule.
- Don't take tolcapone if you have a history of rhabdomyolysis (the dangerous and sometimes fatal disease that destroys muscle tissue) or hyperpyrexia (high body temperature).
- Stop taking this drug if you don't show improvement after three weeks.
- Be careful taking tolcapone if you suffer from severe movement symptoms of Parkinson's.
- Be aware that some side effects may not appear for up to 12 weeks.
- Talk to your doctor before taking this drug if you have severe kidney problems.
- Don't lower your dose or stop taking tolcapone without talking to your doctor.

TOLMETIN

Pregnancy category: C

Brand:

Tolectin   Tolectin DS
Tolectin 600

This nonsteroidal anti-inflammatory drug (NSAID) relieves the symptoms of rheumatoid arthritis, osteoarthritis, and juvenile rheumatoid arthritis.

Possible side effects:

Headache	Swelling
Dizziness	Nausea
Diarrhea	Indigestion
Constipation	Gas
Ulcers	Ringing in the ears
Skin irritation	Inflamed mouth or tongue

Possible interactions:

- Avoid alcohol and aspirin while taking NSAIDs such as tolmetin.
- Tolmetin may increase the effects of the anticoagulant warfarin.
- It may increase levels of the cancer drug methotrexate, possibly to toxic levels.
- If you need to stop taking corticosteroids while you're taking tolmetin, be sure to withdraw slowly from the steroids instead of stopping suddenly.

Other important information:
- Don't take this drug if you are allergic to aspirin or other NSAIDs.
- People with stomach ulcer should not take this drug since it can cause gastrointestinal bleeding.
- Taking tolmetin is more likely to cause kidney problems if you are elderly, if you take diuretics, or if you have lupus, heart failure, or poor liver or kidney function.
- Take this drug with caution if you have liver abnormalities, high blood pressure, blood clotting disorders, or poor heart function.
- It may take several weeks to see improvement.
- Bleeding stomach ulcers and liver or kidney damage are rare but serious reactions to using tolmetin for long periods of time. Warning signs of liver damage include nausea, tiredness, red and itchy skin, yellow eyes and skin (jaundice), and flu-like symptoms.
- Be on the lookout for signs that this drug is depressing your immune system: fever, sore throat, tiredness, weakness, bruising, unusual bleeding.
- If you are having stomach trouble, you can take antacids other than sodium bicarbonate along with tolmetin.

TOLTERODINE TARTRATE

Pregnancy category: C

Brand:
Detrol

Tolterodine tartrate is used to treat overactive bladders that cause the feeling of having to urinate immediately, urinate too often, or the inability to control urination (urinary incontinence).

How to take this drug:
- Tolterodine tartrate can be taken with or without food.

Possible side effects:

Dry mouth	Upset stomach
Dizziness	Headache
Constipation	Dry eyes
Sleepiness	Blurred vision
Urinary retention	Fatigue
Abdominal pain	Back pain
Chest pain	Flu-like symptoms
Diarrhea	Nausea
Upper respiratory infection	Urinary tract infection
Vision problems	

Possible interactions:
- Tolterodine tartrate may interact with certain antibiotics and antifungal medicines. Your doctor may have to adjust your dose.

Other important information:
- Don't take Detrol if you have difficulty urinating due to a bladder blockage, gastric retention (problems emptying the contents of the stomach), or uncontrolled glaucoma.
- If you have liver problems, don't take more than 2 mg of tolterodine tartrate a day.

TRAMADOL HYDROCHLORIDE

Pregnancy category: C
No driving

Brand:
Ultram

Tramadol hydrochloride is prescribed for moderate to severe pain.

How to take this drug:
- You can take this drug with or without food.
- Don't take tramadol hydrochloride more frequently than prescribed.
- Never double a missed dose, instead take it as soon as you remember or skip it and go on with your regular schedule.

Possible side effects:

Dizziness	Nausea or vomiting
Constipation	Headache
Sleepiness	Itching
Nervousness	Weakness
Sweating	Indigestion
Dry mouth	Diarrhea
Tremors	

Possible interactions:
- This drug increases your risk of having a seizure if you are also taking SSRI or tricyclic antidepressants (Paxil, Prozac, Zoloft, Elavil, Norpramin, Tofranil), tricyclics like cyclobenzaprine or promethazine, opioids, MAO inhibitors (Nardil, Parnate), or neuroleptics.
- Tramadol hydrochloride can also have serious interactions with alcohol, narcotic pain relievers (Demerol, morphine, Darvon, Percocet), phenothiazines, tranquilizers (Valium, Xanax), and sleeping pills (Halcion, Dalmane, Restoril).
- Be careful taking it with carbamazepine.

Other important information:
- Doses of this drug may have to be adjusted if you are over 75 years old or have kidney or liver problems.
- If you have epilepsy, a history of seizures, a metabolic disorder, a central nervous system infection, a recent head injury, or are undergoing alcohol or drug withdrawal, your risk of convulsions is increased with this drug.

- If you've had allergic reactions to codeine or other opioids, you are at risk of severely reacting to tramadol hydrochloride.
- This drug can be very addictive. Don't use it if you have a history of drug abuse or dependence.

TRANYLCYPROMINE SULFATE

Pregnancy category: NR
No driving   MAO warning

Brand:
Parnate

Tranylcypromine is an MAO inhibitor used to treat depression.

How to take this drug:
- Don't stop taking this drug suddenly.

Possible side effects:

Anxiety	Sleeplessness
Weakness	Dizziness
Sleepiness	Dry mouth
Nausea	Diarrhea
Abdominal pain	Constipation
Loss of appetite	Swelling
Rapid heartbeat	Vision problems
Chills	Impotence
Headache	Tremors

Possible interactions:
- Do not take this drug with other MAO inhibitors, amphetamines, narcotics, alcohol, high blood pressure drugs, diuretics, weight-loss drugs, antihistamines for colds or allergies, sedatives, pain-relievers, bupropion hydrochloride (Wellbutrin), buspirone hydrochloride (BuSpar), meperidine, or dextromethorphan.
- Avoid these foods while on tranylcypromine: caffeine; broad beans; yeast extracts like Marmite or brewer's yeast; avocado; banana; chocolate; colas; mushrooms; raisins; sour cream; aged cheeses and meats; beer; wine; salted, smoked or pickled fish; chicken livers; or soy sauce.
- SSRIs (Prozac, Zoloft, Paxil) can interact fatally with tranylcypromine sulfate.
- Be careful taking this drug with Antabuse.
- Be careful taking it with drugs for Parkinson's disease.

Other important information:
- Don't take tranylcypromine sulfate if you have heart disease, liver disease, high blood pressure, chronic headaches, or a brain blood vessel disorder (cerebrovascular).
- Stop taking this drug at least 10 days before surgery requiring anesthesia.

- Tell your doctor immediately if you develop headaches, increased heart rate, sweating, dizziness, nausea, vomiting, or a stiff neck. These are the symptoms of dangerously high blood pressure, a sometimes fatal reaction to tranylcypromine sulfate. Have your doctor monitor your blood pressure regularly.
- Tell your dentist you are on this drug.
- Use this drug cautiously if you are epileptic, diabetic, or hyperthyroid.

TRAZODONE HYDROCHLORIDE

Pregnancy category: C
No driving   MAO warning

Brand:
Desyrel

Trazodone is prescribed to treat depression.

How to take this drug:
- Take trazodone after you eat. You will absorb the drug better, and you are less likely to feel dizzy and lightheaded.
- This drug does cause drowsiness, so you may want to take your largest dose at bedtime.

Possible side effects:

Dizziness	Drowsiness
Dry mouth	Nausea
Swelling	Blurred vision
Constipation	Confusion
Headache	Sleeplessness
Achy muscles	Shakiness
Stuffy nose	Ringing in the ears
Weight gain	

Possible interactions:
- Since trazodone can cause low blood pressure, you may need a lower dose of your blood-pressure-lowering drug.
- If you take trazodone along with tranquilizers, alcohol, antihistamines, or muscle relaxers, the combination may dangerously depress your nervous system.
- Trazodone may increase levels of the heart drug digoxin and the seizure drug phenytoin.
- Trazodone may cause increased bleeding if you take it with warfarin.

Other important information:
- Don't take trazodone if you are recovering from a heart attack. If you have heart disease, take the drug very cautiously. It can cause an irregular heartbeat.

- Quit taking trazodone for as long as possible before surgery with general anesthesia.
- It can take up to four weeks for you to notice any improvement.
- If you experience a painful, prolonged penile erection, let your doctor know immediately.

TRETINOIN

Pregnancy category: C

Brand:
Avita   *Retin-A*
Renova

Avita and Retin-A products are prescribed to treat acne. Renova is used to improve fine wrinkles, even out skin tone, and smooth roughness.

How to take this drug:
- Tretinoin comes in a cream, gel, or liquid form.
- Wash your face gently with mild soap and pat dry. Wait about a half hour before applying this product to your skin.
- Don't get this medication in your eyes, ears, nose, or mouth.

Possible side effects:
Warm or stinging skin   Dry or peeling skin
Redness   Itching

Possible interactions:
- Use these skin products cautiously while on tretinoin gel: medicated, drying, or abrasive soaps or cleansers, or cosmetics or cleansers containing alcohol; astringents; spices; lime; benzoyl peroxide; sulfur; resorcinol; or salicylic acid.
- Be careful getting medicated shampoos or hair coloring solutions on your skin while using this product.
- Don't use Renova while taking drugs that make you sensitive to the sun, such as thiazides, tetracyclines, fluoroquinolones, phenothiazines, or sulfonamides.

Other important information:
- Avoid natural or artificial sunlight while using this product. If you must be out in the sun, use sunscreen and wear protective clothing. Extreme wind or cold can also irritate your skin.
- Expect your skin to redden and peel while using this medication, but if it becomes severe or if your skin swells or blisters, see your doctor.
- Don't use this product if you are sunburned or have eczema.
- You may not see improvement for several weeks. Continue using the product regularly.
- Renova has not been proven to work in people over 50, or those with deep wrinkles, extremely dark skin, or with a history of skin cancer.

- Renova has not been tested for use longer than 48 weeks.

TRIAMCINOLONE ACETONIDE

Pregnancy category: C

Brand:

Azmacort	*Nasacort*
Aristocort	*Flutex*
Kenalog	*Triacet*
Triatex	*Triderm*
Trymex	

Triamcinolone is an anti-inflammatory steroid. The forms that you inhale through your mouth are used to treat and control asthma. The forms that you inhale or spray into your nose are used to treat congested, swollen nasal passages, often caused by allergies. They also treat nasal polyps (tumors in your nose). The creams and ointments are used to relieve itchy, inflamed skin.

How to take this drug:

- If you are using the steroid creams or ointments, don't put a bandage or cover over the medicine unless your doctor tells you to.
- Take your medicine at regular intervals.
- For people with asthma, if you use a bronchodilator, you should use it several minutes before the triamcinolone.

Possible side effects:

Inhaled forms:

Hoarseness	Dry mouth
Yeast infections in the mouth and throat (oral thrush)	Wheezing or coughing Facial swelling

Nasal forms:

Nose irritation or infection	Sneezing
Watery eyes	Headache

Cream or ointment forms:

Burning	Itching
Dryness	

Other important information:

- This drug is not meant to treat nonasthmatic bronchitis and won't stop a severe asthma attack.
- If you are switching to triamcinolone from steroid pills or shots, make sure you get off the other drug slowly. Report any signs of corticosteroid withdrawal, including fatigue, weakness, painful joints or muscles, low blood pressure when you stand up, and difficulty breathing.
- If you were taking steroid pills and you are now taking triamcinolone, you may need to get back on the former drug during a severe asthma

attack or during times of stress. Carry a card that says you have used cortisone-related drugs in the past year.
- Take extra care to avoid exposure to people with chicken pox or measles because corticosteroids can weaken your immune system. If you are exposed, let your doctor know right away.
- People with tuberculosis, herpes simplex of the eye, or an untreated infection (fungal, viral, or bacterial) shouldn't use triamcinolone.
- Inhaled, sprayed, or cream steroids are safe compared with steroid pills or shots, but if you use them more often than your doctor recommends, you may suffer some serious side effects: cataracts, osteoporosis, weight gain, high blood pressure, increased blood sugar, easy bruising, slowed growth (in children), muscle weakness, acne, low resistance to infection, water retention, and mood changes.
- You may not get relief until you've used the medication for two or three weeks.
- You can avoid fungal infections in your mouth and throat by rinsing your mouth and gargling with warm water after using your inhaler. Don't swallow the water.

TRIAMTERENE AND HYDROCHLOROTHIAZIDE

Pregnancy category: C

Brand:
Dyazide   *Maxzide*
Maxzide-25

This drug combines two products for people who need a thiazide diuretic but can't afford to risk potassium loss. It is used to treat swelling and high blood pressure.

Possible side effects:
Dizziness when standing suddenly	Jaundice
Nausea	Diarrhea
Rash	Sensitivity to light
Headache	Drowsiness
Sleeplessness	Restlessness
Shortness of breath	Rapid heartbeat
Dry mouth	Muscle cramps
Decreased sexual performance	Weakness

Possible interactions:
- Don't take potassium-containing salt substitutes, other drugs that affect your potassium levels, or eat a potassium-enriched diet while you're on this drug.
- This drug may increase levels of the antipsychotic drug lithium, possibly to toxic levels.
- Taking this drug and NSAIDs at the same time may cause kidney failure.

- Taking this drug along with an ACE inhibitor may increase your risk of dangerously high potassium levels.
- If you have high blood pressure, avoid using over-the-counter cold remedies or diet pills that can increase blood pressure.

Other important information:
- People with kidney problems should not take triamterene and hydrochlorothiazide. Your doctor should monitor your blood, kidney, and liver functions while you are taking this drug.
- It can cause dangerously high levels of potassium, which can be fatal. Some warning signs are a prickling or tingling sensation, muscle weakness, tiredness, and slow heartbeat.
- Weigh daily so you'll know if you're losing too much fluid, which can lead to dehydration and possibly blood clots. Warning signs of dehydration include dry mouth, thirst, drowsiness, weakness, and nausea. Contact your doctor immediately if you stop urinating.
- Hydrochlorothiazide may increase levels of uric acid in the blood (which puts you at risk for gout).

TRIAZOLAM

Pregnancy category: X
No driving

Brand:
Halcion

Triazolam is a sleep-inducing drug used to treat insomnia.

Possible side effects:

Daytime drowsiness	Dizziness
Lightheadedness	Nervousness
Headache	Lack of coordination
Nausea	Memory loss
Aggressiveness	Agitation

Possible interactions:
- If you take triazolam along with a drug that depresses your nervous system, such as tranquilizers, alcohol, antihistamines, or muscle relaxants, the combination may dangerously depress your nervous system.
- Talk to your doctor before drinking grapefruit juice while taking this drug.

Other important information:
- You can become dependent on triazolam. To avoid withdrawal symptoms like seizures, heightened senses, muscle cramps, diarrhea, and blurred vision, quit taking the drug gradually under your doctor's supervision.
- People with poor liver, kidney, or lung function should use triazolam cautiously. The drug may stay in your body longer and increase your risk of side effects.

- It's best not to take sleep-inducing drugs for more than seven to 10 days.
- Triazolam is a short-acting benzodiazepine, which is more likely to cause rebound insomnia (increased sleeping problems, especially during the last third of the night).
- You may have trouble sleeping for the first couple of nights after you stop taking this drug.

TRIFLUOPERAZINE HYDROCHLORIDE

Pregnancy category: NR
No driving

Brand:
Stelazine

This tranquilizer is used to treat anxiety and mental illnesses such as loss of contact with reality or personality disorders.

Possible side effects:
Sleepiness   Dry mouth
Urine retention   Confusion

Possible interactions:
- If you take any phenothiazine along with a drug that depresses your nervous system, such as other tranquilizers, alcohol, antihistamines, or muscle relaxers, the combination may dangerously depress your nervous system.
- Trifluoperazine may decrease the effects of anticoagulants and blood pressure drugs such as guanethidine.
- Taking trifluoperazine and propranolol at the same time can increase the levels of both drugs.
- If you take trifluoperazine with thiazide diuretics, you may have very low blood pressure.
- Trifluoperazine may increase levels of the anticonvulsant phenytoin, possibly to toxic levels.

Other important information:
- People who have depressed central nervous systems, some blood disorders, bone marrow depression, or liver damage shouldn't take trifluoperazine.
- Some people with asthma are sensitive to the sulfites in this drug.
- Take this drug cautiously if you have a history of epilepsy, heart disease, glaucoma, or liver disease.
- Be careful with this drug if you work in extreme heat.
- This drug can cause pregnancy test results to be unreliable.
- Trifluoperazine commonly causes low blood pressure so be careful standing up suddenly.
- If you get a sore throat or other signs of an infection while you're taking this drug, let your doctor know. Trifluoperazine can lower your immunity.

- This drug can cause liver damage. Warning signs include nausea, tiredness, red and itchy skin, yellow eyes and skin (jaundice), and flu-like symptoms.
- Talk to your doctor about the rare possibility of nerve damage, and let him know immediately of any strange side effects.

TRIHEXYPHENIDYL HYDROCHLORIDE

Pregnancy category: NR
No driving

Brand:
Artane

Trihexyphenidyl, combined with levodopa, is used to treat Parkinson's disease. It is also used to treat stiffness and shaking caused by some medicines.

Possible side effects:

Dry mouth	Blurred vision
Dizziness	Nausea
Nervousness	

Possible interactions:
- If you also take phenothiazines, haloperidol, tricyclic antidepressants, or other drugs that have drying side effects, make sure you report to your doctor any signs of fever or stomach complaints or any signs that you can't tolerate heat.

Other important information:
- This drug has drying side effects (for instance, it can keep you from sweating properly). Be very careful in hot weather, and watch yourself for signs of heatstroke.
- People with certain kinds of glaucoma; people with high blood pressure; and people with heart, liver, kidney, or prostate problems should use this drug very carefully.

TRIMETHOBENZAMIDE HYDROCHLORIDE

Pregnancy category: C
No driving

Brand:
Tigan

This drug controls nausea and vomiting.

How to take this drug:
- This drug comes in capsules, suppositories, and injection form.
- Make sure you drink plenty of fluids and eat a balanced diet to replace lost fluids and minerals.

Possible side effects:

Drowsiness	Blood disorders
Convulsions	Diarrhea
Jaundice	Allergic skin reactions
Dizziness	Blurred vision
Disorientation	Headache
Muscle cramps or spasms	

Possible interactions:

- You should be very cautious about taking trimethobenzamide and other depressants such as tranquilizers, sleeping pills and antihistamines at the same time.

Other important information:

- Your doctor should be very cautious in prescribing trimethobenzamide to children.
- Tell your doctor of any side effects you develop.

TRIMETHOPRIM

Pregnancy category: C

Brand:

Proloprim   *Trimpex*

These antibacterial tablets are used to treat urinary tract infections.

How to take this drug:

- Take this drug with food or milk if it upsets your stomach.
- Take all of the prescribed medication.

Possible side effects:

Rash	Itching
Skin eruptions	Fever
Nausea	Inflamed tongue
Upset stomach	

Possible interactions:

- This drug may increase the effects of the seizure drug phenytoin.

Other important information:

- Don't take this drug if you have megaloblastic anemia, a folic acid deficiency.
- People who have poor liver or kidney functions should use it with caution.
- Tell your doctor if you notice any of the symptoms of bone marrow depression, which means your immune system isn't working properly: fever, sore throat, pneumonia, fatigue, weakness, bruising, and bleeding.
- Taking an antibiotic for a long time can cause bacteria or fungus to overgrow, leading to another infection (such as a yeast infection of the

mouth or vagina). If you get one of these "superinfections," you may need to quit taking trimethoprim and start taking another antibiotic for the second infection.

TRIMIPRAMINE MALEATE

Pregnancy category: C
No driving   MAO warning

Brand:
Surmontil

Trimipramine maleate is an antidepressant with an anxiety-reducing sedative.

How to take this drug:
- Never double a missed dose, instead take it as soon as you remember or skip it and go on with your regular schedule.
- Don't take a missed evening dose the next morning. You could experience side effects during the day.

Possible side effects:

Drowsiness	Dizziness when standing suddenly
Vision problems	Dry mouth
Constipation	Urine retention
Rapid heartbeat	Confusion
Nausea	

Possible interactions:
- Trimipramine maleate can block blood pressure drugs like guanethidine (Ismelin).
- It can also interact with cimetidine (Tagamet), decongestants, local anesthetics, tranquilizers, stimulants, and SSRIs like fluoxetine (Prozac), sertraline (Zoloft), and paroxetine (Paxil).

Other important information:
- Be very careful taking this drug if you have heart disease, liver problems, glaucoma, increased pressure within your eye, urinary problems, thyroid disease, or seizures.
- Stop taking trimipramine maleate for a few days before any surgery.
- This kind of antidepressant can affect your blood sugar levels.
- It may be several weeks before you see any improvements.
- Don't take this medication if you've recently had a heart attack.

TRIPELENNAMINE

Pregnancy category: NR
No driving   MAO warning

Brand:
PBZ   *PBZ-SR*

This sedating antihistamine relieves symptoms of food allergies, hay fever, and other allergies. It helps relieve sneezing, runny nose, itching, rashes, hives, swelling, and difficulty breathing. It can be used in addition to epinephrine to treat severe allergic reactions.

How to take this drug:
- The extended-release tablets must be swallowed whole — never crushed or chewed.

Possible side effects:

Sleepiness	Dry mouth
Dizziness	Lack of coordination
Stomach pain	Thickened mucus

Possible interactions:
- While taking tripelennamine, avoid alcohol and other depressants such as sleeping pills and tranquilizers.

Other important information:
- Don't take it if you have some kinds of glaucoma, bladder neck obstruction, obstruction of the pylorus (opening from the stomach to the intestine), stomach ulcer, or an enlarged prostate.
- Don't use tripelennamine if you have a lower respiratory disease such as asthma, bronchitis, or pneumonia.
- Use tripelennamine cautiously if you have increased pressure in the eye, an overactive thyroid, heart disease, or high blood pressure.
- If you are over 60, you're more likely to feel dizzy and sedated and have low blood pressure while taking this drug.

VALPROIC ACID

Pregnancy category: D
No driving

Brand:
Depakene

Valproic acid is used alone or along with other anticonvulsant drugs to treat certain types of seizures.

How to take this drug:
- If your medicine upsets your stomach, make sure you take it with food.
- Don't chew the capsules. They will irritate your mouth and throat.

Possible side effects:

Sleepiness	Nausea
Indigestion	

Possible interactions:
- If you take valproic acid along with a drug that depresses your nervous system, such as tranquilizers, alcohol, antihistamines, muscle relaxers,

and other anticonvulsant drugs, the combination may dangerously depress your nervous system. Barbiturates combined with valproic acid can be especially dangerous. Your doctor should carefully monitor the levels of these drugs in your body.
- Taking valproic acid and aspirin, carbamazepine, dicumarol, or phenytoin at the same time can increase or decrease the levels of any of these drugs in your body.
- Drugs that affect blood clotting (aspirin and warfarin, for instance) should be used cautiously with this drug.
- Valproic acid may make birth control pills less effective.

Other important information:
- People with liver disease or poor liver function should not take this drug. Have your liver tested regularly, and look for the warning signs of liver damage, which include nausea, tiredness, red and itchy skin, yellow eyes and skin (jaundice), and flu-like symptoms. These problems are most likely to show up in the first six months of taking valproic acid.
- Look for unusual bruising, which could mean your blood is not clotting properly, and have regular blood tests.

VALSARTAN HYDROCHLOROTHIAZIDE

Pregnancy category: C/D

Brand:
Diovan HCT

This drug, used to control high blood pressure, is a combination of valsartan and hydrochlorothiazide.

How to take this drug:
- Take this drug with or without food.
- You must take this medication regularly, even if you feel well.
- Never double a missed dose, instead take it as soon as you remember or skip it and go on with your regular schedule.

Possible side effects:

Headache	Tiredness
Dizziness	Viral infection
Sore throat	Coughing
Diarrhea	Nausea
Joint pain	Abdominal pain

Possible interactions:
- Don't take lithium with this medication.
- These drugs may interact with valsartan hydrochlorothiazide: alcohol, barbiturates, narcotics, antidiabetic drugs including insulin, other drugs to lower blood pressure (Cardizem, Lopressor, Procardia), cholestyramine

or colestipol resins (Questran, Colestid), corticosteroids like hydrocortisone and prednisone, pressor amines like norepinephrine, muscle relaxants, and NSAIDs (Advil, Aleve, Motrin).

Other important information:
- If you have severe kidney or liver disease, your doctor may need to adjust your dose of valsartan hydrochlorothiazide.
- Don't take this drug if you have difficulty producing urine or are sensitive to sulfonamides (like Bactrim or Septra).
- Have your doctor regularly measure your electrolyte balance. If you experience dry mouth, thirst, weakness, drowsiness, restlessness, confusion, seizures, muscle pain, nausea, or vomiting, you may be dehydrated. See your doctor immediately.
- If you are diabetic, you may have to adjust your dose of insulin or antidiabetic drugs while on valsartan hydrochlorothiazide.
- Your cholesterol and triglyceride levels may go up while you are on this drug.
- Don't take potassium supplements or potassium-containing salt substitutes without your doctor's permission.
- Be careful when standing up suddenly. You may feel faint or dizzy because of potassium deficiency.
- Be careful taking this drug if you have allergies, bronchial asthma, or lupus erythematosus.

VANCOMYCIN HYDROCHLORIDE

Pregnancy category: C

Brand:
Vancocin HCL

This antibiotic is used to treat various forms of colitis.

How to take this drug:
- Take all of your medicine, even after you begin to feel better.

Possible side effects:
Nausea	Skin rash
Fever	

Possible interactions:
- Check with your doctor before taking this drug with other diarrhea medications.

Other important information:
- Use this drug cautiously if you have poor kidney function, inflammatory disorders of the intestines, or hearing problems.
- Blood levels of this drug should be monitored because it can be toxic to the kidneys.

- Have hearing tests before you begin taking the drug and during long-term treatment. If you feel a sense of fullness in your ears or have ringing in your ears, tell your doctor immediately. Those sensations could indicate nerve damage that could lead to hearing loss.

Venlafaxine Hydrochloride

Pregnancy category: C
No driving   MAO warning

Brand:
Effexor   *Effexor XR*

Venlafaxine hydrochloride is used to treat depression.

How to take this drug:
- This drug is available in regular or extended-release form.
- Take venlafaxine hydrochloride with food.
- Don't break, crush, or chew the extended-release capsule.
- Never double a missed dose, instead take it as soon as you remember or skip it and go on with your regular schedule.

Possible side effects:
Nausea	Constipation
Sleepiness	Dry mouth
Dizziness	Anxiety
Nervousness	Sleeplessness
Loss of appetite	Headache
Weakness	Sweating
Abnormal ejaculation	

Possible interactions:
- If you are elderly or have high blood pressure or liver problems, venlafaxine hydrochloride may interact with cimetidine.
- Talk to your doctor before taking this drug with medications that affect your central nervous system like tranquilizers, sleeping drugs, narcotic painkillers, and other antidepressants.

Other important information:
- If you suffer from liver or kidney disease, your doctor will need to adjust your dose of venlafaxine hydrochloride.
- This drug has not been tested in long-term use (more than six weeks).
- Venlafaxine hydrochloride may increase your blood pressure. Be sure and have it monitored regularly by your doctor.
- Use this drug cautiously if you have a history of seizures.
- Stop taking this drug gradually to avoid withdrawal symptoms.

Verapamil hydrochloride

Pregnancy category: C

Brand:
Verelan

Verelan PM

Calan

Isoptin SR

Verapamil is a calcium channel blocker used to treat angina and irregular heart rhythms.

Possible side effects:
Headache	Dizziness
Tiredness	Nausea
Upset stomach	Constipation
Fluid retention and swelling	Slow or irregular heartbeat

Possible interactions:
- Don't take the heartbeat regulator disopyramide within 48 hours of taking verapamil.
- Taking verapamil along with beta blockers, ACE inhibitors, or diuretics may cause very low blood pressure or heart irregularities.
- Verapamil may increase the levels or effects of muscle relaxers, the seizure drug carbamazepine, the antibiotic cyclosporin, and the heart drug digitalis.
- Levels or effects of verapamil may be decreased by the seizure drug phenobarbital and the tuberculosis drug rifampin.

Other important information:
- People with the following conditions should not use verapamil: sick sinus syndrome (unless using a pacemaker), low blood pressure, heart block (unless using a pacemaker), severe heart failure, dysfunction of the left ventricle of the heart, or atrial fibrillation.
- Your doctor should prescribe this drug cautiously and monitor you carefully if you have heart failure, poor liver or kidney function, or Duchenne's muscular dystrophy.
- In rare instances, verapamil may cause congestive heart failure. Tell your doctor immediately if you have any signs of congestive heart failure such as night cough; swelling and fluid retention in your legs, feet, or hands; or difficulty breathing, especially when lying down or after physical exertion.
- Have your blood pressure tested regularly, especially when you first start taking verapamil.
- If you stop taking calcium channel blockers suddenly, your angina could get worse. Stop taking the drug gradually under your doctor's supervision.
- Have your blood pressure tested regularly, especially when you first start taking verapamil. When you are also taking other drugs to lower your blood pressure, regular tests are even more important.

- Have regular liver function tests while you're taking verapamil.

WARFARIN

Pregnancy category: X

Brand:

Coumadin

Warfarin reduces the ability of the blood to form clots. It is also used to prevent or treat various kinds of clots, especially in people who may be at risk of heart attack or stroke. Warfarin also protects against blood clots after a heart attack.

How to take this drug:

- Take your warfarin dose at the same time every day.

Possible side effects:

Nausea or vomiting	Diarrhea
Stomach cramps	Discolored urine
Swelling	Hair loss
Hives	

Possible interactions:

- If you take warfarin with the anticoagulant ticlopidine, you can get hepatitis.
- The following drugs may increase the effects of warfarin: acetaminophen, the gout drug allopurinol, aspirin, the ulcer drug cimetidine (Tagamet), the blood fat-reducer clofibrate, the antidiabetic drug chlorpropamide, the pain drug diflunisal, the anti-alcoholic drug disulfiram, the anticoagulant heparin, the blood fat-reducer lovastatin, monoamine oxidase (MAO) inhibitors, the blood pressure drug methyldopa, the antibiotic metronidazole, the antifungal miconazole, narcotics, NSAIDs, the seizure drug phenytoin, the cancer drug tamoxifen, the antidiabetic drug tolbutamide, and thyroid drugs.
- The following drugs may decrease the effects of warfarin: antacids, antihistamines, corticosteroids, barbiturates, birth control pills, the seizure drug carbamazepine, the anti-anxiety drug chlordiazepoxide, the antifungal drug griseofulvin, the anti-anxiety drug meprobamate, the seizure drug primidone, the tuberculosis drug rifampin, and the antidepressant trazodone.

Other important information:

- People with blood diseases, intestinal or other bleeding, people who have just had or about to have surgery, and pregnant women shouldn't take this drug.
- Use this drug cautiously if you have poor liver or kidney function, high blood pressure, diabetes, "protein C" deficiency, heart failure, trauma, or infectious disease.

- Fever and skin rash signal a bad reaction to the drug. Tell your doctor immediately.
- Have regular tests to measure clotting time while you're taking this drug.
- Watch yourself for bleeding gums, bruises on your arms or legs, nosebleeds, and blood in your urine. Tell your doctor if you have any of these side effects.
- Eat plenty of leafy green vegetables every day to get a regular, unchanging diet of vitamin K.
- A painful, continuous erection of the penis is a serious side effect you should let your doctor know about immediately.
- This drug can cause liver damage. Warning signs include nausea, tiredness, red and itchy skin, yellow eyes and skin (jaundice), and flu-like symptoms.

YOHIMBINE

Pregnancy category: NR

Brand:
Aphrodyne   *Yocon*

This drug is used to treat certain forms of impotence and male sexual dysfunction. Occasionally doctors prescribe yohimbine to dilate the pupil or to treat low blood pressure and dizziness when you change positions.

Possible side effects:
Nervousness	Irritability
Excitement	Rapid heartbeat
Headache	Dizziness
Tremors	Flushing

Possible interactions:
- Don't take this drug with antidepressants or other mood-altering drugs.

Other important information:
- Don't use this drug if you have kidney disease, heart disease, or a history of stomach or intestinal ulcers.
- This drug is not recommended for use by women, children, the elderly, or people being treated for psychiatric disorders.

ZAFIRLUKAST

Pregnancy category: B

Brand:
Accolate

Zafirlukast is prescribed to prevent and treat asthma in adults and children over 12 years old. It will not help during an acute asthma attack.

How to take this drug:
- Take zafirlukast at least one hour before or two hours after meals.
- Never double a missed dose, instead take it as soon as you remember or skip it and go on with your regular schedule.

Possible side effects:

Headache	Infection
Nausea	Diarrhea
General pain	

Possible interactions:
- If taken with warfarin, this drug could cause dangerous bleeding.
- Zafirlukast may interact with dihydropyridine, calcium-channel blockers (Calan, Cardizem, Procardia), cyclosporin (Sandimmune, Neoral), cisapride (Propulsid), erythromycin, theophylline, and aspirin.

Other important information:
- Don't decrease the dose or stop taking other asthma medications unless your doctor tells you to.
- A rare side effect involves liver function. If you experience abdominal pain in your upper right side, nausea, fatigue, yellow eyes or skin, or flu-like symptoms, contact your doctor.
- Take this drug regularly, even when you don't have any asthma symptoms.
- You can take this medication even if you are using an inhaler to stop an asthma attack.

ZOLPIDEM TARTRATE

Pregnancy category: B
No driving

Brand:
Ambien

Zolpidem is a short-acting, sleep-inducing drug used to treat insomnia.

How to take this drug:
- You will absorb zolpidem more slowly (and fall asleep more slowly) if you take it with or immediately after a meal. Take it without food to fall asleep faster.

Possible side effects:

Daytime drowsiness	Dizziness
Headache	Diarrhea
Nausea	Anxiety
Aggressiveness	Agitation

Possible interactions:

- If you take zolpidem along with a drug that depresses your nervous system, such as tranquilizers, alcohol, antihistamines, or muscle relaxants, the combination may dangerously depress your nervous system. Never drink alcohol while taking sleeping medicines.

Other important information:

- You can become dependent on zolpidem. To avoid withdrawal symptoms like seizures, heightened senses, muscle cramps, diarrhea, and blurred vision, quit taking the drug gradually under your doctor's supervision.
- People with poor liver, kidney, or lung function should use zolpidem cautiously. It may stay in your body longer and increase your risk of side effects.
- Since it is short-acting, it is more likely to cause rebound insomnia (increased sleeping problems, especially during the last third of the night).
- It's best not to take sleep-inducing drugs for more than seven to 10 days.
- You may have trouble sleeping the first night or two after you stop taking zolpidem.

NATURAL ALTERNATIVES

ALLERGIES

Remove as much house dust as possible. Dust mites are tiny insects that live in bedding, carpets, and mattresses. They eat dead, sloughed-off human skin cells and give off waste material that can trigger allergic reactions. And dust mites love dust, so keep it clean. Wash clothes, bedding, and curtains in hot water (at least 130 degrees F). Use washable synthetic materials instead of feather or down pillows, and put dustproof covers on your pillows, mattresses, and box springs.

Use the sun to battle dust mites. Sunlight may help you combat those pesky dust mites. A study in Australia found that leaving mite-infested rugs outside for four hours on a hot, sunny day killed 100 percent of mites and their eggs. This would probably work for bedding, curtains, and pillows as well.

Try tannic acid. For carpets and rugs you can't take outside, a tannic acid solution may be just what you need. Researchers found that one type of this solution, Allersearch ADS, reduced dust mites in carpet by up to 92 percent.

Control the mold. Try to keep your house as dry as possible to limit the growth of mold. Check areas that tend to be damp, like under sinks and around toilets, tubs, and washing machines, and wipe these places down with bleach and water. Houseplants and aquariums can also harbor mold. If you must have houseplants, you can buy mold retardants from your local nursery.

Stay inside. If you're allergic to pollen, staying inside whenever pollen levels are high may help. Spring and fall are the seasons most likely to cause problems. Grass and tree pollen make spring a season of sniffling, and in the fall, ragweed starts the sneezing anew. Pollen levels also tend to be highest in the morning hours, so staying inside until afternoon may help.

Wear a mask. If you have to work in your yard, wear a mask that covers your nose and mouth, especially while cutting grass. It will block out at least some of the allergens. If you're allergic to dust, wear a mask whenever you have to dust or vacuum your house.

Shower up. After outdoor activities, take a quick shower to remove any pollen residue from your skin and hair. Your hair can harbor a lot of pollen, especially if it's long, so it's particularly important to shampoo before going to bed.

Close your windows and turn on the air. Make sure your bedroom windows are closed at night to keep allergens out and help you rest easier. And air conditioners reduce the humidity and pollen levels in your house and allow you to keep your windows closed and still remain comfortable in hot weather.

Keep pets outside. Pet dander (dead skin cells) is a major cause of allergies. The fleas on your pet may also aggravate your hay fever. If you have furry or feathered pets that you can't bear to part with, try to keep them outside. If that's not possible, make sure they are bathed often, and use something to control the fleas.

ANXIETY

Check your medicine cabinet. Prescription drugs such as asthma inhalers, or even over-the-counter drugs such as diet pills and decongestants, can cause anxiety-like symptoms and intensify stress.

Watch the caffeine. Most people know that too much caffeine can make you jittery and irritable. But a new study shows that just a little caffeine may have the opposite effect. Researchers found that caffeine lowered tension while it increased feelings of happiness and calmness. When they tested participants on their ability to recall and process information and solve problems, they performed better with caffeine. So the next time you're feeling tense, a cup of coffee or tea may be just what you need.

Walk and talk. Physical exercise helps relieve tension, and talking with a trusted friend or family member is a time-tested way to work out problems. Doing both together just doubles the benefits.

Try aromatherapy. If you feel like pursuing the ancient practice of aromatherapy, there are several oils recommended for anxiety. These include bergamot, cedarwood, frankincense, geranium, hyssop, lavender, sandalwood, and ylang ylang. Dilute them in your bath or combine them with a massage oil. Some herbalists recommend taking essential oils internally, usually by placing drops on the tongue. Talk to your doctor before doing this, since many oils can be harmful if taken internally.

Get some herbal relaxation. Some people find that herbs help calm their anxieties.

- **Kava.** This herb, also known as kava kava, comes from the South Pacific and has been soothing islanders for generations. It's been shown to improve mood, reduce anxiety, and raise mental alertness. Some studies say it's as effective as a well-known anti-anxiety drug.

- **Valerian.** This herb aids sleep and calms anxiety. As with other herbal treatments, valerian works slowly so it might take more time to see results than with traditional medications.

Take your Bs and C. Stress and anxiety often go hand-in-hand with digestion problems and malabsorption. This means your body may not be able to use all the nutrients you're taking in, and you could become vitamin deficient.

B vitamins, in particular, are quickly used up during times of stress. And studies have found that people who take in the least amount of vitamin B12 are the most likely to suffer from depression and other mental problems, including anxiety. Another important B vitamin is B5, sometimes called the "anti-stress" vitamin. It works to keep your adrenal gland functioning properly. Foods high in B vitamins are peas, beans, lean meat, poultry, fish, whole-grain breads and cereals, bananas, and potatoes.

Stock up on vitamin C during hectic times, too, since your adrenal gland needs it to make stress hormones. Citrus fruits, strawberries, red and green peppers, broccoli, brussels sprouts, and cantaloupe are loaded with vitamin C.

Arthritis

Get plenty of antioxidants. One study in Boston found that people with osteoarthritis of the knee who had a high intake of antioxidants were less likely to have the disease progress any further. The people who had the highest intake of vitamin C, a major antioxidant, were three times less likely to have their arthritis get worse.

Vitamin C helps build and repair all the connective tissues in your body. This includes the ligaments, tendons, and cartilage that surround and cushion your bones. In some forms of arthritis, the cartilage between your joints becomes frayed and worn, leaving a painful bone-grinding connection. The antioxidants vitamin E and beta carotene also helped, though not as much as vitamin C.

Another study found that people with low levels of vitamin E, beta carotene, and selenium were more likely to develop rheumatoid arthritis. Eat plenty of fresh fruits and vegetables every day to get lots of anti-arthritis antioxidants.

Add some B vitamins. A recent study found that people who received a daily supplement containing 6,400 micrograms (mcg) of folic acid (B9) and 20 mcg of cobalamin (B12) had as much gripping power in their hands as people who used NSAIDs like aspirin and ibuprofen. They also had fewer tender joints. To get the most effective dose of these pain-killing B vitamins, ask your doctor for a prescription. You'll pay less for them, and your doctor will be able to monitor any side effects.

Delight in some D. Vitamin D is vital to building healthy bones. That may explain why one large study found that some people with osteoarthritis were three times less likely than others to have their disease get worse. These people took in at least twice as much vitamin D as the study participants who were getting less than the recommended dietary allowance (RDA). If you think you are not getting enough vitamin D, go soak up some sunshine or eat plenty of vitamin D-rich foods like milk and eggs.

Loosen up with glucosamine. Glucosamine is a natural compound of glucose and amino acids. It forms the main ingredient for most of the connective and cushioning tissue in your body. It is the breakdown of these tissues — such as cartilage and synovial fluids — that causes the pain and immobility of arthritis. Several studies have found that glucosamine may be at least as effective as NSAIDs in controlling the pain and stiffness of osteoarthritis, but it may take longer to feel the effect. In one study, people with arthritis were given either ibuprofen or glucosamine. The people taking ibuprofen reported more pain relief in the first and second weeks than the people taking glucosamine, but by the fourth week, both groups had about the same level of pain relief. By the eighth week, glucosamine was slightly more effective than ibuprofen. Glucosamine also caused fewer side effects, like stomach discomfort, than ibuprofen.

You can buy several forms of glucosamine supplements. The most common, and probably most effective, is glucosamine sulfate. The recommended dosage, according to results from studies, is 1,500 milligrams (mg) a day, taken in three doses of 500 mg each.

Feast on fish for pain-free joints. According to researchers, people with rheumatoid arthritis who eat fish containing omega-3 fatty acids have fewer tender joints and less morning stiffness. Adding fatty fish like salmon, sardines, tuna, or herring to your diet regularly may not cure your arthritis, but it could be a delicious way to loosen up your joints. If you choose to take fish oil capsules instead, the effective amount is 3 to 5 grams daily.

Ease arthritis symptoms with veggies. If you don't already love broccoli and spinach, the pain of arthritis may make them seem more appealing. Studies show that many people with rheumatoid arthritis benefit from a vegetarian diet. Researchers aren't sure why vegetarian diets help, but they think it could be because meat affects the types of fatty acids in your blood. Your immune system uses these fatty acids to make substances that can cause inflammation. If you decide to avoid meat, make sure you get enough protein from other sources.

Soothe joints with exotic oils. You may have heard that fish oil is good for arthritis symptoms, but according to recent studies, some unusual oils may also reduce joint inflammation in people with rheumatoid arthritis. These oils include evening primrose, flaxseed, rapeseed, and borage seed oils. They contain a fatty acid similar to omega-3 called gammalinolenic acid (GLA). Because these oils aren't found in foods you normally eat, you have to get them from supplements. The effective dosage is 1 to 2 grams daily.

Water down your joints. If you have arthritis, relaxing in a bathtub full of warm water may ease your aching joints, but drinking a glass of cool water may be even better. Water helps cushion and lubricate your joints. You should drink at least eight glasses of water a day to help keep your joints gliding smoothly along.

Takes the ache out of arthritis. Recent research suggests that ginger may work as a natural anti-inflammatory, reducing the redness, pain, and swelling that often accompanies arthritis. A 2 1/2 year study conducted in Denmark of 56 people who suffered with arthritis or muscle pain found ginger relieved muscle discomfort, pain, and swelling in three-quarters of the study participants. The people who experienced relief with ginger took an average of 5 grams of fresh ginger or 1 gram of powdered ginger daily.

ASTHMA

Keep your house clean. Allergic reactions trigger most asthma attacks. Allergy triggers, or allergens, include pollen, dust, mold, animal hair, and feathers. Clean your house regularly to keep dust and mold to a minimum.

Know which food triggers to avoid. Studies show that certain foods can bring on asthma attacks. Some of the more common foods linked to asthma flare-ups are shellfish, soy, wheat, nuts, eggs, fish, chocolate, and milk.

Search out sulfites. Eating foods with sulfites (food preservatives) and artificial coloring products can also trigger asthma. Some foods that tend to have high sulfite levels are dried apricots, dried peaches, instant mashed potatoes, imported peppers, shrimp, and hominy. Wine is also high in sulfites; just one glass can cause sensitive people to become short of breath. Check food labels for sodium sulfite, sulfur dioxide, or sodium or potassium bisulfite or metabisulfite.

Be wary of benzoates. Benzoates are another type of preservative that can trigger asthma attacks in some people. Check labels for benzoic acid, sodium benzoate, butylated hydroxyanisole (BHA), or butylated hydroxytoluene (BHT). You'll find benzoates in bread, chocolate, fat, instant drink powders, jam, margarine, mayonnaise, oil, and soft drinks.

Eat some soothing chicken soup. Expectorants can ease the after-effects of an asthma attack and soothe your cough. That's because these products help thin and loosen the phlegm in your chest. Scientists have now proven that hot liquids, especially chicken soup, also help break up congestion and nasal mucus. Inhaling the warm vapor definitely helps, but that apparently is not the only benefit. Chicken soup seems to have some unique characteristic that works either through its scent or its taste to thin the phlegm in your chest and head.

Feast on cold-water fish. A study of Eskimo, Japanese, and Dutch populations links a diet high in omega-3 fatty acids, or fish oil, to low instances of asthma. Small amounts of fish oil over a long period of time seem to give the best results. This strategy makes it easier for the average person to work it into their normal diet. The best natural sources are mackerel, salmon, striped bass, lake trout, herring, lake whitefish, anchovy, bluefish, and halibut. If you'd like to try fish oil supplements, check with your doctor first.

Avoid cigarette smoke like the plague. If your friends smoke, ask them politely to take their habit elsewhere. If you smoke, the best and only advice is to quit immediately. One cigarette can hinder your breathing and cause mucus to build up in your lungs. Always ask for the nonsmoking section in restaurants and on airplanes.

Stay away from sick people. Viral infections tend to provoke asthma attacks. Avoid unnecessary exposure to people and situations where you might catch a virus.

Be careful with winter fires. Burning wood gives off tiny particles that can get into your lungs and cause shortness of breath. To enjoy your fireplace in good health, take these precautions: Don't sit close to the fireplace; don't use chemicals, such as kerosene, to light the fire; and keep the chimney clean to prevent fumes. Be sure to air the room out after the fire, and dust and vacuum as soon as possible.

Take a nippy dip. Just the thought of stepping into a cold bath may take your breath away. But if you are bothered by the wheezing and chest-squeezing feelings of asthma attacks, you can take comfort from an icy dip. Research shows cold water baths can improve breathing — but don't stay in there too long. A quick bath in cold water for only one minute or a 30-second cold shower every day showed the greatest results. So turn on the cold water, brace yourself, and jump in — and enjoy easy breathing.

Pour yourself a cup of coffee. You still have your morning coffee or daily soda in spite of all the bad press on caffeine. Well, now you can feel better about it if you have asthma. Scientists report that caffeine can actually help some asthma sufferers by relaxing and expanding the air passages in the lungs. But don't overdo it. Too much caffeine can increase your blood pressure and heart rate and cause insomnia. A moderate amount, especially during an asthma attack, may feel like a breath of fresh air.

Tame wheezing with turmeric. The spice turmeric is a main ingredient of curry powder. It's the pigment in turmeric, called curcumin, that gives curry its yellow color. According to researchers, this pigment can also help prevent asthma attacks. The curcumin curbs the release of substances that cause the symptoms of asthma, like wheezing and chest-tightening. You can get supplements in capsule or liquid form at health food stores. The usual dosage is 1.5 to 3 grams daily. There are no known side effects from turmeric except occasional stomach upsets after prolonged use. But if you have gallstones or a blockage of the bile duct, you shouldn't use it.

Breathe easier with vitamin C. A test group of asthmatics took supplements of 1 to 2 grams of vitamin C, a natural antihistamine. In the majority of cases, breathing symptoms improved. Try to get as much vitamin C as possible from natural sources like citrus fruits and juices, strawberries, broccoli, brussels sprouts, and sweet red peppers. Before taking large doses of any supplement, check with your doctor. Too much vitamin C in your body can cause diarrhea and other side effects.

Lower your risk with E. Low levels of vitamin E may put you at a higher risk of developing asthma. Vitamin E is a powerful antioxidant, which means it protects your cells from damage by free radicals. Some healthy food sources are baked sweet potatoes, sunflower seeds, and fortified cereals. If you're watching your fat intake, you may want to take a supplement, since many foods high in vitamin E are also high in fat. Although vitamin E is relatively safe, large doses — over 400 international units (IU) — taken over a prolonged period of time may cause blurred vision, diarrhea, dizziness, headaches, nausea, or unusual fatigue.

Consider selenium. Several studies show that asthmatics tend to have low levels of selenium, a mineral that functions much like vitamin E in the body. When a test group of asthmatics took 100 micrograms (mcg) of sodium selenite, a selenium supplement, their breathing abilities improved. Good food sources of selenium include liver, kidney, and seafood. If you want to try supplements, talk it over with your doctor. Too much selenium can be toxic.

Open airways with magnesium. A diet rich in magnesium may help your lungs and airways fight the muscle spasms of asthma attacks. In fact, one form of the mineral, magnesium sulfate, has been used by doctors to help asthma sufferers breathe easier. It's best to get the magnesium you need from natural food sources, since this spreads its absorption throughout the day. Eat nuts, legumes, soybeans, seafood, and dark green vegetables to be sure you're getting the recommended dietary allowance (RDA) for magnesium — 280 to 350 milligrams (mg).

Iron out your asthma. Too little iron can cause problems like anemia, but researchers now think too much iron may cause asthma. If you take an iron supplement, make sure you don't take in more than the RDA. The RDA for adults over 50 is 10 mg a day. This is one case where more is definitely not better.

Heal with the power of ginkgo. You have probably heard of ginkgo helping just about every ailment known to man. While that may not be quite true, it certainly seems to have many healing qualities. One is its ability to prevent bronchospasms, a sudden narrowing of the main air passages from the windpipe to the lungs. If you have asthma, a bronchospasm feels like a tightening or squeezing in your chest that makes it difficult to breathe. Ginkgo biloba extract, or GBE, is sold as a food supplement. While no serious side effects have been reported, some people taking ginkgo experience headaches or digestive problems.

Watch what you eat before exercising. If you have a condition called exercise-induced asthma (EIA), you know that vigorous activity can set off a chain reaction in your airways that leaves you dizzy, tired, and wheezing. It's a common problem for asthma sufferers, affecting 80 to 90 percent of them. But did you know that eating certain foods even two hours before you exercise can trigger an episode?

Doctors have discovered that shrimp, celery, peanuts, egg whites, almonds, and bananas are the most common causes of food-related EIA attacks. In some cases, the typical asthma symptoms become worse than usual, even resulting in collapse. So, if you find that even the stairs are giving you trouble, you may have EIA. Watch your diet before you head to the tennis courts, and leave the banana behind.

Beware of royal jelly. Royal jelly is a substance honeybees produce as food for their larvae. It can reportedly boost your energy, rev up your immune system, and improve other aspects of your health. But for some people, it can mean a sudden life-threatening asthma attack or allergic reaction. Allergists and immunologists believe that royal jelly contains something that triggers a reaction in certain people. If you plan on taking royal jelly, watch out for signs of an allergic reaction — coughing or itching on the roof of your mouth, on your palms, or on your feet.

Relieve your heartburn. You probably never thought suffering from heartburn could make it hard to breathe, but doctors have discovered an amazing link between gastroesophageal reflux disease (GERD) and asthma. Studies show that up to 80 percent of asthma sufferers also have GERD, a condition where stomach acid backs up into the esophagus, causing heartburn.

If your breathing problems didn't start until you were an adult and there's no history of asthma in your family, heartburn could be causing your symptoms. Other signs are wheezing or coughing at night or after exercise or meals. If you treat your reflux disorder, you may find asthma relief at the same time. Talk it over with your doctor and follow his advice.

BACK PAIN

Lose weight. If you need to shed a few excess pounds, find a healthy eating plan and stick with it. That extra load around your middle puts a real strain on your back. Give it a break and lighten up.

Stop smoking. Some researchers think that smoking decreases blood flow to your backbone. Less blood flow means greater risk of injury. Others think "smoker's cough" strains the muscles in your back.

Get in shape. Overall fitness makes a big difference in the health of your back. Get out and pump up your heart by walking, biking, or swimming at least 30 minutes three or four times a week. Even a quick 10-minute walk is a good beginning. Before you know it, you'll be up to a half hour or more of healthy, back-strengthening aerobic exercise.

Practice good posture. Try to keep your back straight, not arched, and your shoulders level. Don't slump even when you're relaxing. If you have to stand for long periods, rest one foot on a low stool and shift your weight often. Change positions frequently, no matter what you're doing.

Keep your tummy tight. It may surprise you to learn that the muscles in your abdomen provide some of the main support for your back. Keep them strong with this simple exercise: Pull your stomach muscles up and in, and stand up straight. Hold to a count of 10, then relax and repeat four or five times. Do this several times a day. It's amazing how effective this simple exercise can be. Before you know it, your stomach will be flatter, and your back will be stronger.

Lose the heels. Wearing high-heeled shoes every day can contribute to back problems. Wear comfortable flat shoes with good support for your everyday activities, and save the heels for special occasions.

Lift safely. Always be careful when lifting heavy objects. Keep your spine straight, and either squat, bending your knees, or bend at the hips — not the waist. Use your arms and legs to lift, and keep the object close to your body.

Take a pill and a pillow. Taking aspirin or ibuprofen is a quick way to stop the pain. These over-the-counter painkillers not only attack the discomfort, but also have anti-inflammatory power to help shrink swollen, inflamed muscles. Relax by lying on your back with a pillow under your knees, or on your side with a pillow between your knees.

Cool it or warm it. An ice pack and a gentle back massage may help cool your searing pain. Massage for seven to 10 minutes, repeating as often as once an hour. If heat soothes you better, treat your aching back to a warm heating pad. Just be sure to turn it off before you fall asleep.

Don't overdo the bed rest. A day of bed rest may be needed and deserved when your back is really hurting, but don't overstay your welcome. A recent study showed that back-pain sufferers who went about their daily activities got well faster than those who exercised or stayed in bed. Get up as soon as you feel like it, even for short periods, and start easing back into your normal activities.

Try a chiropractor. Studies have shown that chiropractic care compares well with other types of treatments for back pain, and people are more satisfied with it. Treatments are usually spread out over a longer period of time than traditional treatments.

Relieve pain with magnets. Many people believe therapeutic magnets can help relieve pain, including back pain. In one study at Baylor College of Medicine in Houston, researchers tested magnets on 50 people with post-polio syndrome. Pain decreased in 76 percent of the people treated with real magnets, while only 19 percent of the people treated with fake magnets reported pain relief. Although much of the scientific community is skeptical about magnets, clinical research on the subject is just beginning, and early results look promising.

BRONCHITIS

Rest and relax. Stay in bed until your fever is gone, and get plenty of rest even if you don't think you need it. The more you rest, the more quickly you'll get well. Bronchial infections are usually short-lived — if you get enough rest.

Snuff out the smokes. The most common reasons for getting bronchitis are smoking and breathing secondhand smoke. Continuing to smoke will irritate your lungs and bronchial tubes and make your bout with bronchitis last longer.

Breathe easier. Take frequent hot showers, or stay in a room with a warm vaporizer to give your throat and chest some needed relief. Clean the humidifier daily so that airborne germs collecting in the moist atmosphere won't reinfect you.

Eat well. Nutritious food will help your body fight the infection. Eating junk food may be comforting, but it won't help you get over bronchitis.

Wet your whistle. Every day, drink eight to 10 glasses of water, fruit juice, or tea to make mucus thinner and easier to cough up.

BURSITIS

Give it a rest. Since overuse probably had something to do with your attack of bursitis, resting the joint will go a long way toward fixing it. A few days of being a couch potato will give the swollen bursa a chance to heal, but then get off the couch. Rest is good for a few days, but don't get used to it, or your joints will stiffen up. Stand up, change positions, walk around — just get moving.

Relieve the pain. Take aspirin or ibuprofen to relieve pain and bring down the swelling. If you are experiencing intense pain, try an ice pack or gel-filled cold pack. Never apply ice directly to your skin.

Assess your activities. Are there certain activities that set off your bursitis? Think about what you regularly do that makes you uncomfortable. It may be time to adjust your lifestyle. Yoga, walking, swimming, and gardening are all excellent activities that will gently work and stretch your body.

Don't confuse pain with gain. Despite what some people believe, exercise shouldn't hurt. When it does, stop. Normal, slow joint movement is good therapy for bursitis and will gradually make you more flexible.

Drop some weight. If you are carrying extra pounds, you're placing extra stress on your hips and other joints. Consult your doctor and begin a sensible weight-loss program.

CANCER

Prepare an exotic Indian recipe. Turmeric, a spice used in Indian cooking, contains a substance called curcumin, which gives turmeric its yellow color. Turmeric is found in yellow rice, and it's the main ingredient in curry. Numerous studies find that curcumin may help prevent cancers of the colon, breast, stomach, lung, liver, blood, skin, and mouth. More research is needed to confirm its cancer-fighting abilities, but if you like the flavor of turmeric, eat plenty of it. You could be warding off cancer.

Slash cancer risk with soy. Recent studies show that people who regularly eat soy foods are less likely to get hormone-related cancers, such as breast and prostate cancer. This is because soybean products contain high levels of hormone-like substances called phytoestrogens.

One of these substances, called genistein, is similar enough to human estrogen that it interferes with the cancer-causing activities of your body's own hormones. Although genistein shows some promise as a cancer fighter, it is more effective as a preventive measure. Doctors warn that genistein works 10 times better in preventing cancer growth in healthy cells than in cells already showing cancerous activity.

The American Cancer Society reports that the cancer-inhibiting effects of phytoestrogens in animal testing are encouraging, and recommends soybeans as a good alternative to meat.

Eat less fat. A high-fat diet seems to put you more at risk for certain cancers. Although fat does not actually cause the disease, it helps certain cancers develop faster and earlier. Researchers call fats "promoters" of cancer. If carcinogens, or things that cause cancer, get a foothold in your body, promoters help them enter the cells and multiply. Studies show that a high-fat diet might contribute to ovarian cancer, Non-Hodgkin's lymphoma, skin cancer, prostate cancer, colon cancer and lung cancer.

Make olive oil your fat of choice. While most fats may contribute to cancer risk, olive oil may help protect you from at least one — breast cancer. Harvard researchers studied Greek women to find out if their low breast cancer rate might be the result of their high use of olive oil. They found that women who consumed olive oil more than once a day were less likely to get breast cancer than women who ate it once a day or less. Olive oil is also a good natural source of vitamin E, which may provide additional antioxidant protection against cancer.

Fill up with fiber. A high-fiber diet can lower your risk of cancer, especially colon and rectal cancer. Fiber speeds food through your digestive tract so your body gets less exposure to carcinogens that may be in the food. The National Cancer Institute says most people need to double their amount of daily fiber. It recommends 20 to 30 grams a day rather than the 11 grams the average person takes in. However, to avoid side effects, such as excessive gas, don't get more than 35 grams a day. To take advantage of this easy cancer-thwarting strategy, eat more whole-grain breads, pastas, and cereals; and add some extra fruits and vegetables to your diet.

Soak up some sunshine. If you have prostate cancer, spend some time in the sun. Sunlight helps your body produce vitamin D, and vitamin D seems to slow prostate tumor growth. Studies also show that men with prostate cancer often have low levels of vitamin D in their bodies.

COLDS, COUGHS, AND FLU

Soup it up. Chicken soup is the classic mother's remedy for colds and flu, and research shows that mom was right on the mark. One study found that even when chicken soup was diluted 200 times, it still interfered with the substances that trigger colds. Other studies found that hot soup can break up congestion and thin out mucous secretions.

Drink plenty of fluids. It's important to get plenty of fluids when you have a cold or the flu, particularly if you have a fever. To prevent dehydration, and to thin the mucus in your lungs so you can cough it up, get at least eight to 10 cups of liquid a day.

Make a honey of a cough syrup. Drugstore shelves are crammed with cough syrups, but if you don't like taking medicine, you can make your own natural cough syrup. Mix the juice of one lemon with two tablespoons of glycerine and 12 teaspoons of honey. Take one teaspoon every half hour, stirring before each use. For another soothing and tasty cough reliever, combine 8 ounces of warm pineapple juice and two teaspoons of honey.

Fight cold and flu with echinacea. In Germany, echinacea is listed by the government as a standard, accepted treatment for colds, coughs, sore throats, and flu. Echinacea acts as an antiviral, which is especially important because antibiotics are ineffective against viruses. You might consider taking it as a preventive during cold and flu season.

After symptoms appear, the herb also seems to relieve symptoms and help you get over colds, flu, chronic upper respiratory tract infections, and ear infections faster. Commonly, people report they begin taking echinacea extract at the first sign of a cold and often, to their surprise, they find the cold disappears within 24 hours, sometimes after taking the extract only once.

Calm colds with chamomile. Chamomile can help clear your stuffy nose and sinuses. Pour hot water over a handful of chamomile flower heads in a bowl, place a towel over your head, lean over the bowl, and breathe in the steam. You can also gargle with a cup of tea every hour to soothe a sore throat and relieve a cough.

Ease your symptoms with marshmallow. When you have a cold, just the thought of sipping a warm cup of cocoa with fluffy marshmallows melting on top is probably enough to make you feel better. But did you know marshmallows were originally made from a plant, and this plant may help ease your cold symptoms?

The dried root of the marshmallow plant contains 5 to 10 percent mucilage, which is a substance that becomes a tacky gel when mixed with liquid. Mucilage forms a protective layer over the membranes of your throat, reducing irritation and coughing. Marshmallow is usually taken as a tea or syrup. To make the tea, put one to two teaspoons of ground root in about 5 ounces of cold water. Allow it to sit for about an hour, then warm it and drink it.

Soothe your throat with slippery elm. The inner bark of the slippery elm tree, also called the red elm or sweet elm, is a traditional remedy among Native Americans. They once used it to make a poultice for wounds and burns and to treat stomach problems. The mucilage in slippery elm soothes irritated throats and reduces coughing. You can drink it as a tea, or you can buy slippery elm lozenges. The Food and Drug Administration (FDA) says slippery elm is safe and effective, and it has no known side effects.

Quiet coughs with mullein flower. This plant has been used to treat a multitude of conditions from hemorrhoids to earaches. Its yellow flowers have even been used to make hair dye. This herb's most common use, however, is in the treatment of respiratory ailments. Mullein flowers contain mucilage. This soothes your throat and acts as a mild expectorant, loosening phlegm and mucus, which quiets your cough. To make a tea of mullein flowers, use three to four teaspoonfuls in about 5 ounces of water.

Lick congestion with licorice. The scientific name for licorice — glycyrrhiza — comes from the Greek words for "sweet roots." When you hear the word "licorice," you probably think of candy, but the therapeutic use of this plant dates back to the Roman Empire. It was used to treat coughs because it helps get rid of mucus. If you have high blood pressure though, this is one herb to stay away from. Its active ingredient, glycyrrhizic acid, is similar to an adrenal hormone called aldosterone, and even small amounts can raise your blood pressure dangerously high.

Stop flu short with elderberry. The last time you had the flu, did you think you'd never get over it? Research shows that elderberries may make your next bout with the flu a little shorter. One study gave a standardized elderberry extract, called Sambucol, to people with the flu. Within two days, improvement — including fever reduction — was seen in more than 90 percent of the people taking the elderberry extract. Those who didn't take the extract took six days to improve. Look for elderberry extract as an ingredient in commercial syrups and lozenges.

Don't take antibiotics unless you really need them. Antibiotics can only fight infections caused by bacteria. They are useless against infections caused by a virus. The overuse of antibiotics has contributed to the development of resistant strains of bacteria, so don't ask your doctor to prescribe an antibiotic for a cold or the flu. These are usually caused by viruses, so an antibiotic wouldn't help anyway.

DANDRUFF

Make an herbal oil treatment. Mix together two tablespoons of plain vegetable oil with six drops of burdock root oil. Warm the mixture and gently massage it into your scalp and hair. Put a shower cap over your head. Soak a towel in hot water, wring it out, and wrap around the shower cap.

Keep the towel and shower cap in place for 20 minutes, then wash your hair with a mild shampoo. Rinse thoroughly, two to three times. Style as usual. Other herbal oils that may be mixed with vegetable oil to treat dandruff include rosemary, parsley, chamomile, and licorice.

Rinse with bay laurel tea. Mix three teaspoons of crushed bay laurel leaves into a quart of boiling water. Cover the pot and let the leaves soak for about a half hour. Strain the leaves and pour the "tea" into a plastic container. After shampooing, rinse your hair well and then slowly pour about a cup of the mixture over your head. Distribute it well, all through your hair and over your scalp. Rinse out after one hour. If used regularly, the bay mixture should control common dandruff. Keep the "tea" in your refrigerator for external use.

Try something stronger. If dandruff is a frequent uninvited guest, you may have eczema or psoriasis. You probably should try one of the "medicated" dandruff shampoos. They contain ingredients like salicylic acid or coal tar. A dandruff shampoo will loosen those dry flakes and cleanse your scalp and hair. Always rinse thoroughly, two to three times, and follow up with a hair conditioner.

Wash your hair every day. Dandruff occurs more often in people with oily hair, not dry hair. Frequent washings will help remove the oil.

Alternate your dandruff shampoo with a regular shampoo. Keep both in the shower. Leave the cap flipped up, or turn the bottle upside-down to show which one you used last, in case you forget.

DEPRESSION

Get moving. Numerous studies show that people who get regular exercise are less likely to become depressed than people who don't. Exercise actually stimulates the production of dopamine and serotonin, chemicals in your brain that lift your spirits.

In fact, some studies have shown that exercising regularly is just as effective at treating depression as taking antidepressants and getting counseling. In almost all cases, when people added an exercise program to their drug or counseling treatment, their conditions improved more rapidly and significantly.

Kick the habit. As if you needed another reason not to smoke, depression and tobacco use have been closely linked. One study showed that heavy smokers were almost twice as likely to develop severe depression as people who smoked infrequently. Don't let tobacco bring you down — kick the habit.

Get plenty of sleep. Make sure you get enough shut-eye. Even a slight sleep shortage can cause depression in some people.

Beef up your B vitamins. Even a small deficiency of the B vitamins, such as niacin, folic acid, thiamine, vitamin B2, vitamin B6, and vitamin B12, can send your mood on a downhill slide. To prevent that, eat a balanced diet, or take a multivitamin/mineral supplement that contains at least 100 percent of the recommended daily allowance for these nutrients.

Have some uplifting herbs. More and more people concerned about the side effects of prescription antidepressants are turning to herbal alternatives.

- **St. John's wort.** Studies have proven that this herbal antidepressant works well for many people. This is great news because herbal supplements have fewer and less severe side effects than most antidepressants. Although St. John's wort relieves mild to moderate depression, it doesn't relieve severe depression, manic-depression, or obsessive-compulsive disorder.

- **Kava.** This plant has been used in South Pacific traditional ceremonies for thousands of years. Kava products act as mild tranquilizers — they will relax you and lessen nervousness and depression. You may feel some sleepiness after using kava, so be careful if you must drive or operate machinery.

Put on some music. It is said that music tames the savage beast, but can it do the same for your savage mood? Many mental health professionals seem to think it can. Research shows that relaxing and finding distractions from your problems will keep you in better spirits than if you dwell on them. Those who talk about their frustrations tend to become more negative. Music, art, and other mellow distractions are just the trick for fending off life's daily annoyances that threaten to overwhelm you.

Consider caffeine. If you don't feel like yourself until after your first cup of coffee, you're not alone. Many people say caffeine keeps them alert and improves their mood. Now medical evidence is starting to back this up. In a 10-year study of female nurses, caffeine seemed to make a big difference in the rate of serious depression. Women who were regular coffee drinkers had lower rates of suicide than women who didn't drink coffee.

Caffeine is the most widely used stimulant in the world, and about 75 percent of it is consumed from coffee. While you shouldn't deal with depression by drinking four pots of coffee every morning, how much or how little caffeine you get could be affecting the way you look at the world.

Get plenty of protein. Doctors have found a direct link between depression and low levels of protein in the diet. In one study, not only did depression increase as patients stuck to a low-protein diet, but their lifestyle and quality of life also declined. Most people get more than enough protein, but if you don't, add some meat and dairy products to your diet. Vegetables and grains also contain protein but in lesser amounts.

Go fish. Omega-3 fatty acids, powerful weapons in the fight against heart disease, may also help you win the battle against depression. Research shows that in countries where people eat a lot of fish, a good source of omega-3s, the incidence of depression is low. In one study, Japanese students who took a daily fish oil supplement for three months were less hostile and aggressive than their peers.

Fill up with carbohydrates. That old reliable, oatmeal, may have the power to fill your stomach and warm your soul at the same time. Researchers have learned that complex carbohydrates, found in vegetables, fruits, and grains like oats, can trigger the production of serotonin. Raising the levels of serotonin in your brain can raise your spirits. The increase brought on by just one bowl of oatmeal can improve your mood for several hours.

Escape the blues with a natural supplement. S-adenosyl-methionine — more commonly called SAMe ("sammy") — has been used in Europe for more than 20 years to treat depression and arthritis. It is now available in the United States as well. Studies find that SAMe is effective in treating about 70 percent of depressed people. This is about the same percentage as other treatments for depression, but it doesn't cause the side effects associated with most prescription antidepressants. It also usually works more quickly.

So far, SAMe seems safe and effective, but it needs help from vitamin B12 and folic acid to work properly. If you decide to try SAMe, make sure you're getting enough of those vitamins.

DIABETES

Watch your weight. Even if you have inherited a tendency toward diabetes, you usually need a trigger, like obesity, to develop it. Just look at the statistics — 80 percent of all diabetics are overweight. Obesity has become the single most important cause of type II diabetes. If you already have diabetes, a recent study found that losing as little as five pounds can help reverse type II diabetes. Talk to your doctor about a sensible weight-loss program.

Eat more fiber. Many experts believe soluble fiber, like that found in whole grains, fruits, and vegetables, is your best bet for controlling your glucose levels and weight. Researchers at Harvard recently found that women who eat a diet high in fiber and low in sugar are much less likely to develop diabetes.

Try some chromium. This mineral helps insulin move glucose out of your blood stream and into your cells. If you are at risk for diabetes, get a healthy amount of chromium through foods like beef, liver, seafood, mushrooms, whole grains, asparagus, and nuts.

Get plenty of magnesium. Low levels of this mineral can increase your risk of becoming insulin resistant. To keep your magnesium on track, eat beans, broccoli, corn, shellfish, and skim milk.

Protect yourself with vitamin E. Researchers have found that low levels of vitamin E increase your risk of developing diabetes. In fact, one study found that men with low vitamin E levels were four times more likely to develop this disease. Vegetable oils such as safflower, canola, and corn oils; wheat germ; sunflower seeds; sweet potatoes; and shrimp are good sources of vitamin E.

Beef up your biotin. A relatively unknown B vitamin, it may reduce the amount of insulin your body needs. You can get biotin naturally from liver, egg yolks, and cereals.

Work out for winning health. If you lead a fairly inactive life, your risk of developing diabetes is four times greater than if you exercise, say researchers at the Cooper Institute for Aerobics Research in Dallas, Texas. That makes exercise your most powerful weapon for preventing this disease and the one factor over which you have the most control. A brisk 20-minute walk three or four times a week is a small effort that can bring big results.

Dry skin

Be cool. Wash your skin with warm or cool water — never hot.

Soak up some softness. Baths are actually less drying to your skin than showers — as long as you use warm water and don't soak longer than 10 minutes.

Take a break. Try to bathe every other day or even just a few times a week. This will reduce how often you strip the protective oils from your skin.

Heat the air, not the water. Warm up your bathroom — with a space heater if necessary — so you'll feel more comfortable bathing in cooler water.

Choose a mild soap. Save the strong, antibacterial deodorant soaps for your underarms, feet, and genital area.

Stop scrubbing. Don't rub your skin too hard after bathing. In fact, patting or blotting with a soft towel is best.

Moisturize. Pat on a lotion right after your bath or shower to lock in moisture.

Avoid the elements. Don't expose your skin to too much sun, wind, or cold.

Go tropical. Avoid dry air if possible. Keep a humidifier running in your home or office.

Balance your diet. Eat plenty of foods containing vitamins A and C to keep your skin smooth and supple. For vitamin A, choose dark green and orange fruits and vegetables, meat, and dairy products. To get extra vitamin C, eat citrus fruits, peppers, strawberries, and other fruits and vegetables.

Turn on the tap. Drink lots of water every day — at least three large glasses.

Don't forget your fingers. Wear gloves when you do housework or dishes to protect your hands from drying chemicals and hot water.

Gout

Lose weight and eliminate alcohol. The causes of gout are easy to pinpoint. Being overweight and drinking too much alcohol on a regular basis are known to contribute to the buildup of uric acid that leads to gout.

Go on a low-purine diet. Eating too many foods high in a substance called "purines" could cause gout or worsen its symptoms. The body converts purines into uric acid. Foods high in purines include liver, kidneys, brains, anchovies, sardines, scallops, peas, dried beans, asparagus, cauliflower, mushrooms, and spinach.

Drink six to eight glasses of water daily. Water dilutes uric acid and helps the kidneys remove it.

Check your blood pressure medicine. In some cases, gout may be caused by thiazide diuretics — drugs used to treat high blood pressure. This form of gout usually attacks joints in the hands and knees of older women who may have poor kidney function.

HEADACHE

Don't overdo pain relievers. Over-the-counter pain relievers like aspirin, ibuprofen, and acetaminophen can cause "rebound headaches" if you take them too often. If you're having frequent headaches — more than 15 a month — see your doctor and explore alternatives for pain relief.

Eat regular meals. Skipping meals or going a long time between meals can bring on headaches caused by low blood sugar. By eating at regular times and including some protein food at least three times a day, you may be able to avoid some of the pain.

Keep a food diary. Many foods seem to trigger headaches, but the same ones don't affect everybody the same. To help find out which foods bring on your headaches, make notes about what you eat and drink each day.

Fight back with feverfew. This herb has been used to prevent and treat headaches for more than 2,000 years. Research has found that its leaves contain chemicals that reduce the inflammation and muscle spasms associated with migraine headaches. You can buy feverfew preparations at a health or nutrition store. Check the label to be sure the preparation you buy contains at least 0.2 percent parthenolide, the main ingredient that reduces the pain and frequency of migraines.

Try aromatherapy. If you like the smell of green apples, you may be able to reduce the pain of migraine headaches. A study of 50 "migraineurs" found that those who like the smell of green apples reported less severe headaches when they sniffed this scent.

And researchers in Germany found that peppermint oil was as effective as acetaminophen (Tylenol) in reducing headache pain. A mixture of 10 percent peppermint oil in ordinary alcohol brought pain relief within 15 minutes. The peppermint oil solution was rubbed over the temples and foreheads of people suffering from tension-type headaches. There were no complaints of side effects.

Manage your headache with magnesium. Several studies have shown that migraine sufferers often have low levels of magnesium. Magnesium is sometimes called nature's calcium channel blocker, a drug that is used to prevent migraines. Researchers theorized that since magnesium acts like a calcium channel blocker, it would likely affect migraines the same way.

Several studies support this theory, including a study of 3,000 women who were given 200 milligrams (mg) of magnesium a day. About 80 percent, or 2,400, of those women experienced relief from their migraines.

Ease menstrual migraines with nutrients. If you suffer from menstrually related migraines, studies show that extra doses of vitamin D and calcium may relieve your symptoms.

HEARTBURN

Prop up in bed. Elevate the head of your bed with blocks about four to six inches high, or use a pillow or foam wedge to support your upper body while you sleep. This could help prevent digestive fluids from flowing into your esophagus from your stomach.

Chuck the cigarettes. Smoking increases the production of acid. It also relaxes a little valve between your esophagus and stomach, making it easier for extra acid to back up into your esophagus.

Don't stuff yourself. Use moderation when you eat, and you'll be thankful later. It's a good idea to eat four to six small meals a day instead of two or three big ones, and avoid eating right before bedtime.

Drink lots of water. Water helps wash stomach acid out of your esophagus. On the other hand, many other beverages, like alcohol, caffeinated drinks, acidic fruit and vegetable juices, and carbonated beverages can actually make heartburn worse.

Lose the tight pants or lose the weight. If you've been having unexplained stomach or chest pains lately, the answer could be your pants. Minor abdominal or chest pain sometimes results from wearing pants that are at least 3 inches too small in the waist.

People with this problem, which is called "tight pants syndrome," usually experience pain shortly after meals due to increased pressure on the abdominal area. So buy bigger pants, or better yet, lose weight. Excess weight can also contribute to heartburn.

HIGH BLOOD PRESSURE

Reduce fat. Cutting fat is a good idea if you want to reduce your calories and maintain a healthy weight. Overweight adults have high blood pressure 50 percent more often than those of normal weight. Reducing fat is important to good health whether it affects blood pressure directly or indirectly.

Walk your way to better health. One of the best exercises for people with high blood pressure is walking. It helps you lose weight without temporarily raising your blood pressure the way more strenuous exercises do.

Protect yourself with potassium. Eat your bananas and you'll lower your blood pressure. Bananas are rich in potassium, and scientific studies suggest that a diet high in potassium can help protect against high blood pressure. Potassium appears to work by stimulating the body to get rid of excess sodium, which directly lowers blood pressure. Potassium also may affect the release of certain hormones and chemicals into the blood that can influence blood pressure.

This mineral can have serious side effects if you get too much, especially if you have kidney problems or are taking medications called ACE inhibitors. If you're thinking about taking potassium supplements, talk to your doctor first.

Try bulbs for better blood. Your garden may provide some helpful ingredients to regulate your blood pressure. Both garlic and onions contain certain chemicals that may help lower pressure by relaxing and opening up the blood vessels. Be careful about taking garlic if you are on anti-clotting medications, however. Garlic could intensify the effects of some drugs, such as aspirin or warfarin. It's best to ask your doctor about adding garlic to your diet on a regular basis.

Fight blood pressure battles with fish. If you go fishing to relax, it just might help lower your blood pressure. But whether you catch your own or buy it, eating fish two or three times a week is a good way to battle high blood pressure. It's the omega-3 oil in salmon, mackerel, sardines and other cold-water, fatty fish that makes it so beneficial.

Omega-3 helps keep your blood from becoming too sticky and forming clots that can cause heart attack and stroke. It also lowers your bad cholesterol and triglyceride levels. Eating fish is more likely to help you if your high blood pressure is caused by heart disease, high cholesterol, or atherosclerosis. Apparently, the worse shape you're in, the better fish oil works to lower your pressure. If it's normal to begin with, fish oil doesn't seem to have any effect.

Clear your arteries with calcium. It does more than just give you strong bones and teeth. Studies have shown that this mineral also helps lower high blood pressure, particularly in blacks and white women. For some reason, it doesn't seem to have as much effect on white males.

Calcium is especially helpful to those who are salt sensitive, so if you find salt raises your blood pressure, be sure to get plenty of calcium in your diet. Dairy products, sardines, kale, soybeans, and almonds are good sources. Calcium from supplements does not seem to work as well on lowering blood pressure. But it's easy to get the recommended daily intake of 800 to 1200 milligrams (mg) from your diet.

Relax your blood vessels with magnesium. Found in oysters, baked potatoes, spinach, and black-eyed peas, this mineral seems to relax blood vessels and allow them to open wider. This gives blood more room to flow freely, reducing blood pressure. Magnesium also may help neutralize stress hormones that raise blood pressure.

"C" your way to lower blood pressure. Studies show that people with high amounts of vitamin C in their blood have lower pressure than people with low amounts. It may be that vitamin C strengthens and supports blood vessel walls, making them more resistant to high blood pressure.

The recommended dietary allowance for vitamin C is 60 mg per day. You can easily get that by eating five servings of fruits and vegetables each day. If you think you might benefit from a supplement, check with your doctor. Even though vitamin C is considered one of the safest vitamins, it does cause problems in some people, especially at high doses.

Go slow on salt. You should limit your intake to less than one teaspoon a day if you are salt sensitive, which means your kidneys don't get rid of excess salt very effectively. That doesn't mean you should cut out salt completely. Your body must have about a quarter teaspoon a day to work properly. Surprisingly, eating too little salt can cause your blood pressure to go up as well. It also puts you at risk of heart attack, high cholesterol, sleep disturbances, and loss of important nutrients.

However, if you're like most people, you get more salt than you need, especially if you eat a lot of fast foods or pre-packaged foods. They usually contain large amounts of salt that you might not even taste. Even worse, most of the minerals that help lower blood pressure are lost when fresh foods are processed.

Look before you lick. Black licorice, which is found in some candy and chewing tobacco, may contain glycyrrhizic acid. This can make your body retain salt and lose potassium, leading to higher blood pressure. That ingredient is usually removed from licorice-flavored foods and tobacco produced in this country, but watch for it on the label of imports.

Don't mix coffee and exercise. If you have high blood pressure, you may be better off not drinking coffee before you exercise. In a study of men between the ages of 30 and 45, the heart rates of the men with high blood pressure rose higher during exercise after they drank coffee than when they didn't drink it. Caffeine didn't have the same effect on men with normal blood pressures. During exercise, caffeine may place additional stress on the cardiovascular systems of men with hypertension.

Restrict alcohol. Relaxing with a bottle of wine may seem like a good way to end a stressful day. That should be good for your blood pressure, right? Not necessarily. Having three or more drinks a day may be the sole cause of more than 10 percent of all cases of high blood pressure. If you use alcohol, limit your daily intake to the recommended amounts of 24 ounces of beer, 8 ounces of wine, or 2 ounces of liquor.

HIGH CHOLESTEROL

Eat less saturated fat. Your body manufactures most cholesterol in your liver, but you get dietary cholesterol from animal products such as meat, dairy foods, and eggs. Plant foods, like vegetables, grains, and nuts, don't have any cholesterol.

While eating less cholesterol may help, reducing your intake of saturated fat will be even more beneficial. Animal fats, like butter and lard, and some vegetable fats, like palm oil and coconut oil, are saturated. Substituting a liquid vegetable oil, like canola, when you cook is a good way to lower saturated fat in your diet.

Here's a general guideline — the more saturated a fat is, the more solid it is at room temperature. You don't have to cut fat out of your diet altogether. Researchers say moderate decreases in fat intake can substantially lower cholesterol.

Lose weight. People who are overweight usually have high cholesterol levels. Most can lower their LDL (bad) cholesterol and raise their HDL (good) cholesterol just by dropping a few pounds.

Keep moving. Evidence shows that exercise can lower LDL cholesterol and boost HDL cholesterol. But exercise alone can't perform this magic. People who exercise and still eat high-fat foods may not reap the cholesterol-lowering benefits.

Snack to your heart's content. Don't be afraid to snack several times a day on low-fat foods, such as yogurt, fruit, vegetables, bagels, and whole-grain breads and cereals. As a matter of fact, evidence points to lower cholesterol levels in people who eat small meals several times a day. Eating often keeps hormones like insulin from rising and signaling your body to make cholesterol. Just make sure your total intake of calories doesn't go up when you eat more often.

Avoid egg yolks. One third of Americans are "cholesterol responders." Their blood cholesterol goes up when they eat cholesterol, such as that found in egg yolks. Since you probably don't know if you're a cholesterol responder, the American Heart Association says to play it safe — don't eat more than four egg yolks a week. Remember, though, that it's just the yolk of the egg that contains cholesterol. Some recipes work just as well with egg whites only.

Fill up with fiber. There are two types of fiber — soluble and insoluble. Both can help you improve your cholesterol levels. Soluble fiber softens and forms gels that bind cholesterol and carry it out of your body. It also seems to slow down the liver's production of cholesterol. Oat bran and pectin, which is found in apples and citrus fruits, are soluble fibers.

Insoluble fiber helps move food more quickly through your digestive system. Cellulose, found in the strings of celery and outer skins of corn kernels, is an insoluble fiber. Psyllium, which contains both soluble and insoluble fibers, can help lower cholesterol. You can find it in some cereals and in Metamucil.

Eat more garlic. The cholesterol-lowering effects of garlic have been repeatedly demonstrated in people with normal and high cholesterol. Garlic seems to raise your good HDL levels, too. If the odor bothers you, try it in tablets. These have been shown to be almost as effective as the cooked or raw cloves.

Go a little nutty. If you like nuts, especially walnuts or almonds, add them to your cereal, muffins, pancakes, casseroles, or stir-fries. In one study, eating about

3 ounces of walnuts a day was shown to decrease blood cholesterol levels by 10 percent more than an already low-fat, low-cholesterol diet. Another study showed that about 3 ounces of almonds lowered LDL cholesterol by 9 percent. Be sure to decrease other sources of fat to allow for extra calories from the nuts.

Quench your thirst with fruit juice. A low rate of heart disease in France — despite a high-fat diet — led researchers to investigate the French habit of drinking red wine with meals. They found that both purple grape juice and red wine lower the level of fat in your blood. The cholesterol-lowering effect comes from a naturally occurring compound that helps grapes resist mold. The darker the grape juice, the better.

Try an ancient Chinese remedy. The ancient Chinese believed that red yeast rice, which is made by fermenting a certain type of yeast on a bed of rice, could improve heart health. Modern research indicates that it could indeed have cholesterol-lowering powers. Red yeast rice is available in supplement form under brand names like Cholestin and Cholesterex.

If you decide to try a supplement, don't mix it with your prescription cholesterol-lowering drug. And don't stop taking your prescribed medication without consulting your doctor. Although no serious side effects have been documented with the use of red yeast rice supplements, because they are similar to some cholesterol-lowering drugs, they may cause some of the same side effects.

Have a plate of spaghetti. Some studies have shown that lycopene, which is found naturally in tomatoes, can lower your risk of heart disease and certain types of cancer. Recent research finds that cooked tomatoes provide as much as five times more lycopene than fresh tomatoes. This natural antioxidant protects your heart by preventing the oxidation of bad LDL cholesterol in your arteries.

Lycopene doesn't lessen the amount of cholesterol in your blood. It just keeps the cholesterol from doing any damage. Tomato-based products like ketchup, spaghetti sauce, and tomato juice are rich sources of lycopene. You can also get lycopene from guava, watermelon, rosehip, and pink grapefruit.

Add some avocados to your diet. In a recent study, when people ate avocados as a main source of monounsaturated fat in an otherwise low-fat diet, bad LDL cholesterol levels went down and good HDL cholesterol went up. This could be because avocados contain large amounts of linoleic and linolenic acids. You can only get these two polyunsaturated fatty acids from your diet, yet they are necessary for important heart functions, like controlling blood pressure, blood clotting, and blood fat levels. One avocado provides more than half your daily requirement of linoleic acid.

Enjoy heart-healthy artichokes. In one study, people with high cholesterol received artichoke juice instead of cholesterol-lowering drugs. Their LDL cholesterol, total cholesterol, and triglyceride levels fell an average of 8 percent, while their good cholesterol levels increased. Those on traditional medicines lowered their cholesterol levels only a few percentage points more.

Blast cholesterol with high-fiber additive. Guar gum is a soluble fiber that is added to foods and drugs to improve texture, bind various ingredients together, and improve the stability of many products. Recent research indicates that guar gum also can help lower cholesterol levels by moving food rapidly through your digestive system. It may also affect the cholesterol-binding action of bile.

Studies find that adding gums to your diet can reduce LDL cholesterol by as much as 26 percent. Guar gum is a completely natural product, similar to wheat flour, arrowroot, and cornstarch, and you can find it in most health food stores.

Serve some soy. In a major review of 38 clinical trials involving 730 volunteers, University of Kentucky researchers found that soybean eaters reduced their total cholesterol levels by an average of about 9 percent. Volunteers with the highest cholesterol levels had the most dramatic results. They lowered their total cholesterol levels by nearly 20 percent. It seemed the more soy they ate, the more their cholesterol dropped. Even better, the soy protein reduced only LDL cholesterol. Levels of HDL remained the same and sometimes increased.

Eat two apples a day. Ripe apples contain a soluble fiber called pectin. This substance is used to thicken fruit for making jams and jellies. In the body, pectin absorbs water in your stomach and intestines to form a thick gel. This gel keeps your bowels moving as they should, counteracting constipation and diverticular disease.

A French medical study found that eating two apples a day can lower your cholesterol by as much as 10 to 30 percent — a big payoff for simply choosing a healthy snack. And a recent study at a Minnesota university found additional evidence of pectin's ability to reduce blood cholesterol levels, even in people already on low-fat diets.

Ladle up legumes. You may call them beans or peas, but technically they're legumes, a term that includes hundreds of seed-pod plants like split peas, black-eyed peas, lentils, peanuts, kidney beans, lima beans, and soybeans. Test after test has proven that adding legumes to a healthy diet can make your cholesterol really take a nose-dive.

Researchers think legumes keep your bile acids from circulating through your intestines as freely as usual. Cholesterol is the main ingredient in bile, and if it doesn't circulate, it can't be absorbed into your blood where it can cause artery damage.

Fight cholesterol with flax. It's a proven fact that fiber in grains, like flax, helps lower your bad LDL cholesterol, and it may even raise your good HDL cholesterol. One study found that when people with high cholesterol ate six slices of flaxseed bread a day, their cholesterol levels dropped significantly, even compared with those who ate six slices of wheat bread. And researchers at the University of Toronto found that 50 grams of flaxseed a day (in the form of raw flaxseed, flaxseed flour, or flaxseed oil) lowered LDL cholesterol by as much as 18 percent.

Get plenty of vitamin C. Research indicates that vitamin C may be a particularly effective antioxidant against heart disease. Studies find that vitamin C raises HDL cholesterol, and helps prevent LDL cholesterol from becoming oxidized and turning into artery-clogging plaques. And one large study found that men with the highest intake of vitamin C had almost a 50 percent lower death rate from heart disease.

Be careful with niacin. Niacin, one of the B vitamins, is proven to lower total cholesterol and raise HDL. It is one of the cheapest and most effective cholesterol-lowering drugs around. But without a doctor's supervision, it may not be safe. Doses high enough to lower cholesterol have been shown to cause very high blood sugar or lead to liver damage. If you have very high cholesterol, check with your doctor about niacin.

HYPERTHYROIDISM

Read the label. An overactive thyroid gland can produce too high a rate of metabolism, sending your body into fast forward. If you think you have this problem, ask your doctor to test your thyroid, and then check any nutritional supplements you're taking. Many contain animal thyroid hormones which can send your gland into overdrive. Read the label to see if your supplement contains thyroid or desiccated thyroid, and don't exceed the recommended daily dosage.

Relax. Stress can cause your body to secrete more thyroid hormones.

Eat a high-protein diet. You can lose tissue mass if your thyroid is overactive. To fight the decline, eat protein-rich foods like meats, cheese, dry beans, peas, and whole-grain breads.

Give yourself an "A." In studies of countries with high rates of goiter, or enlarged thyroid, people had low levels of vitamin A. The difference was most significant in young adults. Eating foods rich in vitamin A could lower your risk of a problem thyroid.

IMPOTENCE

Cut the fat. Too much fat in your diet can contribute to high blood pressure or heart disease. These conditions can lead to impotence. Heart disease may interfere with proper blood flow, making impotence more likely. High blood pressure may not cause impotence directly, but many of the medications prescribed for high blood pressure can.

Add some antioxidants. Antioxidants combat free radicals, unstable particles in your body that attack your cells. Some particularly effective antioxidants are vitamin E, vitamin C, and vitamin A. These vitamins interact with free radicals and make them harmless, protecting your precious cells from damage. This includes the cells involved in having an erection, so make sure you get at least the recommended dietary allowance of these important vitamins.

Watch your weight. Excess weight could affect your sex life beyond just having unattractive "love handles." Too much weight can contribute to diabetes and high blood pressure, two major causes of impotence. Forty percent of men who have impotence problems are diabetics.

Limit alcohol. Drinking too much alcohol in one night can cause even a young, healthy man to experience temporary impotence. However, too much alcohol over several years can cause nerve and liver damage. That can lead to impotence that may be irreversible.

Stop smoking. Smoking contributes to blockages in the arteries that lead to the penis. Without adequate blood flow, your penis can't maintain an erection. One study found that smokers had almost double the risk of impotence compared to nonsmokers and past smokers.

Go for ginkgo. This herb has been proven to improve blood flow, so if your impotence is caused by reduced blood flow, ginkgo biloba could be the love potion for you. But be patient, you'll need to take at least 240 mg daily for several months to see an improvement.

Give ginseng a whirl. This herb has an ancient reputation as an aphrodisiac. Although there isn't much scientific evidence to back up its claim to sex fame, some doctors believe it contains compounds that stimulate nerve cells, helping you to maintain an erection.

Try pelvic exercises. Kegel exercises were designed to strengthen the pelvic floor muscles, and pregnant women have been doing them for years. However, Kegels might help reverse impotence, too. To do Kegels, you contract and relax the muscles that control urine flow. Contract slowly, hold for about a count of 10, and then relax.

Then do the same with the anal pelvic muscles. To find these muscles, imagine you're trying to hold back a bowel movement, without tensing your leg, stomach, or buttock muscles. Start with five repetitions of each exercise three to five times a day, gradually working up to 20 or 30 repetitions at once.

INSOMNIA

Make comfort the key. It is much easier to sleep in a comfortable atmosphere. Make sure you have a good mattress, and wear comfortable clothes to bed. The temperature shouldn't be too hot or cold, and your bedroom should be quiet and dark.

Wind down slowly. You're lying in bed unable to sleep, the day's events going round and round in your head. Try to head off this problem by taking about 30 minutes before bedtime to relax and wind down. Read a good book, take a warm bath, or work on a hobby, so you'll be calm and ready to sleep.

Get in a rut. While it may seem boring, getting into a sleep "rut" can help you sleep better. Try to go to bed at the same time every night, and get up at the same time every morning.

Limit your in-bed activities. If you use your bed to eat, read, watch television, or work, you may be asking for trouble. Going to bed should signal your body that it is time to go to sleep. If you use your bed for too many other activities, your body may get confused at bedtime. It won't automatically relax for sleep like it should.

Exercise for sound sleep. Regular exercise can improve your snooze time. About 20 to 30 minutes of exercise three or four days a week should help, but avoid exercising just before bedtime.

Drink decaf at night. Don't drink coffee, tea, or anything else containing caffeine within six hours of bedtime. If insomnia is an ongoing problem, you may want to try eliminating caffeine altogether.

Don't drink alcohol near bedtime. Alcohol may help you drop off, but it also may interfere with your normal sleep patterns and wake you up later.

Help yourself to some warm milk. Why did your grandmother always give you a cup of warm milk before bed? Was it just an old wives' tale that it would help you sleep better? Scientists wondered the same thing and examined all the elements found in milk. They discovered that it contains a group of compounds called beta-casomorphins, which has a soothing effect on your nervous system.

Try melatonin ... maybe. Melatonin somehow controls your sleep cycle, and you produce less of it as you age. For those people whose bodies don't make enough natural melatonin, a supplement could act as a sleeping pill. However, synthetic melatonin has not been tested over the long-term and may cause side effects, including headaches, fatigue, nightmares, and insomnia, the very condition it is supposed to treat.

What may help is boosting your body's level of melatonin through foods, like sweet corn, ginger, barley, bananas, and Japanese radishes. To get the most benefit, experiment with these melatonin-rich foods about an hour before bedtime.

Sleep like a baby with an amazing amino acid. The amino acid L-tryptophan tells your body to produce more melatonin, which helps you sleep better. Eating foods high in this amino acid is the best way to regulate your natural melatonin levels.

Foods especially high in tryptophan are cheddar cheese, cottage cheese, fish, beef, pork, chicken, turkey, beans, eggs, figs, dates, soybean flour, and oatmeal. If you eat tryptophan-rich foods about an hour before bedtime, your melatonin levels may go up and your sleep might be sweeter.

Slip into an herbal slumber. Herbal sleep remedies are almost as old as the herbs themselves, and modern science hasn't come up with anything safer or more natural to send you nodding. Chamomile, valerian, and St. John's wort are examples of herbs that brew up delicious teas to doze by. Or you could sprinkle a little lavender oil on a pillow or in steaming bath water for some heavenly slumber.

But one sleep-inducing herb is sweeping the international health food market like a Pacific typhoon. Kava is made from the root of a certain pepper plant found only on Pacific islands. Kava products have the same effects as mild tranquilizers — they relax muscles and remove sleep barriers. Researchers have found no side effects except a type of scaly rash in heavy users. Talk to your doctor before taking kava and follow label directions carefully.

IRRITABLE BOWEL SYNDROME

Add fiber to your diet. A high-fiber diet may make your colon's job easier and lessen the chances of colon spasms. However, some forms of fiber may actually make IBS symptoms worse. Some people find that bran and certain citrus fruits give them a problem. Try whole-grain products and high-fiber fruits and vegetables. Products that contain psyllium, like Fiberall and Metamucil, may also be helpful.

Learn what foods make your IBS worse. You may need to steer clear of certain foods. Although food triggers may be different for each person, the more common culprits include fatty fried foods and spicy or sugary foods. If lactose intolerance is contributing to your IBS, you need to limit the dairy products you eat.

Cut the caffeine. Caffeine may stimulate you and keep you awake, but it may also stimulate your colon, causing diarrhea.

Eat small. Large meals can set off cramps and diarrhea in people with IBS. You may want to try eating smaller, more frequent meals to avoid these problems.

Exercise. Believe it or not, your bowels work better when you exercise regularly. Exercise is also relaxing, and since stress contributes to IBS, moving your body may ease your IBS in more ways than one.

Lower your stress. Although this is obviously easier said than done, lowering your stress level may help relieve the pain in your gut. Take time out of your busy day to listen to soothing music, read a relaxing novel, or take a brisk walk. If you have a huge amount of stress in your life, counseling may help.

MENOPAUSE

Beat the heat with soy. Researchers around the world say soybean products reduce hot flashes and vaginal dryness in postmenopausal women. Just imagine, two of the most uncomfortable symptoms of menopause eased by a small bean. Soy's healing power may come from phytoestrogens, a group of natural plant estrogens that act like very weak forms of the human hormone estrogen. Whether you bake with soy flour, drink soy milk, or explore the hundreds of ways to add tofu to your own recipes, you'll get a rich source of protein as you relieve the difficulties of menopause.

Fight "flashes" with food. If you suffer from hot flashes, try adding wheat, barley, oat, and rye flour to your shopping list. Or how about green beans, carrots, peas, and potatoes? Cherries, apples, rice, garlic, and alfalfa also sound like the ingredients in some deliciously healthy meals. But these foods also give you something extra — phytoestrogens, the plant compound that can ease your menopausal symptoms, especially hot flashes.

Researchers have even studied grains like red clover sprouts and linseeds and found they have effects similar to hormonal estrogen. Women who supplemented their diets with these grains for six weeks had significant changes in their estrogen levels.

So don't be afraid to experiment with unusual ingredients such as different varieties of grains. They'll not only spice up your recipes — they'll give you extra menopause protection as well.

Practice stress management. During menopausal years, women often find that their unstable hormones lead to more extreme responses to stress. Relaxation techniques practiced for 10 to 20 minutes a day will help you feel calmer and more in control.

Deep breathing is an especially helpful relaxation exercise you can practice anytime, anywhere. Close your eyes and focus on moving your stomach in and out as you breathe through your nose. Breathe in and out 10 times or until you begin to feel yourself relax.

Beat vaginal dryness with water-based lubricants. To combat the vaginal dryness that often accompanies menopause and makes sexual intercourse uncomfortable, use a water-soluble surgical jelly (not petroleum jelly). Water-soluble lubricants help prevent infection, and they aren't as likely to irritate as petroleum-based lubricants.

Exercise your symptoms away. Regular exercise will relieve your hot flashes, improve bladder control, and help you concentrate better, think clearer, and solve problems more effectively. You'll also reduce your risk of osteoporosis and heart disease.

Nail care

Always trim your nails straight across. You don't want the edge to curve down into the skin. When it grows, the nail can become ingrown. This gets even more important as you get older because your nails tend to grow wider.

Clip nails when they're damp and soft. Try clipping your nails immediately after bathing.

Keep your nails short. But never trim them deeper than the tip of your fingers or toes. File down any rough edges that may catch on a surface and cause your nail to tear.

Use moisturizers. Apply lotion regularly to your hands and feet to keep your nails from breaking, splintering, and cracking. Nails become more brittle as you age.

Get natural help for fungal nails. For nails infected with fungus, put 4 to 6 ounces of boric acid in a jar and fill with water. Paint this mixture on your nails twice a day. This method takes a long time to work but is less expensive than prescription drugs.

NARCOLEPSY

Nab naps when you need them. This condition affects the part of the central nervous system that controls sleep and wakefulness. Symptoms include falling asleep at inappropriate times such as while eating or talking, a sudden loss of muscle tone, being unable to move when falling asleep or waking up, unpleasant dream-like experiences as you are dozing off, and waking frequently during the night.

If you notice these symptoms, you should avoid driving or operating heavy machinery. Narcolepsy is a serious condition, and you should see a doctor as soon as possible. The best self-help is to take naps of 15 to 20 minutes at least three times a day.

OSTEOPOROSIS

Get moving! Inactivity increases bone loss. Try to engage in weight-bearing exercises such as walking, bicycling, or aerobics three to four hours a week. Exercising and strengthening your back muscles can help correct or prevent "dowa-ger's hump." Exercise will also strengthen your muscles, making falls less likely.

Call on calcium. If you don't have enough calcium in your diet, your body will draw it from your bones. Dairy products are the best source of calcium, but other good sources include green vegetables like turnip greens, beet greens, and kale, and fish like salmon and sardines (with bones). If you are lactose-intolerant or just don't like dairy products and have trouble getting enough calcium in your diet, supplements can help.

Keep up your vitamin D. Just making sure you eat plenty of calcium-rich foods may not be enough to prevent osteoporosis. You need vitamin D to help absorb calcium so it can do its bone-building duty. Your body can manufacture vitamin D from sunlight, but if you are indoors a lot, you need to get your vita-min D from foods or supplements. About 400 IU of vitamin D daily will help you use your calcium supply to its fullest.

Team up with trace minerals. Other minerals may help your body use calci-um more effectively. One study found that postmenopausal women who were given supplements that included copper, manganese, and zinc lost less bone mass than those who received no supplements. However, too much of some of these minerals, particularly zinc, can actually decrease the amount of calcium you absorb.

To get these minerals from food sources, eat plenty of seafood, potatoes, beans, and whole grains, but don't get more than the RDA, which is 15 mg for zinc. There is no RDA for copper and manganese, but the estimated safe and adequate daily intake is 1 1/2 to 3 milligrams for copper, and 2 to 5 milligrams for manganese.

Skip the sodium. You sit down to eat a well-balanced meal full of calcium, but did you know that shaking too much salt on your potato could cancel out the calcium in your glass of milk? Sodium competes with calcium for absorption, so too much sodium can cause calcium to pass right through your body without being used.

Get your fill of fluoride. You know that fluoride can help you have healthier teeth. It can also help you have healthier bones. Though most people get fluoride through their water supply, if you drink well water or other water without fluoride, you may want to take fluoride supplements.

Can the caffeine. That cup of coffee may help get your bones moving in the morning, but it may keep them from moving when you're older. The caffeine in one cup of coffee can increase your need for calcium by 30 to 50 mg for the day.

Ax the alcohol and toss the cigarettes. If you feel like you need a drink, your bones would prefer that you make it milk instead of liquor. Research finds that alcohol abuse is associated with a greater risk of bone loss and broken bones. However, studies haven't yet provided a clear answer as to whether an occasional drink can increase your risk of osteoporosis.

One study of elderly male twins did find that bone loss increased by 10 percent among those who had an above-average intake of alcohol and cigarettes. Other studies have also found a connection between smoking and a higher risk of bone loss and fractures.

Drop the drug interactions. Certain drugs can interfere with your calcium absorption. For example, antacids that contain aluminum hydroxide may cause calcium loss. Ask your doctor or pharmacist whether any medications you are taking might be stealing calcium right out from under your nose.

PMS (PREMENSTRUAL SYNDROME)

Conquer cravings. It's quite normal to crave foods during PMS, but if you give in to this particular craving, you may feel worse later, and it won't just be from the guilt over the extra pounds. Doctors have discovered that sugar, corn syrup, high-fructose corn syrup, and even molasses all cause water retention, mood swings, and other PMS symptoms.

Stay away from refined foods and convenience foods, which are full of these simple carbohydrates and sugars. Skip the chips or peanuts too, because all that salt spells water retention and bloating.

Exercise. Women who exercise regularly tend to have fewer PMS symptoms. Exercise also cuts down on fluid retention. Try adding 30 minutes a day to your workout the week before your period starts. This should also help you get to sleep more easily.

Get plenty of sleep. PMS sufferers sometimes experience what's called an altered circadian rhythm, leading to insomnia and other sleep disturbances. Try to go to bed and get up at about the same time every day.

Can the coffee and ditch the wine. You may think a quick cup of coffee is just the pick-me-up you need if you're feeling slow, but you couldn't be more wrong. Caffeine is a stimulant, but not only does it pick you up, it throws you back down by increasing your irritability, tension, and insomnia.

And a glass of wine may seem like a good way to relax, but alcohol can exaggerate emotions, so if you're feeling a bit weepy or cranky before that drink, just imagine what you'll feel like after.

Find fishy relief. Fish high in omega-3 oils may reduce symptoms of PMS by helping produce a group of fatty acids that reduce inflammation in the body. Your best source of omega-3 is seafood. Herring, mackerel, salmon, trout, tuna, and whitefish all contain about 1 gram of omega-3 in every 3 or 4-ounce serving. Try to eat fish at least twice a week to receive a good dose of this important nutrient. If you have trouble doing this, try buying some oat germ — it is the best plant source of omega-3.

Believe in vitamin B6. By helping to manufacture certain chemicals called neurotransmitters, vitamin B6 may improve fatigue, depression, breast pain, fluid retention, mood, sleep, and memory. Too much of a good thing, though, isn't good, since high doses of B6 can be harmful. So check with your doctor before you take supplements. Eat green leafy vegetables, chicken, shellfish, and beans for natural doses of B6.

Load up on calcium. You should be doing this already. After all, osteoporosis is so easily avoided with a few dietary safeguards. And here is yet another reason to say yes to calcium — studies have shown that taking anywhere from 1,000 to 1,300 mg of calcium a day can reduce depression, bloating, back pain, irritability, and headaches associated with PMS. Talk to your doctor for a dose that's right for you.

Say goodbye to bothersome symptoms. Can you imagine relieving half a dozen symptoms of PMS with one little mineral? Well, you could say goodbye to nausea, headaches, dizziness, cravings, mood swings, water retention and cramps just by getting more magnesium.

The theory is that too little magnesium in your system lowers certain chemicals in your brain and causes emotions to run amuck. If you decide to take a supplement, take around 350 mg a day. To get more magnesium naturally, eat nuts, peas and beans, spinach, broccoli, and seafood.

Try some herbal comfort. Black cohosh is an herb native to North America, where it was once called squaw root, perhaps because it is helpful in treating a variety of female problems. Scientists have determined that it contains ingredients similar to estrogen. An alcoholic extract of this herb can be helpful in treating the pain, water retention, discomfort, and tensions of PMS.

PSORIASIS

Lay off the bad habits. Several studies reveal that alcohol triggers psoriasis flare-ups. And one study suggests that smoking may account for one-quarter of all cases of a certain type of psoriasis.

Get in shape. If you're overweight, try to lose a few pounds. Maintaining a normal weight should improve your psoriasis. Exercise is one of the greatest natural healers, even for psoriasis. Skin, like all the other body organs, will be healthier if you exercise and eat a healthy diet.

Keep your skin moist. Buy a humidifier for your home. Your skin won't get so dry if the air is moist. Stay away from harsh soaps, cleaners, and long, hot baths. A warm bath with an oatmeal bath product will help heal your skin.

Treat your skin gently. Buy soft clothes so that you don't chafe your skin with rough clothing, and don't scratch or pick at affected areas.

Try mineral baths. Some people believe in the healing powers of natural mineral waters, such as Soap Lake in the state of Washington and the Dead Sea between Israel and Jordan. If you're not lucky enough to have a natural mineral spa near you, look for mineral products to use in your bathtub.

Have fun in the sun. Sunshine or the "sunshine vitamin" may help clear up psoriasis. Some people with psoriasis improve after taking vitamin D supplements, and your doctor may prescribe a cream form of vitamin D that may help. Sitting in the sun for short periods also improves some peoples' conditions, but be careful not to get sunburned.

Zap it with zinc. People who have psoriasis lose more zinc through their skin than other people. Your body needs zinc to absorb linoleic acid, which is necessary for healthy skin. So, keeping up your zinc intake may be especially important if you have this condition.

Lay on the linoleic acid. If you don't get enough of this fatty acid, your skin will become dry, rough, and blotchy. Eat plenty of foods rich in linoleic acid, like nuts, wheat germ, and vegetable oil.

Fight it with fish oil. Some research indicates that a daily fish oil supplement might help control outbreaks of psoriasis. The fatty acids in fish oil help stop inflammation, which may prevent your skin from forming the red, inflamed patches of skin that psoriasis causes.

ULCERS

Ask your doctor for an *H.pylori* test. Although stress and lifestyle can make ulcers worse, the main cause is a tiny, spiral-shaped bacterium called *Helicobacter pylori (H. pylori).* These bacteria penetrate your stomach's protective lining, making it more susceptible to damage from digestive acids. They also cause your stomach to produce more acid, contributing even more to the development of a painful ulcer. Your doctor can do a simple blood test to see if you are infected with *H. pylori.* If you are, he'll probably prescribe antibiotics to kill the bacteria.

Stop smoking. Cigarette smoking increases your risk of developing an ulcer. It also makes existing ulcers heal more slowly and raises the chances that your ulcers will return after they've finally healed.

Can the coffee. Many beverages and foods that contain caffeine, like coffee, tea, and colas, may cause your stomach to produce more acid than usual, making your ulcer pain worse.

Limit stress. Although stress is no longer considered the major cause of ulcers, many people with ulcers say that emotional stress increases the pain. Physical stress, such as surgery or a serious injury, may trigger the formation of ulcers.

Don't overdo NSAIDs. Nonsteroidal anti-inflammatory drugs (NSAIDs) can undermine your stomach's natural protection. Aspirin and ibuprofen are common NSAIDs taken for arthritis, headaches, or just minor aches and pains. If they are causing you stomach pain, ask your doctor about switching to another type of pain reliever.

URINARY TRACT INFECTIONS

Cranberries carry away infection. Cranberry juice may be a tart, delicious way to keep urinary tract infections (UTIs) from cramping your style. For years, cranberries were believed to help prevent urinary problems, and modern research now supports those beliefs. Some doctors think cranberries slow the growth of bacteria by making your urine more acidic. Other studies show that cranberries keep bacteria from clinging to your urinary tract. The bacteria just slip right through and out of your body.

However it works, if you're likely to get UTIs, you may want to add about 3 ounces of cranberry juice cocktail to your diet every day. One study found that the protective effects of cranberry juice appeared only after four to eight weeks, so for the most protection, drink cranberry juice regularly.

Wash it away with water. You can use water to clean almost anything, so it shouldn't surprise you that it may also cleanse your urinary tract. Most doctors agree that water can help wash bacteria out of your body. Drink at least six to eight glasses of water every day. If your urine is pale-colored, you're getting enough. A dark color means you need to visit the water fountain a little more often.

Take some vitamin C. Like cranberry juice, vitamin C supplements may make your urine more acidic, thus making it more difficult for bacteria to grow.

Help yourself to some herbs. Some natural herbs can increase your urine flow, making you less likely to get a urinary tract infection. Among these are goldenrod and parsley. You can find them at your local health food store, or look for fresh parsley in your grocery store. The next time a restaurant puts some decorative parsley on your plate, don't just admire it and set it aside. Try eating it for an extra bit of urinary protection. However, beware of staying outdoors too long afterward. Parsley can increase your sensitivity to the sun.

Cut back on sugar. A sugar-filled diet increases your risk of urinary tract infections. If you suffer frequent infections, reduce your intake of sugar, corn syrup, molasses, and the products made with them. And look for cranberry juice that is artificially sweetened.

WEIGHT LOSS

Exercise. Of course you should exercise if you want to lose weight. Without it, even the best weight-loss plan won't give you the results you're hoping for. Exercise helps you lose weight faster and keep it off longer.

You don't have to become an aerobics expert, however. Walking is one exercise that almost anyone can do, and it has the lowest dropout rate of any form of exercise. It's easy, it doesn't require any special equipment, and it can burn as many calories per mile as running if you walk at a fast pace.

Count calories *and* fat grams. Even though it would be easier to just count one or the other, research suggests you'll get better results from your weight loss efforts if you count both. One study found that overweight people ate about the same amount of calories as lean people. However, the plump people ate more fat and added sugar while the lean people ate more fiber. This suggests that you would lose weight more easily if you change the form of your calories from fat and sugar to fiber.

Don't skip meals. Meal skipping is a big factor in falling off the diet bandwagon and into an eating binge. Giving your body fuel at regular intervals keeps blood sugar levels stable and helps your body burn calories more efficiently.

Eat breakfast. Adults who eat breakfast every day tend to weigh less and have lower cholesterol levels. Also, the body's ability to burn calories is greater in the morning than in the afternoon or evening. People who skip breakfast tend to eat more high-fat snacks, too.

Drink more orange juice. Studies suggest OJ is an effective appetite suppressant. In a Yale University study, overweight men who drank orange juice ate nearly 300 fewer calories at lunch. Overweight women consumed an average of 431 fewer midday calories. Their intakes were compared with similarly overweight men and women who drank plain water before lunch.

To reap theses benefits, drink a glass of OJ a half hour to an hour before a meal. You'll eat fewer calories during the meal and still feel comfortably full. Just don't forget to include that glass of orange juice when figuring total calories for the day.

Savor some psyllium. Researchers think psyllium may work well as an appetite suppressant because it holds water and swells, creating a feeling of fullness. In one small study, women who took psyllium with a glass of water three hours before a meal ate less fat and felt significantly fuller one hour after the meal than women who didn't take it.

Although the evidence to support psyllium as a weight loss aid is scant, it won't harm you unless you take more than the recommended amount or are allergic to it. Other benefits include regularity and cholesterol control. You can find psyllium seeds at most health food stores.

Beat potbelly blahs. Here are four ways to avoid that "Buddha belly" look:

- Don't eat a lot of food at once, especially in the evening. Too much food in your stomach puts pressure on your stomach muscles and pushes them out. When you go to sleep, your abdominal muscles relax, making it even easier for the food to exert pressure on your stomach. Do this often, and you'll soon have a perfect potbelly.

- Suck it in. Consciously holding your stomach in whenever you think of it is one of the best stomach exercises. It also helps you sit and stand straighter and avoid back pain.

- Be sure to stretch your hamstrings (muscles on the back of your thighs) after you run or walk for exercise. Tight hamstrings can cause you to develop a slight swayback and make your potbelly all the more noticeable.

- Exercise your stomach and lower back muscles regularly. Exercise improves posture and helps prevent your stomach from sticking out.